Ankylosing Spondylitis - Axial Spondyloarthritis

Editor
Mohammad Hossein Nicknam
Molecular Immunology Research Center
Tehran University of Medical Sciences
Tehran, Iran

ISBN 978-981-16-4735-2 ISBN 978-981-16-4733-8 (eBook)
https://doi.org/10.1007/978-981-16-4733-8

This Springer imprint is published by the registered company Springer Nature Singapore Pte Ltd.
The registered company address is: 152 Beach Road, #21-01/04 Gateway East, Singapore 189721, Singapore

Preface

In the name of God.

the compassionate, the merciful.

The spondyloarthropathies are a group of chronic autoimmune disorders including ankylosing spondylitis, psoriatic arthritis, reactive arthritis, inflammatory bowel disease-associated spondyloarthropathy, and undifferentiated spondyloarthropathies affecting the spine, large joints, tendons, and small joints in progressive forms.

The prevalence of ankylosing spondylitis, the most common spondyloarthropathy, is approximately 0.2–0.5% in different populations. AS mainly affects young adults causing considerable social and economic damage to their lives, rendering them disabled at older ages if not treated properly.

Despite substantial clinical advances in managing the patients suffering from spondyloarthropathies, the molecular aspects of pathogenesis and the genetic basis of the disease remain mostly unexplained. The most known genetic feature of spondyloarthropathies is HLA-B27 positivity whose contribution to the pathogenesis is still under study and surrounded by unproven hypotheses. Therefore, it is essential to discuss and expand our knowledge about the molecular basis of the pathogenesis of spondyloarthropathies in order to improve diagnosis methods, treatment quality, and preventive strategies for reducing the burden of disease. It might also pave the way for designing more efficient therapeutic agents.

In the present book, we have described the molecular and immunological aspects of spondyloarthropathies in eight elaborated chapters including the detailed role of innate and adaptive immunity, HLA and non-HLA genes, and finally, participation of the environmental factors in disease initiation and progression. Regarding the significance of gut microbiota, nutritional factors as well as mechanical stress in the pathogenesis of spondyloarthropathies, and considering the fact that the environmental risk factors might be more plausible to manipulate than inherent factors, the last chapters could be of special interest for researchers.

Tehran, Iran — Mohammad Hossein Nicknam, MD, PhD

Contents

About the Editor

Nicknam obtained his medical and Ph.D. degree in Clinical Immunology from the Tehran University of Medical Sciences. He also has a fellowship in Clinical Immunology in Pittsburgh University, Pennsylvania. Since 2010, Prof. Nicknam has worked as the head in the Department of Immunology and Biology, School of Medicine, Tehran University of Medical Sciences. He is responsible for a great deal of international affairs of the Tehran University of Medical Sciences and the co-founder and Head of the Molecular Immunology Research Center.

Dr. Nicknam is also an expert on spondyloarthropathies (SpA); in particular, genetics and molecular factors that influence the development of SpA. He is a pioneer in understanding the role of immunologically related gene polymorphisms and describing relevant associations of HLA-B27 subtypes with AS. He is a member of several scientific organizations.

Part I

Introduction

An Overview to Ankylosing Spondylitis and Spondyloarthropathies

1

Sara Assadiasl and Narjes Soleimanifar

1.1 History

Paleopathological studies of Egyptian mummies have shown that the disease, Ankylosing Spondylitis (AS), has been affecting human beings since ancient times [1]. Raldo Colombo presented the anatomical depiction of two skeletons with typical anomalies of AS in his book *De Re Anatomica* which may be the first historical description of AS [2]. Later, in the seventeenth and eighteenth centuries, dramatic phenotypes due to the fusion of sacroiliac, vertebral, and apophyseal joints were detected in postmortem samples. However, the classic clinical description of ankylosing spondylitis was established in the late eighteenth independently by Wladimir von Bechterew in Russia (1893), Adolph Strümpell in Germany (1897), and Pierre Marie in France (1898) [3]. Subsequently, Connor promoted the disease feature description by adding radiographic findings in the 1930s [4]. The hereditary nature of ankylosing spondylitis was demonstrated in the 1960s; at the same time, large-scale studies on AS patients led to the development of AS diagnostic criteria. By the mid-1900s, the term Spondyloarthropathies (SpAs) was coined by Moll as a group of diseases with shared clinical and genetic characteristics including Reiter's disease, psoriatic arthritis, ankylosing spondylitis, juvenile SpA and arthropathies associated with intestinal disease (later modified as undifferentiated forms of SpA (uSpAs)) [5].

S. Assadiasl · N. Soleimanifar (✉)
Molecular Immunology Research Center, Tehran University of Medical Sciences, Tehran, Iran
e-mail: n-soleimanifar@farabi.tums.ac.ir

M. H. Nicknam (ed.), *Ankylosing Spondylitis - Axial Spondyloarthritis*,
https://doi.org/10.1007/978-981-16-4733-8_1

1.2 Epidemiology

Ankylosing spondylitis mainly affects young people (late adolescence and early adulthood) ranging from 12 to 45 years old. The mean age at disease onset is estimated to be between 23 and 31 years old, which has been shown to increase during recent years, especially in developed countries [6, 7]. The prevalence of Ankylosing Spondylitis is slightly variable between different ethnic groups, as it has been calculated to be 0.24% (weighted mean: 0.18%) in Europe, 0.17% (weighted mean 0.18%) in Asia, and 0.10% (weighted mean 0.12%) among Latin American population [8], and to affect 0.32% and 0.07% of North American and African people respectively [9, 10]. A meta-analysis study estimated the prevalence of AS 0.25% for Europe, 0.16% for East Asia, 0.14% for Latin America 0.20% for North America, 0.02% for sub-Saharan Africa and 0.35% in Northern Arctic Communities [11]. Interestingly, the annual incidence rate of AS varies from 0.48/100000 (aged>15) in Japan [12] to 62/100000 in Spain (aged>20) [13], coinciding with the HLA-B27 positivity rate in different ethnic groups. A global study has calculated an overall prevalence of 9 to 30 per 10,000 persons for AS [14]. However, the most reported counts from different centers were ranged from 5.8 to 7.2/10000 [7].

AS has generally been known as a male sex disease according to the former studies indicating nine times more prevalence among men compared to the women [15]; nonetheless, recent analysis describes a 2–3:1 ratio between male and female [16]. Notably, this ratio has been shown to be 1:1 in Switzerland [17]. In case of Non-Radiographic Axial Spondyloarthritis (nr-axSpA) no difference was found between male and female patients' frequency [18]. Actually, it could be merely speculated that in the male sex disease progression is more probable whereas, the female gender plays a protective role against progressive disease [7].

Genetic factors considerably affect the ethnic distribution of SpA. The best example of this could be the HLA-B27 gene which is assumed as a predictive risk factor for AS [19]. In populations with higher rates of HLA-B27 prevalence, more AS cases are detected. Moreover, the familial tendency of AS has been reported as the relative risk of disease development among first-, second-, and third-degree relatives of AS patients is estimated to be 75.5, 20.2, and 3.5, respectively [20]. Interestingly, the risk of nr-axSpA is less associated with HLA-B27 positivity. On the other hand, some HLA-B27 subtypes such as HLA-B27:06 have not been demonstrated to have any correlation with the incidence of AS [21]. Probable mechanisms of HLA-B27 predisposing role and different subtypes' association with the disease will be discussed in other chapters.

The most prominent environmental factors influencing the prevalence of SpA are infections and gut microbiome. Klebsiella has been assumed for years as a trigger factor for AS [22]; nonetheless, recent microbiome studies do not support previous findings strongly. Instead, they introduce a discrete intestinal microbiota in AS and other SpA patients comparing to healthy individuals [23, 24]. Childhood infections, particularly respiratory tract infections and tonsillitis, seem to make the patients prone to AS in adolescence [25]. In addition, reactive arthritis as a subgroup of

SpAs could occur as a consequence of urogenital and gastrointestinal infections by C. trachomatis, Yersinia, Shigella, Salmonella, and Campylobacter [26].

Mechanical stresses such as long-term bending, stretching, trauma, and exposure to vibration have been shown to be associated with functional deficits and radiographic damages, probably through initiating enthesitis at the stress site [27, 28]. In addition, there are findings indicating an association between smoking and hypertension with AS [29]. The implication of environmental factors in Spondyloarthropathies will be described in the last chapter.

A considerable point in SpAs is their progressive nature. In addition to the functional limitations, radiographic worsening, particularly in spine and sacroiliac joints, are considered as reliable tools in patients' follow-up [30]. Some factors have been recognized to accelerate disease progression, for instance, young age onset, male sex, high-risk genetic background (especially HLA-B27 positivity), initial CRP level, positive MRI at disease onset, smoking, and longer disease duration [31, 32].

In contrast to the previous findings, which could not show any significant difference between the survival of AS patients and the normal population [33], recent studies have revealed augmented mortality rate in AS [34] with a standardized mortality rate from 1.33 to 1.80 [35]. At the top of the death causes list stand Amyloidosis, cardiovascular diseases, infections, spinal cord injury, vertebral fracture, and respiratory failure [36–38].

1.3 Clinical Manifestation

1.3.1 General Symptoms, Spondylitis and Arthritis

According to the clinical symptoms, Spondyloarthropathies (SpA) are mainly categorized as axial SpA (axSPA), peripheral SpA (pSpA), and undifferentiated forms of SpA (uSpA). The form axSpA has been further divided into two groups of radiographic (r-axSPA) and non-radiographic (nr-axSpA) axial Spondyloarthropathies regarding absence or presence of radiologic signs [39].

The general symptoms of SpA comprise malaise, anorexia, weight loss, fatigue, and fever. These complaints are more prominent in severe forms and in early-onset disease [40]. The primary specific feature is a dull low back pain felt deep in the buttock representing the inflammation of sacroiliac joint, accompanied by morning stiffness and movement restriction. These symptoms would improve within hours of quotidian activities; however, they could sustain when resting. At initial stages, the pain might be unilateral or alternatively felt in one buttock side or another, but with disease progression, it usually takes a bilateral persistent form. The pain would gradually spread along the spine involving the lumbar, thoracic, and cervical zones, making them tender in touch. Neck pain occurs at advanced stages of the disease [41]. Additionally, one-third of the patients experience hip and shoulder joints involvement during their lives; the hip joint is usually affected in a bilateral and progressive form which results in restricted motion of the hip joint due to the pain and consequent rigidity. Although less severe, enthesitis at the shoulder girdle along with glenohumeral joint inflammation leads to painful shoulders and limited arm movements [40]. Peripheral arthritis other than hip and shoulder joints infrequently occur in SpA patients, but when it happens, it is characterized with asymmetric, mono/oligoarticular features, more affecting lower limbs than upper. Some patients occasionally show knee effusions, but permanent erosive lesions are rare [42]. Enthesitis (inflammation of the entheses, the sites where tendons or ligaments insert into the bone), tendinitis (inflammation of a tendon), bursitis (inflammation of bursa, which are fluid-filled sacs that act as a cushion between bones), tenosynovitis (inflammation of the synovium that surrounds a tendon), and dactylitis (inflammation of finger) mostly affect the patients with concomitant extra-articular manifestations such as psoriasis and celiac disease. Achilles tendinitis accompanied by plantar fasciitis has diagnostic value as seen in one-third of axSpA patients. Dactylitis or sausage digit is the result of simultaneous enthesitis, synovitis and tenosynovitis of the fingers and toes [43].

1.3.2 Extra-Articular Manifestations

Some extra-articular signs and symptoms are frequently seen in SpA patients. The most common findings are anterior uveitis, inflammatory bowel diseases (IBD), psoriasis and with a less frequency cardiovascular diseases. These complications are sometimes considered as diagnostic markers for differentiating SpAs from other rheumatologic disorders and require a multidisciplinary approach to handle the patients [44].

These manifestations are usually accompanied by disease progression as it has been shown that AS patients with uveitis have worse Bath Ankylosing Spondylitis Functional Index (BASFI) scores in comparison to those without uveitis [45]; moreover, IBD or psoriasis symptoms in AS patients are associated with deteriorated function and accelerated disease activity [46].

Uveitis is inflammation of the uvea, which constructs the middle layer of the eye. Uvea consists of anterior (iris and ciliary body) and posterior (choroid) parts [47]. Acute anterior uveitis (AAU) with a mean prevalence of 25.8% is considered as the most common (or first) extra-articular sign of SpA [48]; in addition, its prevalence has a direct correlation with disease duration, as it is observed in approximately 17.5% of patients with a mean disease duration <10 years, while affecting 38.5% of those with a mean disease duration of >20 years; this percentage increases up to 50% if the patient reaches the fortieth year of disease chronicity. There are also geographical differences in extra-articular manifestations of AS;the highest rate of AAU has been reported from North America (35.2%), whereas the lowest incidence is seen in Asia and Latin America with affecting 20 and 21% of patients, respectively [49]. Markedly, AAU is more prevalent in HLA-B27+ patients rather than HLA-B27- ones [50]. Overall clinical evaluations show that uveitis is acute in 88.7% of AS cases, anterior in 90.5%, and unilateral in 87.3% [51]. The prodromal phase includes a vague eye discomfort which is followed by acute onset of ocular pain and photophobia, redness, and pupils' miosis. Visual acuity is usually normal;nonetheless, approximately 5 percent of patients experience visual impairment, and less than 2 percent develop blindness due to severe untreated uveitis [52]. Treatment includes topical corticosteroids application and NSAIDs for preventing recurrence; however, resistant cases need classic therapeutic agents such as mycophenolate, methotrexate and azathioprine or novel drugs like anti-TNF antibodies [49].

The accumulative prevalence of psoriasis and Inflammatory Bowel Disease among SpA cases has been shown to be 9.3% and 6.8%, respectively. Similar to anterior uveitis, the prevalence of IBD and psoriasis differ according to the geographical areas as psoriasis is more prevalent in Europe (10.9%) while less seen in Asia (3.2%). The highest prevalence of IBD in SpA patients has been reported from Latin America (9.6%), and the lowest was observed in Asia (2.9%) [49]. Ulcerative colitis and Crohn's disease could be diagnosed in SpA patients with initial symptoms of chronic abdominal pain, chronic diarrhea, rectal bleeding, weight loss, perianal fistula/abscess and anemia; nevertheless, about 60% of SpA cases are estimated to have microscopic gut lesions [53]. Therefore, a considerable proportion of the SpA patients have subclinical gastrointestinal co-morbidities, which genetic and environmental factors would determine their progression intensity. Recently, the gut microbiota has gained interest in understanding the pathogenesis of inflammatory diseases, and novel therapeutic approaches such as antibiotic therapy, probiotics, and fecal transplant are being investigated in managing the patients. Gut immunity, microbiota, and their implication in SpA-relate IBD will be discussed in a separate chapter of the present book [23]. Due to the known erosive effects of NSAIDs and the adverse effects of corticosteroids on the gastrointestinal tract, treatment of SpA patients with concomitant IBD is fairly challenging. The first-line therapeutic option for gastrointestinal complications consists of sulfasalazine, but the best choice appears to be TNF inhibitors [54].

Psoriasis is the other co-existing complication of Spondyloarthropathies, characterized by excessive proliferation of keratinocyte and consequently scaly patches and plaques formation on trunk, extremities (especially joints), scalp, and face [55]. Studies show that the best choice for treating SpA-related psoriasis is TNF-inhibitors and anti-inflammatory monoclonal antibodies such as secukinumab (IL-17 inhibitor) and ustekinumab (IL-12/23 inhibitor) [56, 57].

1.3.3 Complications and Co-morbidities

Apart from the abovementioned extra-articular manifestations of SpAs, there are some co-morbidities affecting the cardiovascular, pulmonary, renal, reproductive, and nervous systems of patients; for example, cardiovascular complications have been observed in SpA patients, including aortic or mitral regurgitation, aortic-mitral junction, myocarditis, and atrioventricular conduction disorders which are rare but life threatening [58]. Moreover, pulmonary involvement has been shown in SpA patients defined as restrictive ventilatory dysfunction and lowered diffusing capacity [59]. The restrictive pattern at pulmonary function test (PFT) is associated with dorsal spine involvement and decreased thoracic diameter; however, chest imaging evaluation shows nonspecific alterations, mostly linear parenchymal opacities [60]. Kidneys could also be damaged by SpA progression because of excessive deposition of acute-phase reactant protein serum amyloid A in glomeruli which interferes with permselectivity of nephrons and results in proteinuria. This proteinuria could vary from a subclinical form to nephritic syndrome and end-stage renal diseases in different individuals. IgA nephropathy, nephrolithiasis, urolithiasis, and prostatitis are the other urologic disorders which frequently co-exist with Spondyloarthropathies [61]. Besides, osteoporosis, compression fractures and consequent spinal cord injury, as well as atlantoaxial subluxation, Cauda equine syndrome and depression, are neurological co-morbidities that might be seen in SpA patients. Obviously, the most serious complication observed in these patients is spinal fracture, as even minor trauma to the fragile, rigid, inflexible spinal column could result in severe damages. The cervical spine is the most vulnerable site which its fractures could cause quadriplegia [61].

1.4 Diagnosis

SpAs diagnosis, especially at early stages, is fairly difficult due to the unspecific symptoms and common physical examination and laboratory findings in rheumatologic diseases. Joint pain and elevated acute-phase reactants are not exclusive to SpA, but they should be considered as accessory diagnostic factors. In general, physicians have to use a combination of illness history, clinical examination, laboratory indices and imaging facilities to reach a diagnostic conclusion; however, the complicated feature of Spondyloarthropathies makes a quick, definite diagnosis difficult. For that reason, several diagnostic criteria have been developed to help the medical judgment as well as facilitate the follow-up process of the patients.

1.4.1 History and Physical Examination

Apart from the general inflammatory symptoms such as malaise, fatigue, anorexia, weight loss and low-grade fever, usually, the first symptom which brings the AS patient to the health service center is chronic low back pain and with less frequency enthesitis or synovitis. If these complaints are accompanied by certain extra-articular manifestations (e.g., uveitis, psoriatic lesions and intestinal symptoms), SpAs diagnosis should be considered with more probability [62]. The main finding in thephysical examination is loss of spinal mobility, flexion restriction, extension of the lumbar spine, and restricted expansion of the chest [4]. In past medical history, a good response to NSAIDs is a helpful diagnostic clue to SpAs. Nevertheless, regarding the complex feature of Spondyloarthropathies, the diagnosis could not be based on clinical findings, and a string of meticulous para-clinical evaluations are required to confirm the diagnosis.

1.4.2 Lab Test

Although HLA-B27 positivity is present in almost 90% of AS patients, it cannot be considered as a conclusive diagnostic test because a large number of the normal population possess the same allele [63]. On the other hand, the absence of HLA-B27 may not refute the SpA probability as there are numerous HLA-B27-negative individuals with confirmed SpA diseases. The other remarkable point in this context is the association of high-resolution HLA-B27 subtypes with SpA. It has been shown that merely certain HLA-B27 subtypes (e.g., HLA-B27:05) are correlated with increased risk of spondylitis, whereas many others such as HLA-B27:06 show no significant risk; moreover, a subtype could associate with the incidence of AS in an ethnic group but not significantly correlated in another one. Therefore, all HLA-B27-positive individuals are not necessarily at risk for developing spondyloarthropathies [64, 65]. HLA-B27 allele subtypes and their association with SpAs will be discussed in other chapters.

Higher C reactive protein (CRP) levels and raised erythrocyte sedimentation rate (ESR) have been reported to be associated with AS disease activity; however, their serum level has no specific diagnostic value [66].

1.4.3 Imaging

According to the fact that diagnosis, classification, treatment, and follow-up of SpA patients deeply depend on their bone and joint evaluation, the role of radiographic techniques seems to be critical in disease management. Four main methods which are currently applied to evaluate joint lesions and spinal changes of patients with SpA include plain radiography, computed tomography (CT), scintigraphy, and MRI. Sonography is principally used to evaluate the peripheral joints and entheses [67]. CT and MRI are more sensitive to detect early lesions, but it takes too much time to observe plain radiographic features; however, CT and MRI are not routinely used in the clinic due to the repetitive radiation risk and economic reasons [68].

1.4.3.1 Plain Radiography

Plain radiography is of significance in evaluating sacroiliac joint and diagnosis of sacroiliitis as the hallmark of SpAs [69]. axSpA has been classified in the modified New York (mNY) criteria on the basis of radiographic findings of sacroiliitis. Therefore, Ankylosing Spondylitis is diagnosed if (1) grade 3–4 bilateral sacroiliitis associated with at least 1 clinical criterion; or (2) grade 3–4 unilateral or grade 2 bilateral sacroiliitis associated with clinical criterion 1 or with both clinical criteria 2 and 3 are found. Finally, Ankylosing Spondylitis is probable when grade 3–4 bilateral sacroiliitis exists without any convincing clinical sign or symptom (mNY is further described in the diagnostic criteria section) [70].

In fact, radiological changes indicate disease progress. Although radiographic sacroiliitis is usually found at some point during the course of AS, many years of the disease may pass before obvious sacroiliitis becomes evident in radiography. Other than sacroiliac changes, bone remodeling and new bone formations in the spine are considered as valuable diagnostic markers found in plain radiography. On the way to develop so-called "Bambo shape spine" radiographic features of squaring and sclerosis at the vertebral corner are seen, subsequent new bone formation extending vertically from the vertebral corner across the disc space to the adjacent vertebral corner would form syndesmophyte and finally complete ankylosis [69].

1.4.3.2 Computed Tomography

Computed tomography (CT) can detect AS lesions earlier and with greater sensitivity than plain radiography. It is more accurate in identifying sacroiliitis because the overlapping pelvic structures do not interfere with the image [71]. CT has been shown to discover twice more sacroiliitis than plain radiography; moreover, false-positive reports are less prevalent [72]. However, due to the radiation hazard, especially for the young patients at the reproductive age, sufficient cautions should be taken in order to avoid gonadal damage. For this reason, CT is not used routinely in the diagnosis of SpAs unless plain radiology is inconclusive despite clinical findings where MRI is unavailable. Besides, low-dose CT application is becoming more popular as a safer alternative for traditional CT [73].

1.4.3.3 Magnetic Resonance Imaging

MRI is more precise than radiography for detection of early sacroiliitis, it is mainly applied if radiography is negative in patient with clinical signs of AS. At the early stages of SpA, inflammatory lesions are observed in sacroiliac joints on contrast-enhanced MRI along with synovitis, capsulitis, and subchondral bone marrow inflammation. Early spinal abnormalities may also be detected with MRI soon after disease onset presented by bone marrow edema at vertebral corners and adjacent to the vertebral endplate [74]. By disease progression, further inflammation sites are seen, such as facet and costo-transverse joints. Inflammation might also affect sacroiliac and spinal ligaments at the attachment site to the bone. At advanced stages, irreversible structural changes, including bone sclerosis, could be observed in the sacroiliac joints and spine [67].

1.4.4 Classification and Diagnostic Criteria

Until recently, the word "Spondyloarthritis" has been used to illustrate a group of rheumatic diseases showing similar clinical, pathological, and radiological features sharing common genetic background. This group of diseases consists of ankylosing spondylitis (AS), psoriatic arthritis, SpA associated with inflammatory bowel disease, reactive arthritis, and undifferentiated SpA; however, nowadays, this classification has changed into two greater groups defined as axial SpA and non-axial SpA, the first affecting mainly spine and sacroiliac joint while the latter involving peripheral arthritis, enthesitis, and/or dactylitis. This classification is particularly useful in treatment because axial and non-axial SpAs require different management [75]. Ankylosing Spondylitis as the most prominent member of this family, has gained the most interest in classification definition. The first criteria that emerged for the classification of AS were Rome criteria in 1961 which were abandoned soon after due to the lack of specificity. The next criteria established in 1966 by the exclusion of chest pain (for low specificity) and uveitis (for low sensitivity) was the New York classification criteria. Later, in 1984, by improving basic science and widening pathophysiologic knowledge about the inflammatory base of disease symptoms, the modified New York criteria were further developed. Accordingly, the patients with at least one of the clinical findings of inflammatory back pain (present if four of the following five features are present: age at onset <40 years; back pain >3 months; insidious onset; morning stiffness; and improvement with exercise [76]), limited mobility of the lumbar spine, or limitation of the chest expansion together with radiological findings of bilateral grade 2 sacroiliitis or unilateral grade 3–4 sacroiliitis are classified as Ankylosing Spondylitis [77].

In 1990 the Amor criteria were proposed which included a list of clinical, genetic, and radiographic findings. The different clinical items in the Amor criteria contribute 1 point, 2 points, or 3 points, and a total score of 6 or more classifies a patient as SpA case. Some extra-articular clinical items in Amor criteria are urethritis, cervicitis, and diarrhea within 1 month before the onset of arthritis, psoriasis, balanitis, and inflammatory bowel disease. The Amor criteria also included HLA-B27 positivity and familial history of AS, reactive arthritis, psoriasis, uveitis, and IBD as genetic criteria. It was the first to include good response tononsteroidal anti-inflammatory drugs as a criterion, and although the radiographic sacroiliitis was not required to fulfill the diagnostic criteria, it had the highest score (3 points) among all.

The ESSG (European Spondyloarthropathy Study Group) criteria were published in 1991 and concentrated on two predominant symptoms of SpA: (1) inflammatory lumbar pain and (2) synovitis (asymmetric or predominantly in lower limb). In addition to one of these two entry criteria, patients were required to have at least one of the minor criteria, including enthesitis, a positive family history, psoriasis, IBD, urethritis/cervicitis/acute diarrhea within the previous month, buttock pain, and radiographic sacroiliitis [78].

In 2006, Berlin algorithm defined a new system for the early diagnosis of SpA with prominent axial manifestations using clinical, laboratory, and imaging findings. The classic manifestations included inflammatory back pain, peripheral arthritis, enthesitis, dactylitis, anterior uveitis, inflammatory bowel disease, psoriasis, family history of SpA, good response to NSAIDs, HLA-B27 positivity, elevated acute-phase reactants and sacroiliitis on MRI or plain radiographs [79]. Later, a Dutch group modified the Berlin algorithm as they considered a study in which it was demonstrated by two international cohorts of patients with recent axial SpA that inflammatory back pain may not be present in up to 30% of patients with axial SpA. Therefore, in order to avoid missing the diagnosis of patients in early phases, the Assessment of SpondyloArthritis international Society (ASAS) group accepted and applied the proposed modifications to the diagnostic algorithm [80]. The ASAS criteria were published in 2009 for axial SpA and in 2011 for peripheral SpA. This classified patients into two groups according to the predominant manifestations (axial or peripheral) of the disease. The entry criterion for axial SpA is the presence of low back pain for at least 3 months, started before age 45 years; afterward, patients are classified into two categories of imaging and genetics. The imaging category includes the presence of sacroiliitis on radiography or MRI plus at least one SpA feature. The genetic arm consists of the presence of HLA-B27 plus at least two clinical features. The clinical features include enthesitis, dactylitis, uveitis, inflammatory bowel disease, psoriasis, good response to the NSAIDs, family history of SpA, and elevated CRP. In this classification, patients with only peripheral arthritis symptoms are diagnosed as SpA cases if they exhibit arthritis, enthesitis, or dactylitis plus one of the following clinical findings: psoriasis, uveitis, IBD, presence of HLA-B27, preceding infection or sacroiliitis in imaging [81, 82].

Bath Ankylosing Spondylitis Functional Index (BASFI), developed in 1994, was designed to define and monitor physical function in AS patients. BASFI contains ten questions related to quotidian activities, which are scored with a rating scale from 0 (no functional impairment) to 10 (maximal impairment), including eight items about everyday tasks and dependent on functional anatomy (standing, turning, bending, reaching, changing position, and climbing steps) together with two items evaluating the patients' ability to deal with everyday life. Finally, the mean of individual scores is calculated to find the overall index score [83]. Despite feasibility and rapid calculation of BASFI scores, it is not sensitive enough to subtle disease progression without functional impairment [84].

Bath Ankylosing Spondylitis Disease Activity Index (BASDAI) is another patient-reported outcome measurement of disease activity that is routinely used in clinical practice. The questionnaire assesses the severity of fatigue, spinal pain, peripheral joints pain, local tenderness, quantity, and duration of morning stiffness using a 0–10 numeric rating scale (NRS) or 10-cm visual analog scale (VAS) with symptoms ranging from "none" to "very severe" reported by patient. The final score is calculated by summing the first four questions and the average of the last two questions and dividing the result by 5. The score ranges from 0 (no disease activity) to 10 (very active disease). Active disease cutoff is frequently considered to be 4; therefore, scores more than 4 are suggestive of high disease activity which needs changing therapeutic strategy. Similar to BASFI, BASDI also lacks the required accuracy for clinical judgment; additionally, BASDAI scores do not correlate well with imaging results [85].

1.5 Pathogenesis

Both branches of immunity—innate and adaptive—as well as joint tissue cells have been shown to be involved in SpA pathogenesis. The mechanisms of aberrant activation of these cells will be discussed elaborately in the next chapters; however, as a brief introduction, it could be said that the deviant function of antigen-presenting cells triggers auto-reactive T lymphocytes which consequently stimulate B-cells to produce auto-antibodies as well as recruit macrophages, natural killer cells and cytotoxic T cells to attack the self-tissue [86]. Therefore, Dendritic cells (DC) as the principal antigen-presenting cells seem to play a key role in AS pathogenesis. It has been shown that bone marrow transplantation, including DC transfer from the affected donor, could induce AS disease in the recipient [87]. In addition, circulating human CD1c + DCs which induce T helper (Th) 1 and Th2 cells response have been shown to reduce in AS patients while the number of CD14-CD16+ mononuclear cells increased; these cells are capable of inducing CCR6-expressing T cells and IL-6 production which contribute to the Th17 responses and AS manifestations [88]. Moreover, there are some reports indicating altered gene expression in myeloid-derived dendritic cells (MDDCs) of SpA models which result in dysregulated signaling pathways and inflammatory responses [89]. Macrophages also contribute to the inflammation of the synovial membrane as their frequency, especially CD163+ cells, is correlated with disease activity and the number of macrophages in the synovial space diminishes after efficient treatment of SpA patients [90]. Furthermore, in sacroiliac tissue samples from AS patients, there have been a significant number of CD68+ macrophages along with active osteoclasts [91].

AS patients have been shown to possess higher percentages of CD56dim CD16+ NK cells in circulation [92], which is directly associated with BASDAI score of patients [46]. KIR3DL1/3DS1 receptor of NK cells is of particular interest in AS studies because it is a potential ligand for HLA-B27 dimer molecule [93].

Th1 cells activate other immune cells by releasing pro-inflammatory cytokines like interferon-gamma (IFN-γ), IL-2, and tumor necrosis factor-alpha (TNF-α). The number of IFN-γ-producing T CD4+ cells is increased in the blood circulation of AS patients compared to the healthy controls but decreases significantly after TNF-inhibitors administration [94]. There are also findings indicating the importance of IL-23/17 pathway in the pathogenesis of AS; IL-23 is a critical mediator for the development and maintenance of Th17 cells [68]. The IL-17 and IL-23 cytokines level as well as the percentage of Th17 cells have been demonstrated to elevate in AS patients' serum [95]. Recently, targeting Th17 responses has been introduced as a promising approach for the treatment of AS; therefore, several clinical trials have been conducted administrating monoclonal antibodies against IL-17A (secukinumab and ixekizumab), IL-23 (ustekinumab) and IL-17RA receptor (brodalumab) in severe cases [96].

AS patients possess more activated and exhausted B-cells in blood circulation than normal individuals. The B-cell subsets frequency has been demonstrated to associate with disease activity and reduce following efficient treatment [97]; moreover, B lymphocytes' normal activation in response to the stimulants seems to be impaired in vitro, for instance, they produce less IL-10 in the presence of lipopolysaccharide (LPS). Dysregulated p38 expressions and aberrant gene rearrangement have also been observed in B-cells of AS patients [98, 99].

Fibroblast-like synoviocytes (FLS) are directly involved in extending joint inflammation. FLSs have been demonstrated to promote the activation, migration, and survival of NK cells to the synovial space of AS patients. Interaction between NK cells and FLSs results in the increased secretion of pro-inflammatory cytokines and chemokines, in particular IL-15 and matrix metalloproteinase (MMPs) from NK cells which could deteriorate the inflammatory condition of affected joints [100, 101].

1.6 Treatment

The two main goals of treatment in SpAs are disease inactivation and improving the patients' quality of life. In order to achieve these goals, two principal drug groups are applied in the clinic, including synthetic and biological agents. The most commonly used synthetic medications are nonsteroidal anti-inflammatory drugs (NSAIDs) while TNF-inhibitors stay at the top of the biological drugs list. Currently used treatments for axial and peripheral spondyloarthritis are summarized below:

1.6.1 Nonsteroidal Anti-Inflammatory Drugs

NSAIDS, including selective cyclooxygenase-2 (COX-2) inhibitors or antagonists, are used up to the maximal tolerated dosage for controlling the pain and stiffness of SpA patients. They are recognized as the first-line choice and could be used for a long time [102, 103]. Responsiveness to NSAIDs is assumed as a diagnostic criterion in some diagnostic criteria systems.

1.6.2 Glucocorticoids

Glucocorticoids are not considered as routine treatment of SpAs; however, in some situations such as in adult AS patients with isolated unilateral active sacroiliitis or stable axial disease with active enthesitis (despite receiving NSAIDs), local injection of corticosteroids is allowed [102].

1.6.3 Disease-Modifying Anti-Rheumatic Drugs

Conventional Synthetic Disease-Modifying Anti-rheumatic Drugs (csDMARDs) such as methotrexate, sulfasalazine, leflunomide count for the secondary choice in peripheral arthritis; however, their effectiveness for axial SpA has not yet been approved. In adult patients with active AS despite receiving NSAIDs and those who have a contraindication to TNF-inhibitors, treatment with Slow-acting anti-rheumatic drugs (SAARDs) is recommended [102, 103].

In contrast to the csDMARDs, biologic DMARDs (bDMARDs) have been shown to be effective in treating SpAs. The first bDMARD introduced to the clinic were infliximab and etanercept which target the main pro-inflammatory cytokine TNF-α [104]; at present, there are five approved original TNF-inhibitors (TNFi) available for managing active AS. Four of them are monoclonal antibodies directed against TNF-α including adalimumab, infliximab, certolizumab and golimumab, and the fifth one is etanercept, a soluble receptor for TNF-α composed of TNF p75 receptor fused to the human IgG1, acting as a decoy receptor [105]. These agents suppose to improve both signs and symptoms of patients with spondylitis, peripheral arthritis and even extra-articular manifestations. However, etanercept appears to be less effective than monoclonal antibodies in controlling intestinal complications and uveitis [106]. The other biologic DMARDs used for treating SpAs are IL-17 inhibitors. Regarding the role of IL-17/IL-23 cytokines in initiation and development of disease, IL-17 blockers secukinumab, ixekizumab, brodalumab, and bimekizumab have been investigated in the treatment of SpA patients. Secukinumab and ixekizumab target IL-17A, bimekizumab targets both IL-17A and IL-17F, whereas brodalumab is directed against the IL-17 receptor and inhibits all forms of IL-17 [107–109]. Ustekinumab, a humanized monoclonal antibody against p40 subunit of IL-23, has also shown significant clinical improvement in SpAs patients with active arthritis and psoriatic lesions [110].

1.7 Conclusion

In brief, Spondyloarthropathies including several inflammatory diseases present with a wide range of articular and extra-articular manifestations. This group of diseases share distinct genetic and pathophysiologic features, which make them the target of similar treating strategies. The insidious initiation, unpredictable progression, multi-organ involvement and lack of specific diagnostic tests for SpAs create diagnostic difficulties to solve which many diagnostic criteria and scoring systems have been developed, most of them being subjective and inaccurate. Several therapeutic options have already been established for treating SpA patients in different stages and with various clinical manifestations, while many others are under study. It seems that despite all clinical, diagnostic, and pharmacologic progressions, Spondyloarthropathies require further basic and clinical investigations to improve the patient management.

References

1. Ruffer MA. Studies in the Palaeopathology of Egypt. Chicago: University of Chicago Press; 1921.
2. Colombo M. De Re Anatomica. Venice; 1559. This case cited by every French medical writer on hermaphrodites, p. 268–9.
3. Von Bechterew W. Steifigkeit der Wirbelsäule und ihre Verkrümmung als besondere Erkrankungsform. Neurologisches Zentralblatt. 1893;12:426–34.
4. Sieper J, Braun J, Rudwaleit M, Boonen A, Zink A. Ankylosing spondylitis: an overview. Ann Rheum dis. 2002;61(Suppl 3):iii8–iii18.
5. Moll JH, Haslock I, Macrae IF, Wright V. Associations between ankylosing spondylitis, psoriatic arthritis, Reiter's disease, the intestinal arthropathies, and Behcet's syndrome. Medicine (Baltimore). 1974;53:343–64.
6. Rudwaleit M, Haibel H, Baraliakos X, Listing J, Märker-Hermann E, Zeidler H, et al. The early disease stage in axial spondylarthritis: results from the German Spondyloarthritis inception cohort. Arthritis Rheumatism: Official Journal of the American College of Rheumatology. 2009;60(3):717–27.
7. Akkoç N, Khan MA. Chapter 3 – Epidemiology of axial spondyloarthritis. In: Mease P, Khan MA, editors. Axial spondyloarthritis, Amsterdam. Elsevier; 2019. p. 31–56.

8. Dean LE, Jones GT, MacDonald AG, Downham C, Sturrock RD, Macfarlane GJ. Global prevalence of ankylosing spondylitis. Rheumatology (Oxford, England). 2014;53(4):650–7. https://doi.org/10.1093/rheumatology/ket387.
9. Solomon L, Beighton P, Valkenburg HA, Robin G, Soskolne CL. Rheumatic disorders in the south African negro. Part I. rheumatoid arthritis and ankylosing spondylitis. S Afr Med J =uid-Afrikaanse tydskrif vir geneeskunde. 1975;49(32):1292–6.
10. Mikkelsen WM, Dodge HJ, Duff IF, Kato H. Estimates of the prevalence of rheumatic diseases in the population of Tecumseh, Michigan, 1959-60. J Chronic Dis. 1967;20(6):351–69.
11. Stolwijk C, van Onna M, Boonen A, van Tubergen A. Global prevalence of Spondyloarthritis: a systematic review and Meta-regression analysis. Arthritis Care Res. 2016;68(9):1320–31. https://doi.org/10.1002/acr.22831.
12. Hukuda S, Minami M, Saito T, Mitsui H, Matsui N, Komatsubara Y, et al. Spondyloarthropathies in Japan: nationwide questionnaire survey performed by the Japan ankylosing spondylitis society. J Rheumatol. 2001;28(3):554–9.
13. Videm V, Thomas R, Brown MA, Hoff M. Self-reported diagnosis of rheumatoid arthritis or ankylosing spondylitis has low accuracy: data from the Nord-Trondelag health study. J Rheumatol. 2017;44(8):1134–41. https://doi.org/10.3899/jrheum.161396.
14. Wang R, Ward MM. Epidemiology of axial spondyloarthritis: an update. Curr Opin Rheumatol. 2018;30(2):137–43. https://doi.org/10.1097/bor.0000000000000475.
15. Polley HF, Slocumb CH. Rheumatoid spondylitis: a study of 1,035 cases. Ann Intern Med. 1947;26(2):240–9.
16. Bodur H, Ataman Ş, Buğdaycı DS, Rezvani A, Nas K, Uzunca K, et al. Description of the registry of patients with ankylosing spondylitis in Turkey: TRASD-IP. Rheumatol Int. 2012;32(1):169–76.
17. Baumberger H, Khan M. SAT0417 gradual progressive change to equal prevalence of ankylosing spondylitis among males and females in Switzerland: data from the swiss ankylosing spondylitis society (SVMB). London: BMJ Publishing Group; 2017.
18. Rusman T, van Vollenhoven R, van der Horst-Bruinsma I. Gender differences in axial spondyloarthritis: women are not so lucky. Curr Rheumatol Rep. 2018;20(6):35.
19. Schlosstein L, Terasaki PI, Bluestone R, Pearson CM. High association of an HL-A antigen, W27, with ankylosing spondylitis. N Engl J Med. 1973;288(14):704–6.
20. Geirsson AJ, Kristjansson K, Gudbjornsson B. A strong familiality of ankylosing spondylitis through several generations. Ann Rheum Dis. 2010;69(7):1346–8.
21. Nasution A, Mardjuadi A, Kunmartini S, Suryadhana N, Setyohadi B, Sudarsono D, et al. HLA-B27 subtypes positively and negatively associated with spondyloarthropathy. J Rheumatol. 1997;24(6):1111–4.
22. Geczy AF, Alexander K, Bashir HV, Edmonds JP, Upfold L, Sullivan J. HLA-B27, Klebsiella and ankylosing spondylitis: biological and chemical studies. Immunol Rev. 1983;70(1):23–50.
23. Costello ME, Ciccia F, Willner D, Warrington N, Robinson PC, Gardiner B, et al. Brief report: intestinal dysbiosis in ankylosing spondylitis. Arthritis Rheumatol. 2015;67(3):686–91.
24. Breban M, Tap J, Leboime A, Said-Nahal R, Langella P, Chiocchia G, et al. Faecal microbiota study reveals specific dysbiosis in spondyloarthritis. Ann Rheum Dis. 2017;76(9):1614–22.
25. Lindström U, Exarchou S, Lie E, Dehlin M, Forsblad-d'Elia H, Askling J, et al. Childhood hospitalisation with infections and later development of ankylosing spondylitis: a national case-control study. Arthritis Res Ther. 2016;18(1):240.
26. Braun J, Kingsley G, Sieper J. On the difficulties of establishing a consensus on the definition of and diagnostic investigations for reactive arthritis. Results and discussion of a questionnaire prepared for the 4th international workshop on reactive arthritis, Berlin, Germany, July 3–6, 1999. J Rheumatol. 2000;27(9):2185–92.
27. Ward MM, Reveille JD, Learch TJ, Davis JC Jr, Weisman MH. Occupational physical activities and long-term functional and radiographic outcomes in patients with ankylosing spondylitis. Arthritis Care & Research: Official Journal of the American College of Rheumatology. 2008;59(6):822–32.

28. Thorarensen SM, Lu N, Ogdie A, Gelfand JM, Choi HK, Love TJ. Physical trauma recorded in primary care is associated with the onset of psoriatic arthritis among patients with psoriasis. Ann Rheum Dis. 2017;76(3):521–5.
29. Videm V, Cortes A, Thomas R, Brown MA. Current smoking is associated with incident ankylosing spondylitis—the HUNT population-based Norwegian health study. J Rheumatol. 2014;41(10):2041–8.
30. Poddubnyy D, Listing J, Haibel H, Knüppel S, Rudwaleit M, Sieper J. Functional relevance of radiographic spinal progression in axial spondyloarthritis: results from the GErman SPondyloarthritis inception cohort. Rheumatology. 2018;57(4):703–11.
31. Fallahi S, Mahmoudi M, Nicknam MH, Gharibdoost F, Farhadi E, Saei A, Nourijelyani K, Ahmadzadeh N, Jamshidi AR. Effect of HLA-B* 27 and its subtypes on clinical manifestations and severity of ankylosing spondylitis in Iranian patients. Iranian Journal of Allergy, Asthma and Immunology. 2013:321–30.
32. Sepriano A, Rudwaleit M, Sieper J, van den Berg R, Landewé R, van der Heijde D. Five-year follow-up of radiographic sacroiliitis: progression as well as improvement? Ann Rheum Dis. 2016;75(6):1262–3.
33. Khan M, Khan M, Kushner I. Survival among patients with ankylosing spondylitis: a life-table analysis. J Rheumatol. 1981;8(1):86–90.
34. Exarchou S, Lie E, Lindström U, Askling J, Forsblad-d'Elia H, Turesson C, et al. Mortality in ankylosing spondylitis: results from a nationwide population-based study. Ann Rheum Dis. 2016;75(8):1466–72.
35. Mok C, Kwok C, Ho L, Chan P, Yip S. Life expectancy, standardized mortality ratios, and causes of death in six rheumatic diseases in Hong Kong. China Arthritis Rheumatism. 2011;63(5):1182–9.
36. Bakland G, Gran JT, Nossent JC. Increased mortality in ankylosing spondylitis is related to disease activity. Ann Rheum Dis. 2011;70(11):1921–5.
37. Wysham KD, Murray SG, Hills N, Yelin E, Gensler LS. Cervical spinal fracture and other diagnoses associated with mortality in hospitalized ankylosing spondylitis patients. Arthritis Care Res. 2017;69(2):271–7.
38. Fauny M, Albuisson E, Bauer E, Perrier-Cornet J, Chary-Valckenaere I, Loeuille D. Study of vertebral fracture and scanographic bone attenuation coefficient in rheumatoid arthritis and ankylosing spondylitis vs. controls. Sci Rep. 2019;9(1):13323. https://doi.org/10.1038/s41598-019-49712-x.
39. Khan MA. Chapter 2 – Clinical features, physical findings, and diagnosis of axial spondyloarthritis. In: Mease P, Khan MA, editors. Axial Spondyloarthritis. Amsterdam: Elsevier; 2019. p. 9–29.
40. Khan MA. Ankylosing spondylitis. Oxford: Oxford University Press; 2009.
41. Khan MA. Update on spondyloarthropathies. Ann Intern Med. 2002;136(12):896–907.
42. de Winter JJ, van Mens LJ, van der Heijde D, Landewé R, Baeten DL. Prevalence of peripheral and extra-articular disease in ankylosing spondylitis versus non-radiographic axial spondyloarthritis: a meta-analysis. Arthritis Res Ther. 2016;18(1):196.
43. Jacques P, Lambrecht S, Verheugen E, Pauwels E, Kollias G, Armaka M, et al. Proof of concept: enthesitis and new bone formation in spondyloarthritis are driven by mechanical strain and stromal cells. Ann Rheum Dis. 2014;73(2):437–45.
44. El Maghraoui A. Extra-articular manifestations of ankylosing spondylitis: prevalence, characteristics and therapeutic implications. Eur J Intern Med. 2011;22(6):554–60. https://doi.org/10.1016/j.ejim.2011.06.006.
45. Robertson LP, Davis MJ. A longitudinal study of disease activity and functional status in a hospital cohort of patients with ankylosing spondylitis. Rheumatology. 2004;43(12):1565–8. https://doi.org/10.1093/rheumatology/keh386.
46. Brophy S, Pavy S, Lewis P, Taylor G, Bradbury L, Robertson D, et al. Inflammatory eye, skin, and bowel disease in spondyloarthritis: genetic, phenotypic, and environmental factors. J Rheumatol. 2001;28(12):2667–73.

47. Rademacher J, Poddubnyy D, Pleyer U. Uveitis in spondyloarthritis. Ther Adv Musculoskelet Dis. 2020;12:1759720X20951733. https://doi.org/10.1177/1759720X20951733.
48. Krishna U, Ajanaku D, Denniston AK, Gkika T. Uveitis: a sight-threatening disease which can impact all systems. Postgrad Med J. 2017;93(1106):766–73. https://doi.org/10.1136/postgradmedj-2017-134891.
49. Kiwalkar S, Rosenbaum JT, Schwartzman S, Dutz JP, Van den Bosch F. Chapter 11 Extraarticular manifestations uveitis, colitis, psoriasis. In: Axial spondyloarthritis. Amsterdam: Elsevier; 2019. p. 157–82.
50. Khan MA, Haroon M, Rosenbaum JT. Acute anterior uveitis and spondyloarthritis: more than meets the eye. Curr Rheumatol Rep. 2015;17(9):59.
51. Zeboulon N, Dougados M, Gossec L. Prevalence and characteristics of uveitis in the spondyloarthropathies: a systematic literature review. Ann Rheum Dis. 2008;67(7):955–9. https://doi.org/10.1136/ard.2007.075754.
52. Max R, Lorenz H, Mackensen F. Ocular involvement in spondyloarthropathies: HLA B27 associated uveitis. Z Rheumatol. 2010;69(5):397–402.
53. Mielants H, Veys E, Goemaere S, Goethals K, Cuvelier C, De MV. Gut inflammation in the spondyloarthropathies: clinical, radiologic, biologic and genetic features in relation to the type of histology. A prospective study. J Rheumatol. 1991;18(10):1542–51.
54. De Cruz P, Kamm M, Hamilton A, Ritchie K, Gorelik A, Liew D, et al. P342 Adalimumab prevents post-operative Crohn's disease recurrence and is superior to thiopurines: Early results from the prospective POCER study. Journal of Crohn's and Colitis. 2012;6(Supplement_1):S146.
55. Kim WB, Jerome D, Yeung J. Diagnosis and management of psoriasis. Can Fam Physician. 2017;63(4):278–85.
56. Deodhar A, Gensler LS, Sieper J, Clark M, Calderon C, Wang Y, et al. Three multicenter, randomized, double-blind, placebo-controlled studies evaluating the efficacy and safety of ustekinumab in axial spondyloarthritis. Arthritis Rheumatol. 2019;71(2):258–70.
57. Baeten D, Østergaard M, Wei JC-C, Sieper J, Järvinen P, Tam L-S, et al. Risankizumab, an IL-23 inhibitor, for ankylosing spondylitis: results of a randomised, double-blind, placebo-controlled, proof-of-concept, dose-finding phase 2 study. Ann Rheum Dis. 2018;77(9):1295–302.
58. Vinsonneau U, Brondex A, Mansourati J, Saraux A, Cornily JC, Arlès F, et al. Cardiovascular disease in patients with spondyloarthropathies. Joint Bone Spine. 2008;75(1):18–21. https://doi.org/10.1016/j.jbspin.2007.04.011.
59. Jeandel P, Bonnet D, Chouc P, Molinier S, Raphenon G, Martet G, et al. Demonstration of subclinical pulmonary alveolitis in spondylarthropathies. Revue du rhumatisme (Ed francaise: 1993). 1994;61(5):301–9.
60. Sampaio-Barros PD, Cerqueira EMF, Rezende SM, Maeda L, Conde RA, Zanardi VA, et al. Pulmonary involvement in ankylosing spondylitis. Clin Rheumatol. 2007;26(2):225–30.
61. Ward MM. Chapter 12 – Comorbidities*. In: Mease P, Khan MA, editors. Axial Spondyloarthritis. Amsterdam: Elsevier; 2019. p. 183–202.
62. Rudwaleit M, van der Heijde D, Khan MA, Braun J, Sieper J. How to diagnose axial spondyloarthritis early. Ann Rheum Dis. 2004;63(5):535–43. https://doi.org/10.1136/ard.2003.011247.
63. Evans DM, Spencer CC, Pointon JJ, Su Z, Harvey D, Kochan G, et al. Interaction between ERAP1 and HLA-B27 in ankylosing spondylitis implicates peptide handling in the mechanism for HLA-B27 in disease susceptibility. Nat Genet. 2011;43(8):761.
64. Gonzalez-Roces S, Alvarez M, Gonzalez S, Dieye A, Makni H, Woodfield DG, et al. HLA-B27 polymorphism and worldwide susceptibility to ankylosing spondylitis. Tissue Antigens. 1997;49(2):116–23.
65. López-Larrea C, Sujirachato K, Mehra NK, Chiewsilp P, Isarangkura D, Kanga U, et al. HLA-B27 subtypes in Asian patients with ankylosing spondylitis evidence for new associations. Tissue Antigens. 1995;45(3):169–76.

66. Spoorenberg A, van der Heijde D, de Klerk E, Dougados M, De Vlam K, Mielants H, et al. Relative value of erythrocyte sedimentation rate and C-reactive protein in assessment of disease activity in ankylosing spondylitis. J Rheumatol. 1999;26(4):980–4.
67. Maksymowych WP, RGW L. Chapter 10 – Imaging in axial spondyloarthriti. In: Mease P, Khan MA, editors. Axial Spondyloarthritis. Amsterdam: Elsevier; 2019. p. 135–55.
68. Bidad K, Salehi E, Jamshidi A, Saboor-Yaraghi AA, Oraei M, Meysamie A, Mahmoudi M, Nicknam MH. Effect of alltransretinoic acid on Th17 and T regulatory cell subsets in patients with ankylosing spondylitis. The Journal of rheumatology. 2013;40(4):476–83.
69. Bazzocchi A, Aparisi Gomez MP, Guglielmi G. Conventional radiology in Spondyloarthritis. Radiol Clin N Am. 2017;55(5):943–66. https://doi.org/10.1016/j.rcl.2017.04.003.
70. van der Linden S, Valkenburg HA, Cats A. Evaluation of diagnostic criteria for ankylosing spondylitis. A proposal for modification of the New York criteria. Arthritis Rheum. 1984;27(4):361–8. https://doi.org/10.1002/art.1780270401.
71. Geijer M, Göthlin GG, Göthlin JH. The clinical utility of computed tomography compared to conventional radiography in diagnosing sacroiliitis. A retrospective study on 910 patients and literature review. J Rheumatol. 2007;34(7):1561–5.
72. Devauchelle-Pensec V, d'Agostino MA, Marion J, Lapierre M, Jousse-Joulin S, Colin D, et al. Computed tomography scanning facilitates the diagnosis of sacroiliitis in patients with suspected spondylarthritis: results of a prospective multicenter French cohort study. Arthritis Rheum. 2012;64(5):1412–9.
73. de Koning A, de Bruin F, van den Berg R, Ramiro S. Low-dose CT detects more progression of bone formation in comparison to conventional radiography in patients with ankylosing spondylitis: results from the SIAS cohort. Ann Rheum Dis. 2018;77(2):293–9. https://doi.org/10.1136/annrheumdis-2017-211989.
74. Puhakka KB, Jurik AG, Schiottz-Christensen B, Hansen GVO, Egund N, Christiansen JV, et al. Magnetic resonance imaging of sacroiliitis in early seronegative spondylarthropathy. Abnormalities correlated to clinical and laboratory findings. Rheumatology. 2003;43(2):234–7. https://doi.org/10.1093/rheumatology/keh008.
75. Navarro-Compán V, Deodhar A. Chapter 4 – Classification criteria for axial spondyloarthritis. In: Mease P, Khan MA, editors. Axial Spondyloarthritis. Amsterdam: Elsevier; 2019. p. 57–65.
76. Calin A, Porta J, Fries JF, Schurman DJ. Clinical history as a screening test for ankylosing spondylitis. JAMA. 1977;237(24):2613–4. https://doi.org/10.1001/jama.1977.03270510035017.
77. Linden SVD, Valkenburg HA, Cats A. Evaluation of diagnostic criteria for ankylosing spondylitis. Arthritis Rheum. 1984;27(4):361–8.
78. Amor B, Dougados M, Listrat V, Menkes C, Dubost J, Roux H, et al. Evaluation of the Amor criteria for spondylarthropathies and European Spondylarthropathy Study Group (ESSG). A cross-sectional analysis of 2,228 patients. Annales de medecine interne. 1991;142:85–9.
79. Rudwaleit M, Feldtkeller E, Sieper J. Easy assessment of axial spondyloarthritis (early ankylosing spondylitis) at the bedside. Ann Rheum Dis. 2006;65(9):1251–2.
80. van den Berg R, de Hooge M, Rudwaleit M, Sieper J, van Gaalen F, Reijnierse M, et al. ASAS modification of the Berlin algorithm for diagnosing axial spondyloarthritis: results from the SPondyloArthritis caught early (SPACE)-cohort and from the assessment of SpondyloArthritis international society (ASAS)-cohort. Ann Rheum Dis. 2013;72(10):1646–53.
81. Rudwaleit M, Van Der Heijde D, Landewé R, Listing J, Akkoc N, Brandt J, et al. The development of assessment of SpondyloArthritis international society classification criteria for axial spondyloarthritis (part II): validation and final selection. Ann Rheum Dis. 2009;68(6):777–83.
82. Mv R, van der Heijde D, Landewé R, Akkoc N, Brandt J, Chou C, et al. The assessment of SpondyloArthritis international society classification criteria for peripheral spondyloarthritis and for spondyloarthritis in general. Ann Rheum Dis. 2011;70(1):25–31.
83. Calin A, Garrett S, Whitelock H, Kennedy LG, O'Hea J, Mallorie P, et al. A new approach to defining functional ability in ankylosing spondylitis: the development of the Bath ankylosing spondylitis functional index. J Rheumatol. 1994;21(12):2281–5.

84. Magrey MN, Kiltz U. Chapter 9 – clinical assessment of axial spondyloarthritis. In: Mease P, Khan MA, editors. Axial spondyloarthritis. Amsterdam: Elsevier; 2019. p. 121–33.
85. Garrett S, Jenkinson T, Kennedy LG, Whitelock H, Gaisford P, Calin A. A new approach to defining disease status in ankylosing spondylitis: the Bath ankylosing spondylitis disease activity index. J Rheumatol. 1994;21(12):2286–91.
86. Rezaiemanesh A, Abdolmaleki M, Abdolmohammadi K, Aghaei H, Pakdel FD, Fatahi Y, et al. Immune cells involved in the pathogenesis of ankylosing spondylitis. Biomed & Pharmacoth = Biomedecine & pharmacotherapie. 2018;100:198–204. https://doi.org/10.1016/j.biopha.2018.01.108.
87. Stockwin LH, McGonagle D, Martin IG, Blair GE. Dendritic cells: immunological sentinels with a central role in health and disease. Immunol Cell Biol. 2000;78(2):91–102. https://doi.org/10.1046/j.1440-1711.2000.00888.x.
88. Wright PB, McEntegart A, McCarey D, McInnes IB, Siebert S, Milling SWF. Ankylosing spondylitis patients display altered dendritic cell and T cell populations that implicate pathogenic roles for the IL-23 cytokine axis and intestinal inflammation. Rheumatology. 2015;55(1):120–32. https://doi.org/10.1093/rheumatology/kev245.
89. Zambrano-Zaragoza JF, Agraz-Cibrian JM, González-Reyes C, Durán-Avelar M, Vibanco-Pérez N. Ankylosing spondylitis: from cells to genes. Int J Inflamm. 2013;2013:501653.
90. Bresnihan B, Pontifex E, Thurlings RM, Vinkenoog M, El-Gabalawy H, Fearon U, et al. Synovial tissue sublining CD68 expression is a biomarker of therapeutic response in rheumatoid arthritis clinical trials: consistency across centers. J Rheumatol. 2009;36(8):1800–2. https://doi.org/10.3899/jrheum.090348.
91. Braun J, Bollow M, Neure L, Seipelt E, Seyrekbasan F, Herbst H, et al. Use of immunohistologic and in situ hybridization techniques in the examination of sacroiliac joint biopsy specimens from patients with ankylosing spondylitis. Arthritis & Rheumatism: Official Journal of the American College of Rheumatology. 1995;38(4):499–505.
92. Mousavi T, Poormoghim H, Moradi M, Tajik N, Shahsavar F, Soofi M. Phenotypic study of natural killer cell subsets in ankylosing spondylitis patients. Iran J Allergy Asthma Immunol. 2009;8(4):193–8.
93. Boyington JC, Sun PD. A structural perspective on MHC class I recognition by killer cell immunoglobulin-like receptors. Mol Immunol. 2002;38(14):1007–21. https://doi.org/10.1016/S0161-5890(02)00030-5.
94. Limón-Camacho L, Vargas-Rojas MI, Vázquez-Mellado J, Casasola-Vargas J, Moctezuma JF, Burgos-Vargas R, et al. In vivo peripheral blood Proinflammatory T cells in patients with ankylosing spondylitis. J Rheumatol. 2012;39(4):830–5. https://doi.org/10.3899/jrheum.110862.
95. Xueyi L, Lina C, Zhenbiao W, Qing H, Qiang L, Zhu P. Levels of circulating Th17 cells and regulatory T cells in ankylosing spondylitis patients with an inadequate response to anti–TNF-α therapy. J Clin Immunol. 2013;33(1):151–61.
96. Busquets-Perez N, Marzo-Ortega H, Emery P. Emerging drugs for axial spondyloarthritis including ankylosing spondylitis. Expert Opin Emerg Drugs. 2013;18(1):71–86. https://doi.org/10.1517/14728214.2013.752815.
97. Niu X-Y, Zhang H-Y, Liu Y-J, Zhao D, Shan Y-X, Jiang Y-F. Peripheral B-cell activation and exhaustion markers in patients with ankylosing spondylitis. Life Sci. 2013;93(18–19):687–92.
98. Voswinkel J, Weisgerber K, Pfreundschuh M, Gause A. B lymphocyte involvement in ankylosing spondylitis: the heavy chain variable segment gene repertoire of B lymphocytes from germinal center-like foci in the synovial membrane indicates antigen selection. Arthritis Res Ther. 2001;3(3):189.
99. Ge L, Wang J, Zhu BQ, Zhang ZS. Effect of abnormal activated B cells in patients with ankylosing spondylitis and its molecular mechanism. Eur Rev Med Pharmacol Sci. 2018;22(9):2527–33. https://doi.org/10.26355/eurrev_201805_14941.
100. Chan A, Filer A, Parsonage G, Kollnberger S, Gundle R, Buckley CD, et al. Mediation of the proinflammatory cytokine response in rheumatoid arthritis and spondylarthritis by interactions between fibroblast-like synoviocytes and natural killer cells. Arthritis & Rheumatism: Official Journal of the American College of Rheumatology. 2008;58(3):707–17.

101. Barthel C, Yeremenko N, Jacobs R, Schmidt RE, Bernateck M, Zeidler H, et al. Nerve growth factor and receptor expression in rheumatoid arthritis and spondyloarthritis. Arthritis Res Ther. 2009;11(3):R82.
102. Ward MM, Deodhar A, Akl EA, Lui A, Ermann J, Gensler LS, et al. American College of Rheumatology/spondylitis Association of America/Spondyloarthritis research and treatment network 2015 recommendations for the treatment of ankylosing spondylitis and nonradiographic axial spondyloarthritis. Arthritis Rheumatol. 2016;68(2):282–98.
103. van der Heijde D, Ramiro S, Landewé R, Baraliakos X, Van den Bosch F, Sepriano A, et al. 2016 update of the ASAS-EULAR management recommendations for axial spondyloarthritis. Ann Rheum Dis. 2017;76(6):978–91.
104. Braun J, Brandt J, Listing J, Zink A, Alten R, Golder W, et al. Treatment of active ankylosing spondylitis with infliximab: a randomised controlled multicentre trial. Lancet (London, England). 2002;359(9313):1187–93. https://doi.org/10.1016/s0140-6736(02)08215-6.
105. Van den Bosch F, Carron P, Mease P. Chapter 15 – biologic treatment of axial spondyloarthritis. In: Mease P, Khan MA, editors. Axial spondyloarthritis. Amsterdam: Elsevier; 2019. p. 227–42.
106. Carron P, Van Praet L, Jacques P, Elewaut D, Van den Bosch F. Therapy for spondyloarthritis: the role of extra-articular manifestations (eye, skin). Rheum Dis Clin N Am. 2012;38(3):583–600. https://doi.org/10.1016/j.rdc.2012.08.017.
107. Braun J, Baraliakos X, Deodhar A, Poddubnyy D, Emery P, Delicha EM, et al. Secukinumab shows sustained efficacy and low structural progression in ankylosing spondylitis: 4-year results from the MEASURE 1 study. Rheumatology. 2018;58(5):859–68. https://doi.org/10.1093/rheumatology/key375.
108. van der Heijde D, Cheng-Chung Wei J, Dougados M, Mease P, Deodhar A, Maksymowych WP, et al. Ixekizumab, an interleukin-17A antagonist in the treatment of ankylosing spondylitis or radiographic axial spondyloarthritis in patients previously untreated with biological disease-modifying anti-rheumatic drugs (COAST-V): 16 week results of a phase 3 randomised, double-blind, active-controlled and placebo-controlled trial. Lancet (London, England). 2018;392(10163):2441–51. https://doi.org/10.1016/s0140-6736(18)31946-9.
109. Braun J, Kiltz U, Heldmann F, Baraliakos X. Emerging drugs for the treatment of axial and peripheral spondyloarthritis. Expert Opin Emerg Drugs. 2015;20(1):1–14.
110. Ritchlin C, Rahman P, Kavanaugh A, McInnes IB, Puig L, Li S, et al. Efficacy and safety of the anti-IL-12/23 p40 monoclonal antibody, ustekinumab, in patients with active psoriatic arthritis despite conventional non-biological and biological anti-tumour necrosis factor therapy: 6-month and 1-year results of the phase 3, multicentre, double-blind, placebo-controlled, randomised PSUMMIT 2 trial. Ann Rheum Dis. 2014;73(6):990–9.

Part II

Cells and Cytokines

Innate Immune-Related Cells and Cytokines in Spondyloarthropathies

2

Narjes Soleimanifar and Alireza Rezaiemanesh

2.1 Introduction

The innate immune system is considered an evolutionarily conserved system that acts in the first line of the immune system and combats invading foreign agents and endogenous threats. The exact orchestration of the innate immune elements is mandatory for the suitable performance of the immune system in demolishing and removing the pathogens as well as other foreign insults. Among the essential components, dendritic cells (DCs), macrophages, mast cells, and natural killer (NK) cells exert invariant receptors in order to identify the antigens. Furthermore, the non-cell arm of the innate immune system, namely the humoral or soluble agents, includes cytokines, anti-microbial peptides, complement proteins, and cells to improve the overall defensive circumstances. The innate immune system mechanisms initiate not only before the specialized adaptive immune system but also are fundamentally involved in improving and strengthening it to elicit efficient overall effector responses and enduring memory responses [1].

A range of pattern recognition receptors (PRRs) is involved in detecting specific pathogen-associated molecular patterns (PAMPs), predominantly found on the microbes like viruses, bacteria, fungi, and parasites. Additionally, PRRs participate in sensing endogenous "danger" signals by identifying danger-associated molecular patterns (DAMPs). Ligation of PRRs with DAMPs or PAMPs leads to the initiation of inflammatory responses that may include activation of anti-microbial peptides,

N. Soleimanifar
Molecular Immunology Research Center, Tehran University of Medical Sciences, Tehran, Iran

A. Rezaiemanesh (✉)
Department of Immunology, School of Medicine, Kermanshah University of Medical Sciences, Kermanshah, Iran
e-mail: alireza.rezaiemanesh@kums.ac.ir

M. H. Nicknam (ed.), *Ankylosing Spondylitis - Axial Spondyloarthritis*, https://doi.org/10.1007/978-981-16-4733-8_2

production and release of cytokines/chemokines, pyroptotic cell death, and infiltration of effector cells to the site of involvement [2].

Ankylosing spondylitis (AS) is considered the primary type of spondyloarthropathies (SpA) as well as chronic inflammatory arthritis [3]. The disease usually occurs during the young adults life span (20–30 years) and predominantly involves the sacroiliac joints and lower spine. Moreover, other parts of the body like enthesitis, peripheral joints, and extra-skeletal organs (such as eye, skin, gut) and, less likely, the heart and lungs can also be involved [4, 5]. Similar to other autoimmune disorders, the pathogenesis of AS is attributed to the contribution of both genetic and environmental factors that confers an inflammation, despite the fact that the precise cause has not yet been revealed [6, 7]. Among the genetic risk factors for AS, human leukocyte antigen (HLA)-B27, interleukin (IL)-23R, and endoplasmic reticulum aminopeptidase 1 (ERAP1) have been widely implicated [8–10].

During AS development, chronic inflammation occurred in the spinal joints that eventuates in intense and chronic pain and stiffness, leading to new bone formation (ankylosis) [11]. On the other side, aberrant activation of the immune system is considered a significant role as several investigations showed that different immune cells released cytokines, and expressed markers play a critical role in the AS immune-pathogenesis [12, 13].

Up until now, some research has regarded AS as an autoimmune disorder with a concentration on adaptive immune responses implicated in disease pathogenesis [14]. That notwithstanding, recently, SpAs are categorized as polygenic autoinflammatory diseases, in which disruption of the innate immune system has a remarkable role. The intermediate success of T cell and B cell-targeted therapies, male predominance, and the absence of typical autoimmune features result in this autoinflammatory identity [15–17]. Furthermore, accumulation of the innate immune-related cells and cytokines in synovial fluid of psoriatic arthritis (PsA) patients and prosperous treatment through anti-innate cytokines signify the role of innate immunity [15, 18]. This issue is not controversial owing to the fact that chronic irritation of innate immunity can lead to tolerance break toward self-antigens to cause autoimmunity [19]. Other data also offer the involvement of the innate immune responses in the etiopathogenesis of autoimmune disorders. In the case of rheumatoid arthritis (RA), the recruitment of plasmacytoid DCs (pDCs) in perivascular infiltrates is related to the rheumatoid factors in serum. Moreover, signaling of the Toll-like receptors (TLRs) can result in the prolonged stimulation of macrophages in the synovial fluid of such cases [20]. In scleroderma or systemic sclerosis (SSc), another multi-systemic autoimmune disorder, the innate related receptors were overexpressed, and applying strategies for targeting these receptors indicated favorable outcomes [21].

Studies have implicated the alleged role of bacteria [22] as well as the local mechanical stress [23] in the AS pathogenesis. Interestingly, both factors can trigger innate immune activation and are discussed later in the third part of this book. In addition, a substantial amount of the AS predisposing genes recognized from genome-wide association studies (GWAS) and copy number variation (CNV) analyses have been figured out to be encoding the players of the innate immune system

[24, 25]. These data indicate the involvement of the innate immune cells in the etiopathogenesis of AS [26, 27]. In addition, the blockade of innate cytokines with therapeutic applications has demonstrated favorable clinical efficacy in AS cases [28].

2.2 Innate Immunity Components

2.2.1 Pattern Recognition Receptors (PRR)

The potential of innate immune cells to identify self from non-self-components is contingent upon a series of receptors encoded through germ-line. In contrast to the adaptive immune-related receptors dedicated to the specific identification of antigens, receptors of the innate immune system (also called pattern recognition receptors (PRR)) can recognize the shared patterns in microbial pathogens damaged cells. Various subfamilies of such molecules have been identified to date, such as TLRs, NOD-like receptors (NLRs). The signaling of PRRs culminates in inflammatory reactions, which contributes to homeostasis restoration as well. Nonetheless, any disruption in regulatory systems could eventuate in abnormal signaling pathways and, therefore, autoinflammation [29].

2.2.1.1 Toll-Like Receptors (TLRs)

TLRs are the well-characterized members of the PRR family, which were first found in the fruit flies. Currently, ten members of TLRs have been recognized in humans; each of them possesses its specific ligands as well as cellular position. TLRs expressed on the cell surface, including TLR 1, 2, 4, 5, 6, and 10, identify bacterial-derived lipid and protein structures; nonetheless, no ligand has been recognized for TLR10 to date. That notwithstanding, TLRs with intracellular localization, such as TLR 3, 7, 8, and 9, play a role in identifying nucleic acid components, like RNA and DNA molecules. Every TLR comprises three structural domains: leucine-rich domain to recognize ligand, a transmembrane domain, and the Toll/interleukin (IL)-1 receptor (TIR). Various adaptor elements, including myeloid differentiation factor 88(MyD88), TIRAP, TRIF, or TRAM, are found in TLRs signaling pathways that transact with this TIR domain. All TLRs apply MyD88 except TLR 3, which utilizes TRIF to start downstream signaling. Nevertheless, after activation of TLR4, both TRIF and MyD88 are recruited toward the receptor by means of TIR interactions. Such interactions can trigger different transcription factors that ultimately cause the generation of pro-inflammatory or anti-viral mediators [30, 31].

Abnormal TLR signaling is involved in the initiation and progression of several diseases like autoimmune disorders, immunodeficiency syndromes, and atherosclerosis [32–34]. Evaluation of the whole genome expression pattern has shown TLR pathway dysfunction in the mesenchymal stem cells (MSCs) as well as peripheral blood of AS patients [35, 36]. MSCs are first differentiated into chondrocytes during endochondral ossification, which is regarded as a vital mechanism of bone formation in AS subjects [37]. It has been indicated that TLR 2 signaling and four agonists can enhance the conversion of human adipose tissue stromal cells into the bone, while TLR9 signaling may decelerate this process [38]. Considering the importance of gram-negative bacteria in AS [22], investigations have concentrated on the specific receptors that play a role in recognizing them.

The first identified TLR recognizing lipopolysaccharide (LPS) found on the gram-negative bacteria was TLR 4 [39]. The cluster of differentiation (CD)-14 molecule plays a co-receptor role to contribute the ligation of LPS to TLR4 [40]. Another TLR is TLR5 that recognizes the flagellin found in flagellated bacteria [41]. The primary expression evaluation of TLR genes indicated overexpression of TLR4 in the synoviocyte of AS patients [42]. Investigations along with the previous ones on the blood were conducted to reveal the relevant mechanisms.

Similarly, the whole blood gene expression pattern indicated increased expression of TLR4 in AS patients. Furthermore, TLR5 overexpression was also observed in AS patients [35]. In Crohn's disease (CD), it has been found that the flagellin is the most reactive compartment between the antigens of the commensal gut microbiome [43]. Furthermore, it has been shown that a polymorphism in TLR5 stop codon results in CD development resistance [44]. It seems that any alteration in the whole blood might stem from an increase in particular cell subsets.

Nonetheless, compared to healthy controls, TLR5 expression was upregulated in the peripheral blood mononuclear cells (PBMCs) of AS patients [45]. Therefore, the association between TLRs and AS pathogenesis might not be because of a polymorphic association, rather a difference in mRNA levels. Minor studies have addressed this association. Hence, more investigations are mandatory to disclose the status of TLR5 and probable epigenetic mechanisms regulating the expression of signaling molecules during the pathogenesis of AS.

2.2.1.2 NOD-Like Receptors (NLRs)

NLRs are another member of the PRR family. Despite the TLRs which were on the surface of the cells, NLRs are located in the cytoplasm of immune cells. All of the members of NLRs have three structural regions, such as carboxy-terminal leucine-rich repeats (LRR), to detect the ligands, a central oligomerization domain, and an effector domain like caspase activation and recruitment domain (CARD) to transduce the signal through the activation of adaptor molecules. The capability to generate an effective reaction against intracellular bacteria or their elements relies on NOD1 and NOD2, the most common members of the NOD family. The ultimate result of this bacterial detection is signaling cascade activation using CARDs interaction and expression of pro-inflammatory cytokines as well as molecules involved in apoptosis. This signaling pathway plays a vital role in gut immunity [46]. Studies with respect to the expression of NODs are confined in AS context. It has been demonstrated that PBMCs from AS patients were hyperresponsive to NOD2 stimulation, leading to the induction of inflammatory cytokines, including the IL-23/IL-17 axis [47]. The critical role of this axis in AS pathogenesis will be discussed in the text ahead. All in all, these data suggest that PRRs play a pivotal role in developing inflammatory responses in AS. Nonetheless, these pieces of evidence explicitly show that the pathogenic modifications may not be associated with genetic variants and mandate the necessity toward concentration on functional studies concerning the role of transcription factors and epigenetic changes in these signaling pathways.

2.2.2 Innate Cytokines

Cytokine mediators can synchronize immune system responses through their anti- or pro-inflammatory functions like IL-1, IL-10, IL-23, tumor necrosis factor (TNF)-α, and other related players in this family.

2.2.2.1 IL-1 Family

2.2.2.1.1 IL-1 and Receptors

The IL-1 family consists of nine genes that cover sequence homology. The well-studied members in this family are IL-1α and IL-1β, which function as potential inflammatory cytokines, and the naturally arising IL-1 receptor antagonist (IL-1Ra). IL-1β can be released by most mononuclear cells, particularly macrophages, that cause recruitment of other inflammatory cells to work simultaneously for removing infections or evoking adaptive immunity. Nonetheless, IL-1α is commonly found as a membrane-bound or intracellular cytokine [48]. The physiological functions of these cytokines are implemented via binding to type I (IL-1R1) and type II (IL-1R2) receptors. IL-1R1 is considered the pivotal role for IL-1 signaling, while IL-1R2 functions as a decoy receptor to inhibit IL-1R1 function [49]. IL-1Ra competes with IL-1β to avoid the uncontrolled activation of these receptors and regulate its signaling transduction [50]. It is supposed that other members, including IL-1F5 to IL-1F10, obtained from duplication of the gene coding for IL-1Ra (IL-1RN), play antagonistic functions as well. That notwithstanding, recent data indicate pro-inflammatory functions for some of them [51]. IL-1α and IL-1β may stimulate the bone-resorbing osteoclasts in animal models of arthritis resulting in the induction of other joint destruction enzymes [52]. Additionally, data suggest that the patients with PsA have elevated levels of these cytokines in the synovium [53]. The association between AS and IL1A or IL1R single nucleotide polymorphisms (SNPs) along with the reduced levels of IL-1Ra proposes that IL-1 signaling belongs to the critical pro-inflammatory mechanisms that are involved in determining the severity of AS disease [54].

2.2.2.1.2 IL-37

With respect to the other members of the IL-1 family, IL37 dysregulation is related to autoimmunity also. Currently, it is clear that IL-37, known initially as IL-1F7, is a natural suppressor of the innate immune system. Downregulation of pro-inflammatory cytokines has been reported upon treatment of cells with IL-37; however, this reduction was only observed during inflammation and the active phase of the autoinflammatory disease [55]. Current data have indicated that molecular and cellular IL-37 levels were promoted in PBMCs of AS patients. Furthermore, the association of IL-37 with disease severity and inflammatory signatures suggests this cytokine as a new molecule in the AS pathogenesis [56]. The repressing function of IL-37 might describe that its upregulation in various inflammatory disorders like AS could be considered probable negative feedback in the inflammatory conditions. In addition, this research area is newly opened and might supply implications to a prosperous finding to disclose the disease etiopathogenesis.

2.2.2.2 TNF and Receptors

TNF is considered a pleiotropic cytokine generated by several types of cells, primarily by T cells, NK cells, and activated macrophages, to participate in contrary processes like cell survival, proliferation, or cell death and inflammation [57]. Either membrane-bound TNF or the soluble form performs its various biological functions through binding to two types of receptors, including TNF receptor type I (TNFRI) and type II (TNFRII). TNFRI, which is encoded by the TNFRSF1 A gene, is the chief receptor that exerts the pro-inflammatory functions of TNF. The signaling of both receptors culminates in the expression of several cytokines as well as immunoregulatory factors [58–60]. Nonetheless, TNFRI contains a particular intracellular death domain that causes the recruitment of an adaptor molecule called TNFR1-associated death domain (TRADD). Upon TNF-α and TNFRI ligation, the TRADD interaction with the death domain leads to activation of caspase enzymes and, hence, cell death [61]. Several data have pointed out the TNF role in the pathogenesis of AS. Concerning the erosion of the sacroiliac joint as the red flag for AS, evaluation of sacroiliac biopsies revealed that these subjects have an enhanced number of TNF-expressing macrophages [62].

Furthermore, mice with upregulated membrane-bound TNF were shown to demonstrate spinal AS-like symptoms, like a new bone formation found in the axial skeleton joints [63]. In spite of the conflicting observations about the TNF-α levels in the blood, several investigations have reported the enhanced levels of it associated with disease activity in the AS patients [64]. Besides the identified transaction with TNFRI, TRADD also interacts with TLR4. This observation is confirmed by a finding in which TRADD deficient macrophages indicated dysregulated cytokine responses toward TLR signalings [65]. This report can account as a sign that relates the TNF signaling with TLR responses in AS patients. The last evidence was reported in gene encoding TL1A, which is generated upon activation of the antigen-presenting cells (APCs) [66].

Current data show that SNPs in *TNFSF15* gene may confer susceptibility to a higher risk of uveitis and IBD [67, 68]. Moreover, TNFSF15 signaling is a critical pathway for the proliferation and development of T helper (Th) 17 cells [69]. It is supposed that the studies in this field are not enough, and research should concentrate on the role of TL1A in Th17 priming to disclose the processes involved in the pathogenesis of AS.

The TNF gene is placed within the class III region of the major histocompatibility complex (MHC), near the HLA-B locus [70]. It has been proposed that the plausible interpretation for this protection in AS cases relies on the decreased TNF-α production by T cells [71]. In other viewpoints, the IL-1 and TNF signaling partnership can be described in the pathogenesis of AS through the Endoplasmic Reticulum

Aminopeptidase (ERAP) genes function. As a family of aminopeptidases, these genes are located in the endoplasmic reticulum (ER) that trims antigenic peptides for presentation by HLA molecules, particularly HLA-B27. ERAP1 is known as one of the non-MHC genes considered the second most important gene, after HLA-B27, related to AS risk. It has been proposed that SNPs in ERAP1 gene (such as rs30187 and rs10050860) can modulate the peptidase function of this enzyme to construct unusual peptides to be presented on APCs [24, 72]. Currently, some replicated studies have been performed indicating the association of ERAP with AS susceptibility in different populations [73]. Above the known action in trimming antigenic peptides for presentation by HLA-B27, this enzyme is likewise involved in cleaving cytokine receptors from the cell surfaces. The shedding function of the ERAP1 can decrease the signaling pathways downstream of these cytokine receptors, such as TNFRI and IL-1R2 [74, 75]. Nonetheless, investigations from ERAP1 knock-out mice and AS patients have not led to the validation of this function in ERAP enzymes [72, 76]. Therefore, it seems that the ERAP association as one of the critical AS susceptibility genes is more linked to its activity in HLA-B27 processing instead of shedding cytokine receptors.

2.2.2.3 IL-23 and Receptor

IL-23 is considered the master regulator of immune responses mainly generated by monocytes, macrophages, and activated DCs [77]. Aside from the shared p40 subunit with IL-12, IL-23 has a distinct chain known as p19. The biological function of IL-23 is implemented by ligation to a specific IL-23 receptor (IL-23R) to make a signaling complex [78]. Following IL-23 binding, the signaling pathway would be initiated downstream of IL-23R through a specific kinase, called Janus kinase 2 (JAK2), leading to recruitment and phosphorylation of the signal transducer and activator of transcription 3 (STAT3) transcription factor. Similar to other transcription factors, activated STAT3 is translocated into the nucleus to trigger the transcription of pro-inflammatory cytokine genes [79]. Very first reports have proposed that IL-23 is enough to stimulate the particular subset of inflammatory Th cells, namely Th17 [80]. These cells are categorized by producing IL- 21 and IL-17 involved in the protection of the host against fungal and extracellular infections. IL-23R expression on Th17 cells enables the potential to generate cytokines when ligated with IL-23.

Nonetheless, IL-23 is not needed to develop Th17 cells but confers the highly pathogenic characteristic to these cells [81, 82]. This condition can result in uncontrolled immune responses and intense autoimmunity settings [83]. Information from human and experimental studies has suggested the involvement of the IL-23 signaling pathway dysregulation in the pathogenesis of multiple chronic inflammatory disorders. In mice, systemic upregulation of IL23 via injection of mini-circle DNA could trigger the clinical signs of SpA [84]. Nevertheless, because of interspecies variations, it might be conflicting to rely only on animal findings. A raised number of IL-23 positive cells in the sites of bone formation have been observed in the histological analysis of the affected joints in AS patients. It has been proposed that macrophages and myeloperoxidase-positive cells are the major causes of IL-23 generation and release in these sites [85]. Currently, most approaches about the origin of IL-23 production are according to the aberrant folding of the HLA-B27 as one of the suggested hypotheses in AS pathogenesis [86].

The misfolded protein triggers a particular stress response in the ER, named unfolded protein response (UPR). This induction contributes to homeostasis restoration as well as cell survival. That notwithstanding, another essential part of the innate immune response against infections is referred to as autophagy. Autophagy, other than involvement in the host defense, can play a role in targeting and degrading the misfolded proteins. Data propose that autophagy, instead of UPR, plays a role in the regulation of the IL-23 generation [87].

Additionally, after activation, AS macrophages can release a high rate of IL-23 without the prominent UPR stimulation [88]. These findings are at odds with what has been reported in the transgenic rats [89]. On the other hand, similar to rats, another investigation reported that increased production of IL-23 has relied on the activation of UPR. This incongruent finding can be described through the sufficiency of disease-modifying drugs to prevent the upregulation of the UPR-related genes in macrophages from AS [90].

2.2.3 Soluble Components of Innate Immunity

2.2.3.1 Defensins

Defensins are the primary host anti-microbial peptides expressed predominantly in innate immune cells that contribute to the early defense as a core host-protective component against viral, fungal, and bacterial infection [91]. Paneth cells which are located at the bottom of intestinal crypts are the particular secretory cells that account for generating human α-defensin HD-5 and HD-6 subtypes. In humans, there are only α- and β-defensins that both molecules possess chemotactic and anti-microbial functions [92, 93]. This chemotactic function facilitates the recruitment and triggering of APCs, which can also incline adaptive immunity through activation of naive T cells. In fact, they are substantially involved in linking innate and adaptive immune responses. Paneth cells play a role in the protection of intestinal cells through generating HD-5, HD-6, and other anti-microbial components [94]. Evidence shows dysregulation of HD-5 in the affected ileal biopsies taken from AS and CD patients [95]. Even though the variations in NOD2 enhanced the risk of ileal Crohn in AS, not all of the variations affect defensin production.

Consequently, HD-5 deficiency results from epithelium loss in the acute phase of inflammation, and it seems to be acquired [17]. Currently, minor studies have evaluated the status of defensins in AS. All the investigations in this field have been limited to CNVs. The β-defensin gene is one of the most copy number variable regions found in the human genome [96]. Given the association of β-defensin genes CNV with some autoimmune diseases [97, 98], two investigations are heading for probing a parallel association with AS [99, 100]. Ding N et al. have reported that more than two copies of DEFB4 fragment 2 (human β-Defensin-2 encoding gene) confer a protective sign in AS development. Nonetheless, the Cai G et al. study proposed the lack of DEFB103 CNV contribution in AS risk. These CNV analyses suggest more evaluations in AS. To date, no possible association between AS and IBD predisposing factors, including defensins and NOD2, has been demonstrated. This can be described as one of the possible hypotheses for discussing the conundrums in the field of AS research.

2.2.3.2 Complement System

Complement proteins are considered as a different class of soluble elements involved in innate immune responses. These components encompass C1-C5 proteins and the membrane attack complex (MAC) activated by various triggers. Complement system activation contributes to the processes such as inflammation, chemotaxis, and MAC-dependent cell lysis to eliminate microbial pathogens, especially bacteria [101]. Investigations have reported the complement proteins contribution in AS patients as well as other autoimmune rheumatic disorders [102, 103]. Two studies have investigated the genetic variations association and uveitis in complement encoding genes. The earliest has identified no significant association between AS and copy number variation of the C4 gene in simultaneous analysis of AS and Behcet disease (BD), another uveitis-associated disorder. Nonetheless, cases harboring more than two copies of the C4 gene demonstrated an increased risk of BD proneness. The considerable importance is that BD is regarded as an inflammatory vascular disorder with the involvement of immune complexes in its etiopathogenesis [104]. The latest, evaluation of SNPs in C3 and C5 genes indicated that the GG genotype in C5 SNP (rs2269067) was strongly associated with uveitis. This genotype was found to be responsible for increased levels of IL-17 [105]. That notwithstanding, a similar investigation is required to evaluate the rs2269067 SNP genotype frequencies and function in AS disease in various races. Inhibition of complement in a mouse model of AS has resulted in the deceleration of the disease progression. Nonetheless, this inhibition was not complete since the pharmacological features of the inhibitor were not satisfying. AS-like arthritis and bone fusion were induced through the administration of proteoglycan in mice. In order to validate the activation of complement pathways, considerable levels of C3b and MAC were detected. Consequently, cellular, histological, and *in vitro* analyses were carried out, resulting in no manifestations of anyone fusion or inflammation upon treatment via complement inhibitor [106]. Despite a less potency of the complement system in mice compared with humans [103], it confers a promising approach to be targeted for therapeutic goals.

2.2.4 Innate Immune Cells

2.2.4.1 Dendritic Cells (DC)

DCs play critical roles in the immune system through initiation and regulation of the immune responses. Different types of DCs are identified upon their surface markers, tissue location, and functions [107]. DCs in humans are found in both the lymphoid and non-lymphoid organs that are divided into conventional DC1 ($CD1c^+$) and conventional DC2 (CD141$^+$) subsets [107–109]. CD1c$^+$ cells express myeloid antigens, such as CD11b, CD11c, CD13, CD33, CD45RO, and CD172 (SIRPa) markers on their surfaces. Conversely, CD141$^+$ DCs express less amount of CD11c and CD11b markers [110]. Other subtypes of DCs are called monocyte-derived DCs (Mo-DC, or MD-DC) [111]. It has been reported that Mo-DC plays a critical function in both innate and adaptive immunity because of their potential in triggering CD4+ and CD8+ T cell responses, as well as their involvement in the immunoglobulin generation by plasma cells [111].

CD56+ plasmacytoid dendritic cell (pDC) is another subset of DCs with plasma cell morphology and express markers like derived dendritic cell antigen-2 (BDCA-2), CD4, CD123, HLA-DR, TLR7, and TLR9. These cells do not express CD14 and CD11c, distinguishing them from monocytes and conventional DCs, respectively [112]. Other defined subtypes of DCs are inflammatory DCs and Langerhans cells [107, 108]. Some of these DCs participate at tolerance to self-antigens, while others develop immune responses to nonself-antigens [108]. Langerhans cells do not express several important TLRs; however, they are able to induce IL-22 production and regulatory T (Treg) development. The CD14+ monocytes have been recognized as the precursors of inflammatory DCs [110].

Several investigations have implicated the role of DCs in the etiopathogenesis of AS. Allegedly, DCs are the primarily involved cells during disease transferring through bone marrow transplantation [113].

CD1c$^+$ DCs are able to induce Th1 and Th2 responses. Previous investigations have reported that the number of circulating CD1c$^+$ DCs has decreased in AS patients, which were concurrent with an enhanced frequency of CD14- CD16+ mononuclear cells with the potential of triggering CC chemokine receptor (CCR) 6-expressing T cells and the generation of IL-6 and IL-1β. These occurrences may help the Th17-mediated immune reactions and, hence, associate with AS disease presentations [107, 114].

In addition, other investigations have reported a modified feature of the function as well as gene transcription in MD-DCs from HLA-B27+ axial SpA patients. AS such, a number of signaling cascades of MD-DCs have been dysregulated in SpA patients resulting in the launch of inflammation associated with Th17 cells [115, 116]. MD-DCs obtained from AS patients were shown to express reduced levels of class II MHC molecules (especially HLA-DR) that probably cause a disturbed function of these cells [117].

Data from B27 transgenic mice have proposed that SpA development is contingent upon the HLA-B27 overexpression on APCs and CD4+ T cells. Moreover, the immunological synapse of these mice DCs was disrupted, stemming from some molecular aberrancies. An investigation proposed that modified MHC class II expression, impaired cytoskeletal dynamics, and increased apoptotic cell death were the significant causes accounting for this dysfunction [118]. The same abnormal DCs are recognized in the patients of AS, which treatment with LPS compensated the downregulation of MHC molecules [119]. The loss of tolerogenic CD103+ subset accompanies this impaired function which induces Th17 proliferation in these transgenic mice [120, 121]. Nonetheless, the analogous CD141+ subset decreased frequency does not seem to trigger AS in human cases [122]. More investigations are required to reveal if this functional disruption in DCs is observed in AS patients. Transcriptional analysis in DCs from B27 transgenic mice [123] shows that dysregulated gene expression profile is regarded as another plausible approach of Th17 bias. Downregulation of TLR-associated genes and downmodulated IFN pathways have been detected as well. A class of innate immune controllers, called suppressor of cytokine signaling (SOCS), account for this converse IFN mark. A reduced expression of SOCS1 in PBMCs from AS patients has been reported. Furthermore, it was observed that SOCS1 was inversely correlated with serum levels of IL-17 in AS patients [124]. IFN impairment, accompanied by reduced IL-10/IL-17 ratio, might contribute to the polarization of Th17 cells.

2.2.4.2 Macrophage Cells

Macrophages play critical functions in innate immunity and host protection, mainly through phagocytosis and presenting antigens to adaptive immune cells. Macrophages are involved in wound healing through modulation of the extracellular matrix [125]. Macrophages are classified into two significant populations based on the response to several signals and environments, namely classic (M1) or alternative (M2) macrophages [126]. Microbial antigens and cytokines like IFN-γ and TNF-α lead to the promotion of the M1 macrophage development. On the contrary, complement proteins, immune complexes, and cytokines or mediators like macrophage colony-stimulating factor (M-CSF), IL-13, IL-33, and IL-4 stimulate the development of M2 cells. In the inflammatory phase, M1 macrophages generate IL-23, IL-1, and TNF-α to implement the direct eradication of microbial pathogens. Whereas M2 macrophages produce immunoregulatory cytokines like IL-10 in the resolution phase of immune system activation, resulting in inflammation attenuation [127, 128].

Synovial membrane inflammation exhibits similar macroscopic manifestations in RA and SpA patients. Studies have reported that the inflammation circumstances and the number of inflammatory cells infiltrated into the synovial membrane are analogous in both these pathologic conditions [129, 130]. A number of studies revealed that CD163+ macrophages are the most frequent cells in the inflamed peripheral joints in SpA patients [131, 132]. Evidence indicated that macrophages play a pivotal part in the inflammation of the synovial membrane and their numbers associated with the disease activity. Moreover, upon efficient therapies in SpA, the frequency of the macrophages is reduced [133]. An abundance in the CD68+ macrophages and osteoclasts has been reported in the sacroiliac tissues from AS patients [134].

According to the animal arthritis models, depletion of macrophages results in reduced inflammatory settings [135, 136]. In an AS mouse model, IL-4 treatment decreased the intensity as well as the incidence of arthritis. Additionally, the treatment eventuated in the polarization of mouse macrophages from M1 to M2 subtype both *in vivo* and *in vitro*. As such, IL-4 treatment mitigated the expression of receptor activator of nuclear factor kappa-B ligand (RANKL) in the macrophages [137].

Studies on the HLA-B27/human β2-microglobulin transgenic rats indicated an indispensable role of HLA-B27+ macrophages in the inflammation of entheses. In this setting, macrophages generate pro-inflammatory cytokines, particularly IL-23 [138]. Several pieces of research divulged a high level of IL-23 in the serum as well as the tissues from AS patients [139]. It has been well established that IL-23 has the potential to stimulate the IL-23/17 axis, which plays a pivotal role in AS pathogenesis [140].

Histological observation of the inflammatory tissues has established the accumulation of innate related immune cells, particularly macrophages [141, 142]. The morphology of another subset, named the resolution phase, emphasizes the macrophages capability for phenotypes modulating at the inflammation zone. Such cells are characterized through the expression of M1 markers and releasing the M2-associated cytokines, including IL-10 [143]. Many investigations in this regard have highlighted the CD163 marker on M2 macrophages as a unique receptor. CD163 which belongs to the scavenger superfamily is mainly the haptoglobin receptor, a protein involved in preserving iron released from hemoglobin [144]. The frequency of the CD163-positive macrophages has been increased in the colonic biopsies and inflamed synovial obtained from SpA patients. Upregulation of CD163 in the synovium has been observed to be related to the disease activity and disturbed function of lymphocytes in the SpA patients [141, 145]. In line with the upregulation of CD163, reduced M1-associated cytokines in the damaged joints imply that M1 macrophages cannot account for the inflammation source in SpA [146]. Additionally, assessing the affected ileum from AS patients has indicated that even a gentle enhancement in the frequency of M1 macrophages resulting from incubation with intestinal bacteria is covered up through the elevated amounts of M2 macrophages [145]. Therefore, it seems that M2 macrophages are the chief players blamed in the etiopathogenesis of AS.

Furthermore, IL-4, an anti-inflammatory cytokine that is also a significant trigger of M2 macrophages, can decelerate the occurrence and intensity of arthritis in an AS mouse model. Moreover, IL-4 attenuates the osteoclasts activation and differentiation in favor of reducing bone destruction [147]. Analogous studies with replicating outcomes in human subjects could hopefully confer promising therapeutic targets in AS.

It is suggested that the macrophages obtained from AS patients can express a smaller amount of IFN-γ, which leads to overexpression of genes commonly downregulated through this cytokine conversely. This occurrence, which is named as reversed IFN signature, may result in impaired removal of the intracellular bacteria, a suggested hypothesis characterizing the etiopathogenesis of reactive arthritis (ReA) [148, 149]. Considering that IFN-γ regulates Th17 cell proliferation and differentiation negatively [150], decreased expression of IFN-γ might promote the Th17 cell polarization and, hence, confers a pivotal role in AS pathogenesis.

2.2.4.3 Natural Killer (NK) Cells

Natural Killer (NK) cells are vital members of the innate immune system and confer immune surveillance at the front line defense against virus, intracellular bacteria, and tumor cells. These cells construct 5 to 15% of the PBMCs and are found in the secondary lymphoid tissues, such as tonsils, spleen, and lymph nodes, as well as other organs like liver, skin, intestine, and lung [151, 152]. NK cells are identified through the expression of CD56 and CD16 molecular markers and lack of the CD3 complex expression. These cells are categorized into two main subsets according to the CD56 expression [153]. $CD56^{dim}$ NK cells comprise about 90% of circulating NK cells in the periphery and express inhibitory killer immunoglobulin-like receptors (KIRs) as well as perforin [154]. In contrast, $CD56^{bright}$ NK cells exist predominantly in the secondary lymphoid tissues, like tonsils and lymph nodes [155].

Although an impaired function or reduced frequency of NK cells has been related to autoimmune disorders, such as RA, systemic lupus erythematosus (SLE), multiple sclerosis (MS), and psoriasis [156–158], there is a remarkably higher amount of NK cells (predominantly $CD56^{dim}$ CD16+ subset) in AS patients with a significantly higher expression of carcinoembryonic antigen-related cell adhesion molecule 1 (CEACAM1) molecule [159, 160]. Additionally, this promoted frequency of NK cells is associated with the disease severity with respect to Bath AS Disease Activity Index (BASDAI) score in the patients [161].

HLA molecules are ligands for NK cell receptors. Concerning the importance of HLA-B27 in the AS etiopathogenesis [162, 163], the KIR3DL1/3DS1 locus has been reported to be particularly important in AS setting as it recognizes HLA-B27 [159, 164]. The lysis of NK cells is prevented upon the interaction of inhibitory receptors with HLA class I molecules. According to the reports, HLA-B27 subtypes, including B*2701, *2703, *2704, *2705, and *2706 confer inhibitory impressions on NK cells, while the B*2702 subtype does not possess inhibitory effects [165]. As an inhibitory receptor, KIR3DL1 interacts with HLA-Bw4 serotype (including HLA-B27) to repress the cytolytic potential of T or NK cells, whereas KIR3DS1 confers merely an activating property.

Even though the KIR3DL1 frequency is approximately 79%, numerous investigations have reported the KIR3DS1 enrichment in HLA-B27+ AS patients [166, 167]. As such, decreased frequency of KIR3DL1 was reported in AS patients in relation to HLA-B27+ healthy individuals [168, 169]. Due to the ligand specificity of KIR3DS1, a plausible interaction of KIR3DS1 and HLA-B27 in AS disease requires more addressing. According to reports, *KIR2DL1*, *KIR3DL1*, *KIR3DS1*, *KIR2DL5*, and *KIR2DS5* genes have been associated with AS risk across various populations [170, 171]. Interestingly, the role of NK cells as biosensors in responding to Etanercept has been implicated in AS patients [172].

It has been shown that the combined inheritance of special KIR and HLA alleles (HLA-KIR haplotypes) governs the susceptibility risk to autoimmune diseases [173–175]. The significance of KIR molecules in the context of AS is noticeable in various aspects. Foremost, KIR3DL1 is the exclusive KIR that recognizes HLA-B alleles [176]. KIR3DL1 and KIR3DS1 (the activating equivalent of KIR3DL1) alleles are located in the same locus [177]. As mentioned above, the Bw4 epitope as a common KIR3DL1 ligand is found in all HLA-B27 subtypes other than B2708 [178, 179]. Compared with healthy subjects, a large number of circulating NK cells in SpA have a cytotoxic phenotype that predominantly expresses KIR3DL1 [180,

181]. Second, there is a consensus that AS patients express higher amounts of activating receptors compared with the healthy controls. Overexpression of activating receptors on NK cells from AS patients results in the transduction of activating signals, leading to the recruitment of further immune cells to the site of inflammation. This condition leads to an intensified immune context in AS disease [182]. Several replicated studies have been performed in various ethnicities concerning the significance of KIR3DL1/KIR3DS1 in AS disease [183]. It has been shown that *KIR3DL1* and *KIR3DS1* are found in little and higher quantity in AS patients from Caucasian [179, 184, 185] and Asian [182, 186] ethnicities, respectively.

Among the KIRs, KIR2DL5 has been shown to be an exclusive inhibitory receptor that takes a particular function in innate immune responses [187, 188]. Studies are controversial with respect to the KIR2DL5 status in AS patients. Two investigations have reported higher frequency of KIR2DL5 in East Asian populations [182]. Nonetheless, a protective role of KIR2DL5 was identified in the Iranian AS patients.

Regarding the relations of the KIRs with the clinical presentations of AS patients, it has been reported that KIR2DL5 was frequently found in patients manifesting uveitis episodes. Moreover, higher KIR2DL5 levels were identified in patients diagnosed at age below 17 years. The activating KIR2DS5 has also been identified to have higher frequencies in patients with AS. Increased levels of HLA-C group 2 have been reported in the AS patients, which is in line with the increased related receptor, namely KIR2DS1 [182]. The third point of KIR significance in AS is attributable to HLA-B27 potential for generating the homodimers of the heavy chain [189, 190]. Researches have indicated the expression of HLA-B27 dimers (B272) in SpA patients. KIR3DL2 has been identified as the receptor for free-β2m disulfide-bonded molecules [191]. On the other side, overexpression of KIR3DL2 has been detected on the CD4+ T and NK cells in the blood as well as the mononuclear cells from the synovium of SpA patients. These NK and CD4+T cells that are KIR3DL2 positive present phenotypic signatures that imply an already activation in the gut [192].

Furthermore, upon interaction with B272-expressing cells, KIR3DL2+ T cells have been reported to be able to proliferate and release IL-17 [193]. The specific promoter region of the *KIR3DL2* gene permits its temporary transcription. The later interactions with B272 result in transcription of the Th17-associated markers as well as anti-apoptotic molecules [194]. Since B272 confer a stronger affinity to bind to KIR3DL2, it can cause intensified stimulation in comparison with the other HLA class I molecules [195].

References

1. Ragu S, Matos-Rodrigues G, Lopez BS. Replication stress, DNA damage, inflammatory cytokines and innate immune response. Genes. 2020;11(4):409.
2. Wang JX, Vasta GR. Introduction to special issue: pattern recognition receptors and their roles in immunity in invertebrates. Dev Comp Immunol. 2020;109:103712.
3. Dougados M, Baeten D. Spondyloarthritis. Lancet (London, England). 2011;377(9783):2127–37.

4. Rudwaleit M. New approaches to diagnosis and classification of axial and peripheral spondyloarthritis. Curr Opin Rheumatol. 2010;22(4):375–80.
5. Sieper J, Poddubnyy D. Axial spondyloarthritis. The Lancet. 2017;390(10089):73–84.
6. Sieper J, Braun J, Rudwaleit M, Boonen A, Zink A. Ankylosing spondylitis: an overview. Annals Rheumat Dis. 2002;61(Suppl 3):iii8.
7. Soleimanifar N, Nicknam MH, Bidad K, Jamshidi AR, Mahmoudi M, Mostafaei S, et al. Effect of food intake and ambient air pollution exposure on ankylosing spondylitis disease activity. Adv Rheumatol. 2019;59(1):9.
8. Brown MA. Non-major-histocompatibility-complex genetics of ankylosing spondylitis. Best Pract Res Clin Rheumatol. 2006;20(3):611–21.
9. Mahmoudi M, Jamshidi AR, Amirzargar AA, Farhadi E, Nourijelyani K, Fallahi S, et al. Association between endoplasmic reticulum aminopeptidase-1 (ERAP-1) and susceptibility to ankylosing spondylitis in Iran. Iran J Allergy Asthma Immunol. 2012;11(4):294–300.
10. Wtccc T. Association scan of 14,500 nsSNPs in four common diseases identifies variants involved in autoimmunity. Nat Genet. 2007;39(11):1329–37.
11. Maksymowych WP. Disease modification in ankylosing spondylitis. Nat Rev Rheumatol. 2010;6(2):75–81.
12. Madej M, Nowak B, Świerkot J, Sokolik R, Chlebicki A, Korman L, et al. Cytokine profiles in axial spondyloarthritis. Reumatologia. 2015;53(1):9–13.
13. Sveaas SH, Berg IJ, Provan SA, Semb AG, Olsen IC, Ueland T, et al. Circulating levels of inflammatory cytokines and cytokine receptors in patients with ankylosing spondylitis: a cross-sectional comparative study. Scand J Rheumatol. 2015;44(2):118–24.
14. Kenna TJ, Brown MA. Immunopathogenesis of ankylosing spondylitis. Int J Clin Rheumatol. 2013;8(2):265–74.
15. Ambarus C, Yeremenko N, Tak PP, Baeten D. Pathogenesis of spondyloarthritis: autoimmune or autoinflammatory? Curr Opin Rheumatol. 2012;24(4):351–8.
16. Chyuan IT, Chen JY. Role of interleukin- (IL-) 17 in the pathogenesis and targeted therapies in spondyloarthropathies. Mediators Inflamm. 2018;2018:2403935.
17. Ciccia F, Bombardieri M, Rizzo A, Principato A, Giardina AR, Raiata F, et al. Over-expression of paneth cell-derived anti-microbial peptides in the gut of patients with ankylosing spondylitis and subclinical intestinal inflammation. Rheumatology. 2010;49(11):2076–83.
18. Leijten EF, van Kempen TS, Boes M, Michels-van Amelsfort JM, Hijnen D, Hartgring SA, et al. Brief report: enrichment of activated group 3 innate lymphoid cells in psoriatic arthritis synovial fluid. Arthritis Rheumatol (Hoboken, NJ). 2015;67(10):2673–8.
19. Stoll ML. Interactions of the innate and adaptive arms of the immune system in the pathogenesis of spondyloarthritis. Clin Exp Rheumatol. 2011;29(2):322–30.
20. Gierut A, Perlman H, Pope RM. Innate immunity and rheumatoid arthritis. Rheum Dis Clin North Am. 2010;36(2):271–96.
21. Fullard N, O'Reilly S. Role of innate immune system in systemic sclerosis. Semin Immunopathol. 2015;37(5):511–7.
22. Asquith M, Elewaut D, Lin P, Rosenbaum JT. The role of the gut and microbes in the pathogenesis of spondyloarthritis. Best Pract Res Clin Rheumatol. 2014;28(5):687–702.
23. Jacques P, Lambrecht S, Verheugen E, Pauwels E, Kollias G, Armaka M, et al. Proof of concept: enthesitis and new bone formation in spondyloarthritis are driven by mechanical strain and stromal cells. Ann Rheum Dis. 2014;73(2):437–45.
24. Cortes A, Hadler J, Pointon JP, Robinson PC, Karaderi T, Leo P, et al. Identification of multiple risk variants for ankylosing spondylitis through high-density genotyping of immune-related loci. Nat Genet. 2013;45(7):730–8.
25. O'Rielly DD, Uddin M, Rahman P. Ankylosing spondylitis: beyond genome-wide association studies. Curr Opin Rheumatol. 2016;28(4):337–45.
26. Rezaiemanesh A, Abdolmaleki M, Abdolmohammadi K, Aghaei H, Pakdel FD, Fatahi Y, et al. Immune cells involved in the pathogenesis of ankylosing spondylitis. Biomed Pharmacother. 2018;100:198–204.
27. Zambrano-Zaragoza JF, Agraz-Cibrian JM, González-Reyes C, Durán-Avelar MDJ, Vibanco-Pérez N. Ankylosing spondylitis: from cells to genes. Int J Inflam. 2013;2013:501653.

28. Sieper J. New treatment targets for axial spondyloarthritis. Rheumatology (United Kingdom). 2016;55:ii38–42.
29. Mullen LM, Chamberlain G, Sacre S. Pattern recognition receptors as potential therapeutic targets in inflammatory rheumatic disease. Arthritis Res Ther. 2015;17(1):122.
30. Chen JQ, Szodoray P, Zeher M. Toll-Like Receptor Pathways in Autoimmune Diseases. Clin Rev Allergy Immunol. 2016;50(1):1–17.
31. Lim KH, Staudt LM. Toll-Like receptor signaling. Cold Spring Harb Perspect Biol. 2013;5(1):a011247.
32. Duffy L, O'Reilly SC. Toll-like receptors in the pathogenesis of autoimmune diseases: recent and emerging translational developments. Immuno Targets Therapy. 2016;5:69–80.
33. Maglione PJ, Simchoni N, Cunningham-Rundles C. Toll-like receptor signaling in primary immune deficiencies. Ann N Y Acad Sci. 2015;1356(1):1–21.
34. Falck-Hansen M, Kassiteridi C, Monaco C. Toll-like receptors in atherosclerosis. Int J Mol Sci. 2013;14(7):14008–23.
35. Assassi S, Reveille JD, Arnett FC, Weisman MH, Ward MM, Agarwal SK, et al. Whole-blood gene expression profiling in ankylosing spondylitis shows upregulation of Toll-like receptor 4 and 5. J Rheumatol. 2011;38(1):87–98.
36. Li Y, Wang P, Xie Z, Huang L, Yang R, Gao L, et al. Whole genome expression profiling and signal pathway screening of MSCs in ankylosing spondylitis. Stem Cells Int. 2014;2014:913050.
37. Lories RJ, Luyten FP, de Vlam K. Progress in spondylarthritis. Mechanisms of new bone formation in spondyloarthritis. Arthritis Res Ther. 2009;11(2):221.
38. Hyun HC, Yong CB, Jin SJ. Role of toll-like receptors on human adipose-derived stromal cells. Stem Cells. 2006;24(12):2744–52.
39. Medzhitov R, Preston-Hurlburt P, Janeway CA Jr. A human homologue of the Drosophila toll protein signals activation of adaptive immunity. Nature. 1997;388(6640):394–7.
40. Wright SD, Ramos RA, Tobias PS, Ulevitch RJ, Mathison JC. CD14, a receptor for complexes of lipopolysaccharide (LPS) and LPS binding protein. Science. 1990;249(4975):1431–3.
41. Hayashi F, Smith KD, Ozinsky A, Hawn TR, Yi EC, Goodlett DR, et al. The innate immune response to bacterial flagellin is mediated by Toll-like receptor 5. Nature. 2001;410(6832):1099–103.
42. De Rycke L, Vandooren B, Kruithof E, De Keyser F, Veys EM, Baeten D. Tumor necrosis factor α blockade treatment down-modulates the increased systemic and local expression of Toll-like receptor 2 and Toll-like receptor 4 in spondylarthropathy. Arthritis Rheum. 2005;52(7):2146–58.
43. Lodes MJ, Cong Y, Elson CO, Mohamath R, Landers CJ, Targan SR, et al. Bacterial flagellin is a dominant antigen in Crohn disease. J Clin Investig. 2004;113(9):1296–306.
44. Gewirtz AT, Vijay-Kumar M, Brant SR, Duerr RH, Nicolae DL, Cho JH. Dominant-negative TLR5 polymorphism reduces adaptive immune response to flagellin and negatively associates with Crohn's disease. Am J Physiol Gastrointest Liver Physiol. 2006;290(6):G1157–G63.
45. Almasi S, Aslani S, Poormoghim H, Jamshidi A, Poursani S, Mahmoudi M. Gene expression profiling of toll-like receptor 4 and 5 in peripheral blood mononuclear cells in rheumatic disorders: ankylosing spondylitis and rheumatoid arthritis. Iran J Allergy Asthma Immunol. 2016;15(1):87–92.
46. Motta V, Soares F, Sun T, Philpott DJ. Nod-like receptors: versatile cytosolic sentinels. Physiol Rev. 2015;95(1):149–78.
47. Vanaki N, Golmohammadi T, Jamshidi A, Akhtari M, Vojdanian M, Mostafaei S, et al. Increased inflammatory responsiveness of peripheral blood mononuclear cells (PBMCs) to in vitro NOD2 ligand stimulation in patients with ankylosing spondylitis. Immunopharmacol Immunotoxicol. 2018;40(5):393–400.
48. Palomo J, Dietrich D, Martin P, Palmer G, Gabay C. The interleukin (IL)-1 cytokine family – balance between agonists and antagonists in inflammatory diseases. Cytokine. 2015;76(1):25–37.

49. Garlanda C, Dinarello CA, Mantovani A. The interleukin-1 family: back to the future. Immunity. 2013;39(6):1003–18.
50. Bresnihan B, Cunnane G. Interleukin-1 receptor antagonist. Rheum Dis Clin North Am. 1998;24(3):615–28.
51. Laurincová B. Interleukin-1 family: from genes to human disease. Acta Univ Palacki Olomuc Fac Med. 2000;143:19–29.
52. Loo FAJVD, Joosten LAB, Van Lent PLEM, Arntz OJ, Van Den Berg WB. Role of interleukin-1, tumor necrosis factor α, and interleukin-6 in cartilage proteoglycan metabolism and destruction effect of in situ blocking in murine antigen- and zymosan-induced arthritis. Arthritis Rheum. 1995;38(2):164–72.
53. Ritchlin C, Haas-Smith SA, Hicks D, Cappuccio J, Osterland CK, Looney RJ. Patterns of cytokine production in psoriatic synovium. J Rheumatol. 1998;25(8):1544–52.
54. Nossent JC, Sagen-Johnsen S, Bakland G. IL-1A gene variation in relation to cytokine levels and clinical characteristics in ankylosing spondylitis. European J Rheumatol. 2019;6(2):67.
55. Xu WD, Zhao Y, Liu Y. Insights into IL-37, the role in autoimmune diseases. Autoimmun Rev. 2015;14(12):1170–5.
56. Chen B, Huang K, Ye L, Li Y, Zhang J, Zhang J, et al. Interleukin-37 is increased in ankylosing spondylitis patients and associated with disease activity. J Transl Med. 2015;13(1):36.
57. Vassalli P. The pathophysiology of tumor necrosis factors. Annu Rev Immunol. 1992;10:411–52.
58. Dembic Z, Loetscher H, Gubler U, Pan Y-CE, Lahm H-W, Gentz R, et al. Two human TNF receptors have similar extracellular, but distinct intracellular, domain sequences. Cytokine. 1990;2(4):231–7.
59. Tartaglia LA, Weber RF, Figari IS, Reynolds C, Palladino MA, Goeddel DV. The two different receptors for tumor necrosis factor mediate distinct cellular responses. Proc Natl Acad Sci. 1991;88(20):9292.
60. Black RA, Rauch CT, Kozlosky CJ, Peschon JJ, Slack JL, Wolfson MF, et al. A metalloproteinase disintegrin that releases tumour-necrosis factor-∅ from cells. Nature. 1997;385(6618):729–33.
61. Hsu H, Xiong J, Goeddel DV. The TNF receptor 1-associated protein TRADD signals cell death and NF-κB activation. Cell. 1995;81(4):495–504.
62. Braun J, Bollow M, Neure L, Seipelt E, Seyrekbasan F, Herbst H, et al. Use of immunohistologic and in situ hybridization techniques in the examination of sacroiliac joint biopsy specimens from patients with ankylosing spondylitis. Arthritis Rheum. 1995;38(4):499–505.
63. LMv D, Ambarus CA, Masdar H, MNv T, Tak PP, Yeremenko NG, et al. A2.15 relative overexpression of transmembrane versus soluble tnf in human and experimental spondyloarthritis. Annals Rheumat Dis. 2013;72(Suppl 1):A9.
64. Asadbeik M, Farazmand A, Vanaki N, Mostafaei S, Jamshidi AR, Ahmadzadeh N, et al. Gene expression profile of pro-inflammatory cytokines in Iranian patients with ankylosing spondylitis. Rheumatol Res. 2017;2(1):31–8.
65. Chen N-J, Chio IIC, Lin W-J, Duncan G, Chau H, Katz D, et al. Beyond tumor necrosis factor receptor: TRADD signaling in toll-like receptors. Proc Natl Acad Sci. 2008;105(34):12429.
66. Aiba Y, Nakamura M. The role of TL1A and DR3 in autoimmune and inflammatory diseases. Mediators Inflamm. 2013;2013:9.
67. Li H, Hou S, Yu H, Zheng M, Zhang L, Zhang J, et al. Association of genetic variations in TNFSF15 with acute anterior uveitis in chinese hanassociation of TNFSF15 with AAU. Invest Ophthalmol Vis Sci. 2015;56(8):4605–10.
68. Zucchelli M, Camilleri M, Nixon Andreasson A, Bresso F, Dlugosz A, Halfvarson J, et al. Association of TNFSF15 polymorphism with irritable bowel syndrome. Gut. 2011;60(12):1671.
69. Pappu BP, Borodovsky A, Zheng TS, Yang X, Wu P, Dong X, et al. TL1A–DR3 interaction regulates Th17 cell function and Th17-mediated autoimmune disease. J Exp Med. 2008;205(5):1049.
70. Campbell RD, Trowsdale J. Map of the human MHC. Immunol Today. 1993;14(7):349–52.

71. Rudwaleit M, Siegert S, Yin Z, Eick J, Thiel A, Radbruch A, et al. Low T cell production of TNFα and IFNγ in ankylosing spondylitis: its relation to HLA-B27 and influence of the TNF-308 gene polymorphism. Ann Rheum Dis. 2001;60(1):36–42.
72. Evans DM, Spencer CC, Pointon JJ, Su Z, Harvey D, Kochan G, et al. Interaction between ERAP1 and HLA-B27 in ankylosing spondylitis implicates peptide handling in the mechanism for HLA-B27 in disease susceptibility. Nat Genet. 2011;43(8):761–7.
73. Bettencourt BF, Rocha FL, Alves H, Amorim R, Caetano-Lopes J, Vieira-Sousa E, et al. Protective effect of an ERAP1 haplotype in ankylosing spondylitis: investigating non-MHC genes in HLA-B27-positive individuals. Rheumatology. 2013;52(12):2168–76.
74. Cui X, Hawari F, Alsaaty S, Lawrence M, Combs CA, Geng W, et al. Identification of ARTS-1 as a novel TNFR1-binding protein that promotes TNFR1 ectodomain shedding. J Clin Investig. 2002;110(4):515–26.
75. Cui X, Rouhani FN, Hawari F, Levine SJ. Shedding of the type II IL-1 decoy receptor requires a multifunctional aminopeptidase, aminopeptidase regulator of TNF receptor type 1 shedding. J Immunol. 2003;171(12):6814.
76. Haroon N, Tsui FWL, Chiu B, Tsui HW, Inman RD. Serum cytokine receptors in ankylosing spondylitis: relationship to inflammatory markers and endoplasmic reticulum aminopeptidase polymorphisms. J Rheumatol. 2010;37(9):1907.
77. Trinchieri G, Pflanz S, Kastelein RA. The IL-12 family of heterodimeric cytokines: new players in the regulation of t cell responses. Immunity. 2003;19(5):641–4.
78. Parham C, Chirica M, Timans J, Vaisberg E, Travis M, Cheung J, et al. A receptor for the heterodimeric cytokine IL-23 Is composed of IL-12Rβ1 and a novel cytokine receptor subunit, IL-23R. J Immunol. 2002;168(11):5699.
79. Cho M-L, Kang J-W, Moon Y-M, Nam H-J, Jhun J-Y, Heo S-B, et al. STAT3 and NF-κB signal pathway is required for IL-23-mediated IL-17 production in spontaneous arthritis animal model IL-1 receptor antagonist-deficient mice. J Immunol. 2006;176(9):5652.
80. Aggarwal S, Ghilardi N, Xie MH, de Sauvage FJ, Gurney AL. Interleukin-23 promotes a distinct CD4 T cell activation state characterized by the production of interleukin-17. J Biol Chem. 2003;278(3):1910–4.
81. Langrish CL, Chen Y, Blumenschein WM, Mattson J, Basham B, Sedgwick JD, et al. IL-23 drives a pathogenic T cell population that induces autoimmune inflammation. J Exp Med. 2005;201(2):233.
82. McGeachy MJ, Chen Y, Tato CM, Laurence A, Joyce-Shaikh B, Blumenschein WM, et al. The interleukin 23 receptor is essential for the terminal differentiation of interleukin 17–producing effector T helper cells in vivo. Nat Immunol. 2009;10:314.
83. Croxford AL, Mair F, Becher B. IL-23: one cytokine in control of autoimmunity. Eur J Immunol. 2012;42(9):2263–73.
84. Sherlock JP, Joyce-Shaikh B, Turner SP, Chao C-C, Sathe M, Grein J, et al. IL-23 induces spondyloarthropathy by acting on ROR-γt+ CD3+CD4−CD8− entheseal resident T cells. Nat Med. 2012;18:1069.
85. Appel H, Maier R, Bleil J, Hempfing A, Loddenkemper C, Schlichting U, et al. In Situ analysis of interleukin–23– and interleukin-12–positive cells in the spine of patients with ankylosing spondylitis. Arthritis Rheum. 2013;65(6):1522–9.
86. Mear JP, Schreiber KL, Münz C, Zhu X, Stevanović S, Rammensee HG, et al. Misfolding of HLA-B27 as a result of its B pocket suggests a novel mechanism for its role in susceptibility to spondyloarthropathies. J Immunol. 1999;163(12):6665–70.
87. Ciccia F, Accardo-Palumbo A, Rizzo A, Guggino G, Raimondo S, Giardina A, et al. Evidence that autophagy, but not the unfolded protein response, regulates the expression of IL-23 in the gut of patients with ankylosing spondylitis and subclinical gut inflammation. Ann Rheum Dis. 2014;73(8):1566.
88. Zeng L, Lindstrom MJ, Smith JA. Ankylosing spondylitis macrophage production of higher levels of interleukin-23 in response to lipopolysaccharide without induction of a significant unfolded protein response. Arthritis Rheum. 2011;63(12):3807–17.

89. DeLay ML, Turner MJ, Klenk EI, Smith JA, Sowders DP, Colbert RA. HLA–B27 misfolding and the unfolded protein response augment interleukin-23 production and are associated with Th17 activation in transgenic rats. Arthritis Rheum. 2009;60(9):2633–43.
90. Rezaiemanesh A, Mahmoudi M, Amirzargar AA, Vojdanian M, Jamshidi AR, Nicknam MH. Ankylosing spondylitis M-CSF-derived macrophages are undergoing unfolded protein response (UPR) and express higher levels of interleukin-23. Mod Rheumatol. 2017;27(5):862–7.
91. Zasloff M. Antimicrobial peptides of multicellular organisms. Nature. 2002; 415(6870):389–95.
92. Boniotto M, Jordan WJ, Eskdale J, Tossi A, Antcheva N, Crovella S, et al. Human β-defensin 2 induces a vigorous cytokine response in peripheral blood mononuclear cells. Antimicrob Agents Chemother. 2006;50(4):1433.
93. Chaly YV, Paleolog EM, Kolesnikova TS, Tikhonov II, Petratchenko EV, Voitenok NN. Human neutrophil α-defensin modulates cytokine production in human monocytes and adhesion molecule expression in endothelial cells. Eur Cytokine Netw. 2000;11(2):257–66.
94. Keshav S. Paneth cells: leukocyte-like mediators of innate immunity in the intestine. J Leukoc Biol. 2006;80(3):500–8.
95. Simms LA, Doecke JD, Walsh MD, Huang N, Fowler EV, Radford-Smith GL. Reduced α-defensin expression is associated with inflammation and not NOD2 mutation status in ileal Crohn's disease. Gut. 2008;57(7):903.
96. Hardwick RJ, Machado LR, Zuccherato LW, Antolinos S, Xue Y, Shawa N, et al. A worldwide analysis of beta-defensin copy number variation suggests recent selection of a high-expressing DEFB103 gene copy in East Asia. Hum Mutat. 2011;32(7):743–50.
97. Zanetti M, Gennaro R, Romeo D. Cathelicidins: a novel protein family with a common proregion and a variable C-terminal anti-microbial domain. FEBS Lett. 1995;374(1):1–5.
98. Zhou X-J, Cheng F-J, Lv J-C, Luo H, Yu F, Chen M, et al. Higher DEFB4 genomic copy number in SLE and ANCA-associated small vasculitis. Rheumatology. 2012;51(6):992–5.
99. Ding N, Yang X, Zhang L, Cai G, Xia Q, Fan D, et al. Association of β-defensin gene copy number variations with ankylosing spondylitis in Chinese population: a case–control study. Mod Rheumatol. 2016;26(1):146–50.
100. Cai G, Xia Q, Fan D, Li X, Ding N, Hu Y, et al. Association between DEFB103 gene copy number variation and ankylosing spondylitis: a case–control study. Tissue Antigens. 2015;86(3):195–8.
101. Noris M, Remuzzi G. Overview of complement activation and regulation. Semin Nephrol. 2013;33(6):479–92.
102. Brinch L, Vinje O, Teisberg P, Mellbye OJ, Aakesson I. The in-vivo metabolism of C3 in ankylosing spondylitis. Ann Rheum Dis. 1982;41(1):86.
103. Trouw LA, Pickering MC, Blom AM. The complement system as a potential therapeutic target in rheumatic disease. Nat Rev Rheumatol. 2017;13:538.
104. Hou S, Qi J, Liao D, Zhang Q, Fang J, Zhou Y, et al. Copy number variations of complement component C4 are associated with behçet's disease but not with ankylosing spondylitis associated with acute anterior uveitis. Arthritis Rheum. 2013;65(11):2963–70.
105. Xu D, Hou S, Jiang Y, Zhang J, Cao S, Zhang D, et al. Complement C5 gene confers risk for acute anterior UveitisC5 polymorphisms are associated with AAU. Invest Ophthalmol Vis Sci. 2015;56(8):4954–60.
106. Yang C, Ding P, Wang Q, Zhang L, Zhang X, Zhao J, et al. Inhibition of complement retards ankylosing spondylitis progression. Sci Rep. 2016;6:34643.
107. O'Keeffe M, Mok WH, Radford KJ. Human dendritic cell subsets and function in health and disease. Cell Mol Life Sci: CMLS. 2015;72(22):4309–25.
108. Shortman K, Liu YJ. Mouse and human dendritic cell subtypes. Nat Rev Immunol. 2002;2(3):151–61.
109. Guilliams M, Ginhoux F, Jakubzick C, Naik SH, Onai N, Schraml BU, et al. Dendritic cells, monocytes and macrophages: a unified nomenclature based on ontogeny. Nat Rev Immunol. 2014;14(8):571–8.

110. Collin M, McGovern N, Haniffa M. Human dendritic cell subsets. Immunology. 2013;140(1):22–30.
111. Qu C, Brinck-Jensen NS, Zang M, Chen K. Monocyte-derived dendritic cells: targets as potent antigen-presenting cells for the design of vaccines against infectious diseases. Int J Infect Dis: IJID: Official Publication of the International Society for Infectious Diseases. 2014;19:1–5.
112. McKenna K, Beignon A-S, Bhardwaj N. Plasmacytoid Dendritic Cells: linking Innate and Adaptive Immunity. J Virol. 2005;79(1):17–27.
113. Stockwin LH, McGonagle D, Martin IG, Blair GE. Dendritic cells: immunological sentinels with a central role in health and disease. Immunol Cell Biol. 2000;78(2):91–102.
114. Wright PB, McEntegart A, McCarey D, McInnes IB, Siebert S, Milling SW. Ankylosing spondylitis patients display altered dendritic cell and T cell populations that implicate pathogenic roles for the IL-23 cytokine axis and intestinal inflammation. Rheumatology (Oxford, England). 2016;55(1):120–32.
115. Zambrano-Zaragoza JF, Agraz-Cibrian JM, Gonzalez-Reyes C, Duran-Avelar Mde J, Vibanco-Perez N. Ankylosing spondylitis: from cells to genes. Int J Inflam. 2013;2013:501653.
116. Talpin A, Costantino F, Bonilla N, Leboime A, Letourneur F, Jacques S, et al. Monocyte-derived dendritic cells from HLA-B27+ axial spondyloarthritis (SpA) patients display altered functional capacity and deregulated gene expression. Arthritis Res Ther. 2014;16(4):417.
117. Slobodin G, Kessel A, Kofman N, Toubi E, Rosner I, Odeh M. Phenotype of resting and activated monocyte-derived dendritic cells grown from peripheral blood of patients with ankylosing spondylitis. Inflammation. 2012;35(2):772–5.
118. Dhaenens M, Fert I, Glatigny S, Haerinck S, Poulain C, Donnadieu E, et al. Dendritic cells from spondylarthritis-prone HLA–B27–transgenic rats display altered cytoskeletal dynamics, class II major histocompatibility complex expression, and viability. Arthritis Rheum. 2009;60(9):2622–32.
119. Slobodin G, Kessel A, Kofman N, Toubi E, Rosner I, Odeh M. Phenotype of resting and activated monocyte-derived dendritic cells grown from peripheral blood of patients with ankylosing spondylitis. Inflammation. 2012;35(2):772–5.
120. Glatigny S, Fert I, Blaton MA, Lories RJ, Araujo LM, Chiocchia G, et al. Pro-inflammatory Th17 cells are expanded and induced by dendritic cells in spondylarthritis-prone HLA–B27–transgenic rats. Arthritis Rheum. 2012;64(1):110–20.
121. Utriainen L, Firmin D, Wright P, Cerovic V, Breban M, McInnes I, et al. Expression of HLA–B27 causes loss of migratory dendritic cells in a rat model of spondylarthritis. Arthritis Rheum. 2012;64(10):3199–209.
122. Wright PB, McEntegart A, McCarey D, McInnes IB, Siebert S, Milling SWF. Ankylosing spondylitis patients display altered dendritic cell and T cell populations that implicate pathogenic roles for the IL-23 cytokine axis and intestinal inflammation. Rheumatology. 2015;55(1):120–32.
123. Fert I, Cagnard N, Glatigny S, Letourneur F, Jacques S, Smith JA, et al. Reverse interferon signature is characteristic of antigen-presenting cells in human and rat spondyloarthritis. Arthritis Rheum. 2014;66(4):841–51.
124. Chen CH, Chen HA, Liao HT, Liu CH, Tsai CY, Chou CT. Suppressors of cytokine signalling in ankylosing spondylitis and their associations with disease severity, acute-phase reactants and serum cytokines. Clin Exp Rheumatol. 2016;34(1):100–5.
125. Wynn TA, Barron L, Thompson RW, Madala SK, Wilson MS, Cheever AW, et al. Quantitative assessment of macrophage functions in repair and fibrosis. Current protocols in immunology. 2011;Chapter 14:Unit14.22. https://doi.org/10.1002/0471142735.im1422s93.
126. Okabe Y, Medzhitov R. Tissue-specific signals control reversible program of localization and functional polarization of macrophages. Cell. 2014;157(4):832–44.
127. Mantovani A, Biswas SK, Galdiero MR, Sica A, Locati M. Macrophage plasticity and polarization in tissue repair and remodelling. J Pathol. 2013;229(2):176–85.
128. Murray Peter J, Allen Judith E, Biswas Subhra K, Fisher Edward A, Gilroy Derek W, Goerdt S, et al. Macrophage activation and polarization: nomenclature and experimental guidelines. Immunity. 2014;41(1):14–20.

129. Baeten D, Demetter P, Cuvelier CA, Kruithof E, Van Damme N, De Vos M, et al. Macrophages expressing the scavenger receptor CD163: a link between immune alterations of the gut and synovial inflammation in spondyloarthropathy. J Pathol. 2002;196(3):343–50.
130. Kruithof E, Baeten D, De Rycke L, Vandooren B, Foell D, Roth J, et al. Synovial histopathology of psoriatic arthritis, both oligo- and polyarticular, resembles spondyloarthropathy more than it does rheumatoid arthritis. Arthritis Res Ther. 2005;7(3):R569–80.
131. Mulherin D, Fitzgerald O, Bresnihan B. Synovial tissue macrophage populations and articular damage in rheumatoid arthritis. Arthritis Rheum. 1996;39(1):115–24.
132. Bruhl H, Cihak J, Plachy J, Kunz-Schughart L, Niedermeier M, Denzel A, et al. Targeting of Gr-1+,CCR2+ monocytes in collagen-induced arthritis. Arthritis Rheum. 2007;56(9):2975–85.
133. Bresnihan B, Pontifex E, Thurlings RM, Vinkenoog M, El-Gabalawy H, Fearon U, et al. Synovial tissue sublining CD68 expression is a biomarker of therapeutic response in rheumatoid arthritis clinical trials: consistency across centers. J Rheumatol. 2009;36(8):1800–2.
134. Braun J, Bollow M, Neure L, Seipelt E, Seyrekbasan F, Herbst H, et al. Use of immunohistologic and in situ hybridization techniques in the examination of sacroiliac joint biopsy specimens from patients with ankylosing spondylitis. Arthritis Rheum. 1995;38(4):499–505.
135. Barrera P, Blom A, van Lent PL, van Bloois L, Beijnen JH, van Rooijen N, et al. Synovial macrophage depletion with clodronate-containing liposomes in rheumatoid arthritis. Arthritis Rheum. 2000;43(9):1951–9.
136. Kashiwagi N, Nakano M, Saniabadi AR, Adachi M, Yoshikawa T. Anti-inflammatory effect of granulocyte and monocyte adsorption apheresis in a rabbit model of immune arthritis. Inflammation. 2002;26(4):199–205.
137. Lin S, Qiu M, Chen J. IL-4 modulates macrophage polarization in ankylosing spondylitis. Cell Physiol Biochem. 2015;35(6):2213–22.
138. Rezaiemanesh A, Mahmoudi M, Amirzargar AA, Vojdanian M, Jamshidi AR, Nicknam MH. Ankylosing spondylitis M-CSF-derived macrophages are undergoing unfolded protein response (UPR) and express higher levels of interleukin-23. Mod Rheumatol. 2017;27(5):862–7.
139. Mei Y, Pan F, Gao J, Ge R, Duan Z, Zeng Z, et al. Increased serum IL-17 and IL-23 in the patient with ankylosing spondylitis. Clin Rheumatol. 2011;30(2):269–73.
140. Jethwa H, Bowness P. The interleukin (IL)-23/IL-17 axis in ankylosing spondylitis: new advances and potentials for treatment. Clin Exp Immunol. 2016;183(1):30–6.
141. Baeten D, Kruithof E, De Rycke L, Boots AM, Mielants H, Veys EM, et al. Infiltration of the synovial membrane with macrophage subsets and polymorphonuclear cells reflects global disease activity in spondyloarthropathy. Arthritis Res Ther. 2005;7(2):R359.
142. Gordon S, Taylor PR. Monocyte and macrophage heterogeneity. Nat Rev Immunol. 2005;5(12):953–64.
143. Bystrom J, Evans I, Newson J, Stables M, Toor I, van Rooijen N, et al. Resolution-phase macrophages possess a unique inflammatory phenotype that is controlled by cAMP. Blood. 2008;112(10):4117–27.
144. Ritter M, Buechler C, Langmann T, Orso E, Klucken J, Schmitz G. The scavenger receptor CD163: regulation, promoter structure and genomic organization. Pathobiology. 1999;67(5-6):257–61.
145. Ciccia F, Alessandro R, Rizzo A, Accardo-Palumbo A, Raimondo S, Raiata F, et al. Macrophage phenotype in the subclinical gut inflammation of patients with ankylosing spondylitis. Rheumatology. 2013;53(1):104–13.
146. Vandooren B, Noordenbos T, Ambarus C, Krausz S, Cantaert T, Yeremenko N, et al. absence of a classically activated macrophage cytokine signature in peripheral spondylarthritis, including psoriatic arthritis. Arthritis Rheum. 2009;60(4):966–75.
147. Lin S, Qiu M, Chen J. IL-4 Modulates Macrophage Polarization in Ankylosing Spondylitis. Cell Physiol Biochem. 2015;35(6):2213–22.
148. Smith JA, Barnes MD, Hong D, DeLay ML, Inman RD, Colbert RA. Gene expression analysis of macrophages derived from ankylosing spondylitis patients reveals interferon-γ dysregulation. Arthritis Rheum. 2008;58(6):1640–9.

149. Inman RD, Chiu B. Early cytokine profiles in the joint define pathogen clearance and severity of arthritis in Chlamydia-induced arthritis in rats. Arthritis Rheum. 2006;54(2):499–507.
150. Chu C-Q, Swart D, Alcorn D, Tocker J, Elkon KB. Interferon-γ regulates susceptibility to collagen-induced arthritis through suppression of interleukin-17. Arthritis Rheum. 2007;56(4):1145–51.
151. Shi FD, Ljunggren HG, La Cava A, Van Kaer L. Organ-specific features of natural killer cells. Nat Rev Immunol. 2011;11(10):658–71.
152. Tian Z, Gershwin ME, Zhang C. Regulatory NK cells in autoimmune disease. J Autoimmun. 2012;39(3):206–15.
153. Cooper MA, Fehniger TA, Turner SC, Chen KS, Ghaheri BA, Ghayur T, et al. Human natural killer cells: a unique innate immunoregulatory role for the CD56(bright) subset. Blood. 2001;97(10):3146–51.
154. Caligiuri MA. Human natural killer cells. Blood. 2008;112(3):461–9.
155. Fehniger TA, Cooper MA, Nuovo GJ, Cella M, Facchetti F, Colonna M, et al. CD56bright natural killer cells are present in human lymph nodes and are activated by T cell-derived IL-2: a potential new link between adaptive and innate immunity. Blood. 2003;101(8):3052–7.
156. Aramaki T, Ida H, Izumi Y, Fujikawa K, Huang M, Arima K, et al. A significantly impaired natural killer cell activity due to a low activity on a per-cell basis in rheumatoid arthritis. Mod Rheumatol. 2009;19(3):245–52.
157. Park YW, Kee SJ, Cho YN, Lee EH, Lee HY, Kim EM, et al. Impaired differentiation and cytotoxicity of natural killer cells in systemic lupus erythematosus. Arthritis Rheum. 2009;60(6):1753–63.
158. Cameron AL, Kirby B, Griffiths CE. Circulating natural killer cells in psoriasis. Br J Dermatol. 2003;149(1):160–4.
159. Azuz-Lieberman N, Markel G, Mizrahi S, Gazit R, Hanna J, Achdout H, et al. The involvement of NK cells in ankylosing spondylitis. Int Immunol. 2005;17(7):837–45.
160. Mousavi T, Poormoghim H, Moradi M, Tajik N, Shahsavar F, Soofi M. Phenotypic study of natural killer cell subsets in ankylosing spondylitis patients. Iran J Allergy Asthma Immunol. 2009;8(4):193–8.
161. Akalın N, Soy M. Natural killer and natural killer T cells as a prognostic factor for rheumatoid arthritis and ankylosing spondylitis. Int J Bio Res. 2015;6:301–08.
162. Baeten D, Kruithof E, Van den Bosch F, Demetter P, Van Damme N, Cuvelier C, et al. Immunomodulatory effects of anti-tumor necrosis factor alpha therapy on synovium in spondylarthropathy: histologic findings in eight patients from an open-label pilot study. Arthritis Rheum. 2001;44(1):186–95.
163. Nicknam MH, Mahmoudi M, Amirzargar AA, Ganjalikhani Hakemi M, Khosravi F, Jamshidi AR, et al. Determination of HLA-B27 subtypes in Iranian patients with ankylosing spondylitis. Iran J Allergy Asthma Immunol. 2008;7(1):19–24.
164. Boyington JC, Sun PD. A structural perspective on MHC class I recognition by killer cell immunoglobulin-like receptors. Mol Immunol. 2002;38(14):1007–21.
165. Luque I, Solana R, Galiani MD, Gonzalez R, Garcia F. Lopez de Castro JA, et al. Threonine 80 on HLA-B27 confers protection against lysis by a group of natural killer clones. Eur J Immunol. 1996;26(8):1974–7.
166. Diaz-Pena R, Vidal-Castineira JR, Alonso-Arias R, Suarez-Alvarez B, Vicario JL, Solana R, et al. Association of the KIR3DS1*013 and KIR3DL1*004 alleles with susceptibility to ankylosing spondylitis. Arthritis Rheum. 2010;62(4):1000–6.
167. Lopez-Larrea C, Blanco-Gelaz MA, Torre-Alonso JC, Armas JB, Suarez-Alvarez B, Pruneda L, et al. Contribution of KIR3DL1/3DS1 to ankylosing spondylitis in human leukocyte antigen-B27 Caucasian populations. Arthritis Res Ther. 2006;8(4):R101-R.
168. Mousavi T, Poormoghim H, Moradi M, Tajik N, Shahsavar F, Asadifar B. Inhibitory killer cell immunoglobulin-like receptor KIR3DL1 in combination with HLA-B Bw4iso protect against ankylosing spondylitis. Iranian J Immunol: IJI. 2010;7(2):88–95.

169. Wang S, Li G, Ge R, Duan Z, Zeng Z, Zhang T, et al. Association of KIR genotype with susceptibility to HLA-B27-positive ankylosing spondylitis. Mod Rheumatol. 2013;23(3):538–41.
170. Harvey D, Pointon JJ, Sleator C, Meenagh A, Farrar C, Sun JY, et al. analysis of killer immunoglobulin-like receptor genes in ankylosing spondylitis. Ann Rheum Dis. 2009;68(4):595–8.
171. Jiao YL, Zhang BC, You L, Li JF, Zhang J, Ma CY, et al. Polymorphisms of KIR gene and HLA-C alleles: possible association with susceptibility to HLA-B27-positive patients with ankylosing spondylitis. J Clin Immunol. 2010;30(6):840–4.
172. Schulte-Wrede U, Sörensen T, Grün J, Syrbe U, Sieper J, Häupl T, et al. A6.09 Nk cells as biosensors for responsiveness to etanercept in ankylosing spondylitis (Morbus Bechterew). Ann Rheum Dis. 2016;75(Suppl 1):A50–A1.
173. Parham P. MHC class I molecules and kirs in human history, health and survival. Nat Rev Immunol. 2005;5(3):201–14.
174. Fusco C, Guerini FR, Nocera G, Ventrella G, Caputo D, Valentino MA, et al. KIRs and their HLA ligands in remitting–relapsing multiple sclerosis. J Neuroimmunol. 2010;229(1):232–7.
175. Podhorzer A, Paladino N, Cuarterolo ML, Fainboim HA, Paz S, Theiler G, et al. The early onset of type 1 autoimmune hepatitis has a strong genetic influence: role of HLA and KIR genes. Genes Immun. 2016;17(3):187–92.
176. D'Andrea A, Chang C, Franz-Bacon K, McClanahan T, Phillips JH, Lanier LL. Molecular cloning of NKB1 a natural killer cell receptor for HLA-B allotypes. J Immunol. 1995;155(5):2306–10.
177. Wilson MJ, Torkar M, Haude A, Milne S, Jones T, Sheer D, et al. Plasticity in the organization and sequences of human KIR/ILT gene families. Proc Natl Acad Sci U S A. 2000;97(9):4778–83.
178. Gumperz JE, Litwin V, Phillips JH, Lanier LL, Parham P. The Bw4 public epitope of HLA-B molecules confers reactivity with natural killer cell clones that express NKB1, a putative HLA receptor. J Exp Med. 1995;181(3):1133–44.
179. Lopez-Larrea C, Blanco-Gelaz MA, Torre-Alonso JC, Armas JB, Suarez-Alvarez B, Pruneda L, et al. Contribution of KIR3DL1/3DS1 to ankylosing spondylitis in human leukocyte antigen-B27 Caucasian populations. Arthritis Res Ther. 2006;8(4):R101.
180. Szanto S, Aleksza M, Mihaly E, Lakos G, Szabo Z, Vegvari A, et al. Intracytoplasmic cytokine expression and T cell subset distribution in the peripheral blood of patients with ankylosing spondylitis. J Rheumatol. 2008;35(12):2372–5.
181. Scrivo R, Morrone S, Spadaro A, Santoni A, Valesini G. Evaluation of degranulation and cytokine production in natural killer cells from spondyloarthritis patients at single-cell level. Cytometry B Clin Cytom. 2011;80B(1):22–7.
182. Jiao Y-L, Ma C-Y, Wang L-C, Cui B, Zhang J, You L, et al. Polymorphisms of KIRs gene and HLA-C alleles in patients with ankylosing spondylitis: possible association with susceptibility to the disease. J Clin Immunol. 2008;28(4):343–9.
183. Harvey D, Pointon JJ, Sleator C, Meenagh A, Farrar C, Sun JY, et al. Analysis of killer immunoglobulin-like receptor genes in ankylosing spondylitis. Annals Rheumat Dis. 2009;68(4):595.
184. Zvyagin IV, Mamedov IZ, Britanova OV, Staroverov DB, Nasonov EL, Bochkova AG, et al. Contribution of functional KIR3DL1 to ankylosing spondylitis. Cell And Mol Immunol. 2010;7:471.
185. McCappin J, Harvey D, Wordsworth BP, Middleton D. No association of KIR3DL1 or KIR3DS1 or their alleles with ankylosing spondylitis. Tissue Antigens. 2010;75(1):68–73.
186. Wang S, Li G, Ge R, Duan Z, Zeng Z, Zhang T, et al. Association of KIR genotype with susceptibility to HLA-B27-positive ankylosing spondylitis. Mod Rheumatol. 2013;23(3):538–41.
187. Estefania E, Flores R, Gomez-Lozano N, Aguilar H, Lopez-Botet M, Vilches C. Human KIR2DL5 is an inhibitory receptor expressed on the surface of NK and T lymphocyte subsets. J Immunol (Baltimore, Md: 1950). 2007;178(7):4402–10.

188. Vilches C, Gardiner CM, Parham P. Gene structure and promoter variation of expressed and nonexpressed variants of the KIR2DL5 gene. J Immunol (Baltimore, Md: 1950). 2000;165(11):6416–21.
189. Allen RL, O'Callaghan CA, McMichael AJ, Bowness P. Cutting edge: HLA-b27 can form a novel β2-microglobulin-free heavy chain homodimer structure. J Immunol. 1999;162(9):5045–8.
190. Khare SD, Luthra HS, David CS. Spontaneous inflammatory arthritis in HLA-B27 transgenic mice lacking ß2-microglobulin: a model of human spondyloarthropathies. J Exp Med. 1995;182(4):1153–8.
191. Kollnberger S, Bird L, Sun MY, Retiere C, Braud VM, McMichael A, et al. Cell-surface expression and immune receptor recognition of HLA-B27 homodimers. Arthritis Rheum. 2002;46(11):2972–82.
192. Chan AT, Kollnberger SD, Wedderburn LR, Bowness P. Expansion and enhanced survival of natural killer cells expressing the killer immunoglobulin-like receptor KIR3DL2 in spondylarthritis. Arthritis Rheum. 2005;52(11):3586–95.
193. Bowness P, Ridley A, Shaw J, Chan AT, Wong-Baeza I, Fleming M, et al. Th17 cells expressing KIR3DL2+ and responsive to HLA-B27 homodimers are increased in ankylosing spondylitis. J Immunol (Baltimore, Md: 1950). 2011;186(4):2672–80.
194. Ridley A, Hatano H, Wong-Baeza I, Shaw J, Matthews KK, Al-Mossawi H, et al. Activation-induced killer cell immunoglobulin-like receptor 3DL2 binding to HLA–B27 licenses pathogenic T cell differentiation in spondyloarthritis. Arthritis Rheumatol. 2016;68(4):901–14.
195. Wong-Baeza I, Ridley A, Shaw J, Hatano H, Rysnik O, McHugh K, et al. KIR3DL2 binds to HLA-B27 dimers and free H chains more strongly than other HLA class I and promotes the expansion of T cells in ankylosing spondylitis. J Immunol (Baltimore, Md: 1950). 2013;190(7):3216–24.

Adaptive Immune-Related Cells and Cytokines in Spondyloarthropathies

3

Maryam Akhtari

Abbreviations

AHR	Aryl hydrocarbon receptor
AS	Ankylosing spondylitis
BASDAI	Bath Ankylosing Spondylitis Disease Activity Index
bDMARDs	Biological disease-modifying anti-rheumatic drugs
BMP	Bone morphogenetic protein
CCL	Chemokine C-C motif ligand
CCR4	C-C chemokine receptor type 4
CLIP	Class II-associated invariant chain peptide
CRP	C-reactive protein
CTL	Cytotoxic T lymphocyte
DCs	Dendritic cells
ER	Endoplasmic reticulum
ESR	Erythrocyte sedimentation rate
FLS	Fibroblast-like synoviocytes
FOXP3	Forkhead box protein P3
GM-CSF	Granulocyte-macrophage colony stimulating factor
HLA	Human leukocyte antigen
IBD	Inflammatory bowel disease
IFN	Interferon
IL	Interleukin
IL-23R	IL-23 receptors
ILC3	Type 3 innate lymphoid cells
IP-10	IFN-gamma-inducible protein-10

M. Akhtari (✉)
Rheumatology Research Center, Tehran University of Medical Sciences, Tehran, Iran
e-mail: m.akhtari@ut.ac.ir

M. H. Nicknam (ed.), *Ankylosing Spondylitis - Axial Spondyloarthritis*,
https://doi.org/10.1007/978-981-16-4733-8_3

M-CSF	Macrophage colony-stimulating factor
MCV	Mutated citrullinated vimentin
MDC	Macrophage-derived chemokine
MSCs	Mesenchymal stem cells
MFI	Mean fluorescence intensity
MMP	Matrix metalloproteinase
NKT	Natural killer T cells
NSAID	Nonsteroidal anti-inflammatory drug
OA	Osteoarthritis
PBMCs	Peripheral blood mononuclear cells
PGE2	Prostaglandin E2
PPM1A	Protein phosphatase magnesium-dependent 1A
PsA	Psoriatic arthritis
RA	Rheumatoid arthritis
RANKL	Receptor activator of nuclear factor-kappa B ligand
ReA	Reactive arthritis
RORγt	RAR-related orphan receptor gamma isoform t
ROS	Reactive oxygen species
SF	Synovial fluid
SFMC	Synovial fluid mononuclear cells
SpAs	Spondyloarthropathies
TARC	Thymus and activation-regulated chemokine
TCR	T cell receptor
TGF	Transforming growth factor
Th	Helper T
TNF-α	Tumor necrosis factor-alpha
Treg	Regulatory T lymphocyte
UPR	Unfolded protein response
uSpA	Undifferentiated Spondyloarthropathy
Wnt	Wingless protein

3.1 Adaptive immunity in autoimmune disorders

The immune system is typically divided into two pillars: the innate, which mediates rapid nonspecific immune responses following antigen's appearance; and the adaptive, which induces "non-self" antigen-specific responses during the antigen presentation process and develops memory [1]. The interaction of the innate and adaptive immune cells is crucial to generate effective responses [2].

Adaptive immunity is composed of specialized T and B cell lineage lymphocytes and includes both cell-mediated and humoral immune mechanisms [3]. The hallmark of autoimmunity is the breakdown of immunologic tolerance to self-antigens [4, 5]. In autoimmune diseases, abnormal recognition mechanisms of self and non-self by lymphocytes leads to inflammatory responses, tissue injury, and dysfunction [6].

The reasons that lead to breaking immune tolerance in autoimmune diseases are multiple and the initial trigger is not clear [4]. Some pathogens express epitopes that have the potential to display antigenic homology to host tissue-derived peptides and induce both autoreactive T or B cell responses [3, 7]. Thus, it is suggested that antibody or T cell receptor (TCR) cross-reactivity can trigger pathogenic pathways in autoimmune diseases. Although autoreactive lymphocytes are eliminated and silenced in a series of multiple checkpoints in the body, a low level of these cells still found in healthy individuals. Therefore, de-novo generation or the lack of intensity in the elimination of self-reactive lymphocytes is other important feature of autoimmune diseases [3].

Among autoimmune diseases, some rheumatic diseases are associated with autoantibody production and human leukocyte antigen (HLA) class II molecules including subgroups of rheumatoid arthritis (RA). Some other rheumatic diseases are associated with certain HLA-class I molecules including spondyloarthropathies (SpAs) which indicated the involvement of adaptive immunity in their pathogenesis [7].

3.2 The Pathogenic Role of Adaptive Immune Lymphocytes in SpAs

SpAs including ankylosing spondylitis (AS), inflammatory bowel disease (IBD) associated arthritis, psoriatic arthritis (PsA), reactive arthritis (ReA), and undifferentiated spondyloarthropathies (uSpAs) are a subset of disorders with strong adaptive and inflammatory innate immunity overlap. The immunopathology of this group of rheumatic diseases is related to MHC class-I molecule and adaptive immune responses [7, 8]. Other factors that are also contributed to the MHC-I antigen presentation pathway are highly significant in their pathogenesis. However, the adaptive immunity of SpAs has been rarely considered [9].

HLA-B27 as an MHC-I molecule appears to play the most important role in AS susceptibility. It is a polymorphic molecule that binds to peptides and presents them for $CD8^+$ T cell recognition. It has been also proposed that $CD4^+$ T lymphocytes are also be involved in class I-restricted immune responses [8, 10].

It has been found that various HLA-B27 subtypes with different sequences, conferring variation in protein stability and peptide binding ability, influence the incidence and contribute to the development of AS. The HLA-B27 misfolding may cause endoplasmic reticulum (ER) stress, then unfolded protein response (UPR), and IL-23 production, resulting in Th17 cell activation and type 3 immunity induction in AS (the UPR hypothesis) [11, 12].

However, two other different HLA-B27 hypotheses, the arthritogenic peptide and free heavy chained hypotheses have been proposed to explain how HLA-B27 might induce disease development in AS. The first one suggested that cross-reactivity or molecular mimicry between bacterial and pathogenic antigens and different joint-specific peptides which are presented by AS-associated HLA-B27 subtypes to autoreactive T cells resulted in a self-tolerance break. In 1993, it was found that cytotoxic

T cells from AS patients are activated by both pathogens infected and non-infected cells, however, a definitive arthritogenic peptide that can activate T cells and trigger immune responses in AS patients has not been recognized by peptidome analysis in recent years. The second hypothesis suggested that homodimers of the HLA-B27 heavy chain in the absence of the β2M light chain can also be presented on the cell surface and activate adaptive immune responses in AS [11].

There are numerous evidence that showed the involvement of adaptive immunity in the pathogenesis of AS in animal models [13, 14]. Expanded clonal T lymphocyte populations have been reported in the SpA patients especially in their synovium [15–17]. Histological data has also demonstrated infiltrated and presence of T lymphocytes in the synovium and sacroiliac joints of AS patients [18–20]. Besides, the elevated level of IgA antibodies has been reported in the serum sample of SpA patients and is correlated with the patient's disease activity [21–23].

Here we have reviewed the involvement and the pathogenic role of adaptive immune responses, related cells, and cytokines in SpA pathogenesis.

3.3 T Cell Activation, Signaling, and Cytokines in SpAs

Autoreactive T lymphocytes have been involved in many aspects of autoimmunity and inflammation and play a decisive role in the break of immune tolerance [24]. T lymphocytes participate in the induction and development of arthritis, AS, and related SpAs. It is demonstrated that athymic animals are resistant to arthritis induction [25–28]. Various alternation in the T cells population and their cytokines have been described in the different rheumatic diseases and contributed to the disease progression and severity [29].

Based on the surface receptors, T lymphocytes are divided into the following subsets: CD4$^+$ (helper T) and CD8$^+$ (cytotoxic T) cells. Helper T cells are sorted into Th1, Th2, Th17, Th22, and regulatory T lymphocytes (Treg) and cytotoxic T cells (CTL) are sorted into Tc1, Tc2, and Tc17, based on their secretory cytokines [30]. While Th1 and Tc1 contribute to Type 1 immunity, secrete inflammatory interleukin (IL)-2, tumor necrosis factor-alpha (TNF-α), and interferon-gamma (IFN-γ) and induced M1 macrophage polarization, Th2 and Tc2 participate in the type 2 immunity, secrete IL-4, IL-5 and IL-13 cytokines and induced M2 macrophages polarization [31]. The immunological imbalance in T lymphocyte subsets and their function is correlated with SpAs incidence and progression. Here we discuss the pathogenic role of distinct subsets of T lymphocytes in the pathogenesis of SpA diseases.

3.3.1 Th1 and Th2 role in SpAs

Mounting evidence demonstrates a crucial role of helper T cells in the initiation, progression, and maintenance of auto-inflammatory responses in AS and other SpA patients. It is observed that SpA-like disorders are mediated by CD4$^+$ T rather than CD8$^+$ T lymphocytes in HLA-B27 transgenic animals [26, 27, 32]. It is also demonstrated that the peripheral blood CD4^{+} CD28^{-} T cells are aggregated in patients with AS and their level is correlated with disease status [33].

The imbalance in the proportion of Th1 and Th2 and their cytokines is a fundamental step in the progression of rheumatic diseases [34]. Th1 secretes pro-inflammatory cytokines and induced anti-sepsis and pro-inflammatory immune responses which may lead to cellular immunity and autoimmune reactions in different organs. Whereas, Th2 cells mainly participate in the humoral immune responses and tissue repair and remodeling. They secrete cytokines that mostly contribute to the pathogenesis of asthma and allergic disorders [35–37]. Therefore, the balance in Th1/Th2 responses determines immune responses; however, its role and function in the pathogenesis of AS and other SpAs need more investigation.

Some studies have investigated the frequency and activity of Th1 and Th2 lymphocytes in patients with PsA, ReA, and uSpA. Herrera et al. evaluated the Th1 and Th2 cytokine profiles in 50 PsA and 30 controls. The results have shown an increase in *TNFA* expression, Th1 and Th17 cytokine profiles in PsA patients. They did not find a significant difference in Th2 cytokine profiles in patients [38]. These results suggest that Th1 and Th17 could have major roles in inflammatory responses in PsA patients.

The level of produced cytokines by helper T cells was analyzed in synovial fluid (SF) and paired serum sample of 51 patients with ReA or uSpA, by Singh et al. It has been demonstrated that the level of transforming growth factor-beta (TGF-β), IL-17, IL-6, IFN-γ, and the ratio of IFN-γ/IL-10 are significantly upregulated in SF of ReA/uSpA patients compared to whom with RA [39]. The results implicate a possible role of Th1 immunity in ReA. By contrast, in a study by Yin et al., the cytokine pattern of helper T cells was investigated in the synovial fluid mononuclear cells (SFMCs) of 11 individuals with ReA following infection. Their finding showed that SFMC secreted a low amount of Th1-related cytokines such as IFN-γ and TNF-α and a high amount of IL-10 Th2 cytokine upon infection [40]. In addition, Braun et al. found diminished TNF-α production by peripheral blood mononuclear cells (PBMCs) and T cells from 53 ReA patients compared to RA patients, which was followed with longer disease duration [41]. However, Simon et al. have reported that the level of both IFN-γ as a Th1 and IL-4 as a Th2 cytokine is significantly altered in synovial tissue from ReA patients [42]. In addition, Cañete et al. found that IFN-γ was expressed significantly lower in T cells from synovial tissue of SpA patients (including 10 uSpA, two AS, and two PsA) compared to the RA group and the Th1/Th2 cytokine ratio was fivefold higher in RA than in SpA group [43]. Altogether it seems that IFN-γ has a fundamental function in the ReA and uSpAs pathogenesis and the role of Th1 or Th2 immunity needs more investigations.

Results regarding AS is more complicated. In a study by Szalay et al., the phenotype, frequency, and function of T cells were analyzed in 13 AS patients. They have shown that the prevalence of CD4^{+} lymphocytes rised in the AS group. They also found an increase in the prevalence of Th2 and Th17 cells in patients that results in an imbalance in the Th1/Th2 ratio toward Th2. C-C chemokine receptor type 4 (CCR4) is one of the major Th2 chemokine receptors. Due to the increased CCR4^{+} Th2 cells in AS patients, their results suggested an increased Th2 activity in patients [24]. In a study by Szanto et al., the subset of peripheral blood lymphocytes and their intracellular cytokine have been investigated in 42 AS patients compared to 52 healthy individuals. The results showed that $CD4^+$ T lymphocytes have an increased frequency in the case group. The frequency of undifferentiated helper T cells was significantly elevated in the patients in contrast to the control group; however, there were no remarkable differences in the Th1/Th2 ratio between patients and controls and the proportion of IL-10 producing T helper cells did not differ in patients in comparison to healthy individuals [44]. In another study the PBMCs from 46 AS patients were analyzed by contrast to the RA patients and control group. The amount of $CD3^+$ $CD4^+$ IFN-γ^+ T helper cells (Th1) was significantly upregulated in AS than in healthy individuals. However, they did not find any substantial differences in Th2 percentage between patients and healthy groups. In addition, in their study, the elevated serum levels of Th1 related pro-inflammatory cytokines containing IFN-γ, TNF-α, IL-6, and IL-12 were found in AS patients. They found that the level of Th1 cell population and their cytokines such as IFN-γ were significantly diminished in patients who were treated with TNF-α inhibitors [45]. Previous studies showed that TNF-α is associated with AS inflammation and is highly expressed in sacroiliac joints of AS patients [46].

In a study by Wang et al., the correlation of the disease progression with the T cells subset from lesions and serum of 55 AS patients (23 moderate and 22 severe) in comparison to 20 healthy controls has been assessed. The results implicated that the percentage of Th1 cells and the proportion of Th1/Th2 were notably elevated in patients and contributed to the elevated level of IFN-γ expression in lesion and serum of patients. Although they did not report any meaningful differences in the Th2 proportion of AS patients, the expression levels of IL-4 and TGF-β were upregulated in lesions of the mild and severe AS patients [10].

Yang et al. analyzed the proportion of $CD4^+$ $CCR4^+$ T lymphocytes in AS patients. They found that the proportion of $CD4^+$ $CCR4^+$ T cells is remarkably increased in individuals who suffer from AS, which can indicate enhanced Th2 activity and responses in the disease. Besides they observed that AS patients have an increased IL-10 and IFN-γ serum levels (but not TNF-α), and the level of $CD4^+$ $CCR4^+$ T cells was directly associated with IL-10 level in AS patients [47].

Rudwaleit et al. reported that the percentage of TNF-α^+ IFN-γ^+ T cells is notably lower in AS patients while the percentage of IL-10^+ T cells is higher in patients in comparison to control groups which suggesting Th2 dominance in AS [48].

However, in a study by Wang et al., it is suggested that dysregulation in both Th1 and Th2 chemoattractant is contributed to the pathogenesis of AS. The serum level of cytokines from Th1 (TNF-α and IFN-γ) and Th2 (IL-4 and IL-10) were measured in 42 AS patients and 25 healthy individuals. Chemokines are a fundamental factor for the recruitment of leukocytes to the inflamed tissues, therefore, the serum level of key chemokines contributes to the migration of Th1 including IFN-gamma-inducible protein-10 (IP-10/CXCL10) and Th2 including thymus and activation-regulated chemokine (TARC) or chemokine C-C motif ligand (CCL)-17 and macrophage-derived chemokine (MDC/CCL22) were also evaluated between patients and controls [49]. The result showed that serum IFN-γ and TNF-α cytokines level and IP-10, CCL17, and CCL22 chemokine levels are significantly higher in AS patients. They did not see significant differences in IL-4 level between groups.

They found that the level of IP-10 as a Th1 chemokine is correlated with the level of TNF-α, erythrocyte sedimentation rate (ESR), and C-reactive protein (CRP) in patients, and both Th1 and Th2 chemokines reduced by blocking TNF-α. It seems that anti-TNF therapy improved AS patient's conditions by altering lymphocyte activity rather than the proportion of Th cells subsets [24, 49]. The alternations of Th1, Th2, Th17, and Th22 lymphocytes subsets and related cytokines in SpA disorders have been summarized in Table 3.1.

There are conflicting results regarding Th1 and Th2 ratio and cytokines in AS patients. However, altogether the results suggested that imbalance in Th1 and Th2 cytokines contributed to AS pathogenesis. It seems that recruitment and functional

Table 3.1 The alternations of Th1, Th2, Th17, and Th22 lymphocytes subsets and related cytokines in patients with SpA disorders

Authors	Patients	Sample	Th1 pathway alternation in patients	Th2 pathway alternation in patients	Th17/Th22 pathway alternation in patients	References
Herrera et al.	50 PsA patients compared to healthy controls	Serum sample	Increased mRNA expression of Th1 (IFN-γ, TNF-α) cytokine profiles	No significant difference in Th2 cytokine profiles	Increased mRNA expression of Th17 (IL-17, IL-22) cytokine profiles	[38]
Wang et al.	95 PsA patients compared to healthy controls	Peripheral blood	No significant difference in Th1 cell numbers	No significant difference in Th2 cell numbers	Increased absolute number of Th17 cells	[50]
Menon et al.	33 PsA patients	Mononuclear cells from SF	–	–	Increased $IL\text{-}17^{+}CD4^{-}$ and $IL\text{-}17^{+}CD4^{+}$ T cells	[51]
Benham et al.	12 PsA patients compared to healthy controls	Peripheral blood and SF	–	–	Increased frequencies of $IL\text{-}17^{+}$ $CD4^{+}$ T and $IL\text{-}22^{+}$ $CD4^{+}$ T cells and elevated IL-17 and IL-22 secretion	[52]
Mitra et al.	15 PsA patients compared to OA patients	SF	–	–	Elevated IL-22 level	[53]

(continued)

Table 3.1 (continued)

Authors	Patients	Sample	Th1 pathway alternation in patients	Th2 pathway alternation in patients	Th17/Th22 pathway alternation in patients	References
Ezeonyeji et al.	83 PsA patients compared to healthy controls	Peripheral blood	No significant differences in IFN-γ^+ $CD4^+$ T cells Increased ratio of IFNγ/IL-22 in $CD4^+$ T cells following activation	–	Reduced frequency of IL-22^+ $CD4^+$ T cells following activation	[54]
Yin et al.	11 ReA patients following infection	SFMCs	Secreted low amounts of IFN-γ and TNF-α upon infection	Secreted high amounts of IL-10 upon infection Higher number of IL-4^+ cells	–	[40]
Braun et al.	53 ReA patients compared to RA patients	PBMCs and T cells	Diminished TNF-α production	No significant differences in IL-4 and IL-10 production	–	[41]
Simon et al.	9 ReA patients compared to RA patients	Synovial tissue	Increased IFN-γ positive samples	Increased IL-4 positive samples	–	[42]
Shen et al.	8 ReA patients compared to healthy controls	PBMCs and SFMCs	–	–	Increased percentages of IL-17^+ $CD4^+$ T cells in SFMCs	[55]
Singh et al.	50 ReA/uSpA patients compared to OA patients	Synovial fluid	–	–	Upregulated IL-17A level	[56]
Singh et al.	51 ReA/uSpA patients compared to RA patients	SF and paired serum sample	Upregulated TGF-β, IL-6, and IFN-γ secretion	Upregulated the ratio of IFN-γ/IL-10	Upregulated IL-17 secretion	[39]

Table 3.1 (continued)

Authors	Patients	Sample	Th1 pathway alternation in patients	Th2 pathway alternation in patients	Th17/Th22 pathway alternation in patients	References
Jandus et al.	10 PsA and 10 AS patients compared to RA patients and healthy controls	Peripheral blood	–	–	Increased numbers of circulating Th17 cells	[57]
Cañete et al.	14 SpA patients (10 uSpA, 2 AS, and 2 PsA) compared to RA patients	Synovial tissue	Diminished IFN-γ level	Increased Th2/Th1 ratio	–	[43]
Szalay et al.	13 AS patients compared to controls	Peripheral blood	Decreased Th1/Th2 ratio	Higher prevalence of Th2 cells and increased $CCR4^+$ Th2 cells	Higher prevalence of Th17 cells	[24]
Szanto et al.	42 AS patients compared to healthy controls	Peripheral blood	No significant differences in the Th1/Th2 ratio Decreased Tc1 cells	Increased $IL\text{-}10^+$ Tc cells	–	[44]
Limon-Camacho et al.	46 AS patients compared to RA patients and healthy controls	PBMCs and serum sample	Increased percentage of Th1 cells and elevated serum level of IL-6, IL-12, and TNF-α	No significant differences in Th2 percentage	Increased percentage of Th17 cells and elevated serum level of IL-17A level	[45]
Wang et al.	55 AS patients compared to healthy controls	Lesions and the serum sample	Increased percentage of Th1 cells and the Th1/Th2 ratio and upregulated IFN-γ and TGF-β expression	No significant differences in Th2 proportion and increased IL-4 expression	Increased percentages of Th17 cells and the Th17/Treg ratio Upregulated IL-17 expression	[10]

(continued)

Table 3.1 (continued)

Authors	Patients	Sample	Th1 pathway alternation in patients	Th2 pathway alternation in patients	Th17/Th22 pathway alternation in patients	References
Yang et al.	11 AS patients compared to healthy controls	Circulating lymphocytes and serum samples	Increased IFN-γ serum level (but not TNF-α)	Increased proportion of $CD4^+$ $CCR4^+$ T cells and IL-10 level	–	[47]
Rudwaleit et al.	25 HLA-$B27^+$ AS patients compared to healthy controls	PBMCs	Reduced percentage of TNF-α^+ IFN-γ^+ T cells	Increased percentage of IL-10^+ $CD8^+$T cells	–	[48]
Wang et al.	42 axial AS patients compared to healthy controls	Serum samples	Increased IFN-γ, TNF-α, and IP-10 serum levels	Increased CCL17 and CCL22 serum levels No significant differences in IL-4 level	–	[49]
Shen et al.	20 AS patients compared to healthy controls	PBMCs	No significant differences in IFN-γ^+ $CD4^+$ T cells	No significant differences in IL-10^+ $CD4^+$ T cells	Increased percentages of IL-17^+ $CD4^+$ T and IL-22^+ $CD4^+$ T cells and elevated level of IL-17 in the supernatants	[58]
Wang et al.	57 AS patients compared to healthy controls	Serum and supernatants of cultured PBMCs	–	–	Elevated level of IL-17	[59]
Zhang et al.	32 AS patients compared to healthy controls	Peripheral blood and plasma sample	–	–	Increased frequencies of Th22 cells and Th17 and elevated IL-22 level	[60]

PsA psoriatic arthritis, *ReA* Reactive arthritis, *AS* Ankylosing spondylitis, *uSpA* Undifferentiated spondyloarthropathies, *Th*: Helper T, *IFN-γ* Interferon-gamma, *TNF-α* Tumor necrosis factor-alpha, *TGF-β* Transforming growth factor-beta, *IL* Interleukin, *SF* Synovial fluid, *Treg* regulatory T cell, *RA* Rheumatoid arthritis, *SFMC* Synovial fluid mononuclear cells, *PBMC* Peripheral blood mononuclear cells, *CCR4* Chemokine receptor type 4, *Tc* T cytotoxic, *CCL* Chemokine C-C motif ligand activity of T lymphocytes have more pivotal roles in the AS inflammatory responses than the proportion of them.

3.3.2 Th17 and IL-17 in SpAs

IL-23/IL-17 signaling pathway and Th17 immunity play an essential role in SpA disorders immuno-pathogenesis. Several genetic polymorphisms in this axis have been found in association with SpA disease [61–64]. IL-23 acts through IL-23 receptors (IL-23R) on the surface of Th17 cells and resulted in Th17 cells differentiation, expansion, and proliferation. Th17 cells are one of the T helper subsets and the main source of IL-17; however, they can produce different inflammatory cytokines such as IFN-γ, IL-26, IL-22, and IL-21. IL-17 superfamily includes 6 members (IL-17A-F) which attach to the 5 receptors (IL-17R A-E) and contribute to host defense against pathogens and participates in epithelial and mucosal immunity as well as inflammatory responses and bone resorption. IL-17A plays the most important role in auto-inflammatory responses and seems to be associated with skin and joints manifestations of SpA [65, 66].

A raised amount of Th17 lymphocytes and elevated level of IL-17 cytokine have been found in blood and synovial tissue of PsA and AS patients [45, 52, 55, 57–59, 67]. It is reported that Th17/Treg cells ratio and the mRNA and protein expression level of IL-17A were remarkably higher in AS patients regarding the control group [10]. In a study by Xueyi et al., the level of Th17 and serum inflammatory cytokine were investigated before and after anti-TNF-α therapy. They showed that anti-TNF-α therapy reduced Th17 cell frequency and IL-17 level in 168 patients who respond to treatment. However, the level of Th17 and IL-17 was significantly increased in patients after anti-TNF-α therapy in the non-responder group of patients [68].

Menon et al. showed that the IL-17$^+$ CD3$^+$ T lymphocytes were notably enriched in synovial fluid of PsA patients. The proportion of IL-17$^+$ CD4$^-$ T cells (predominantly CD8+) synovial fluid was meaningfully associated with CRP level, joint damage development, and disease activity in the case group [51]. In addition, previous researches showed that the level of IL-17 was considerably elevated in ReA/uSpA patients comparing to RA patients or individuals with non-inflammatory osteoarthritis (OA) [39, 56].

In addition to Th17 cells, IL-17 producing CD8$^+$ T lymphocytes (Tc17) and some of the innate leukocytes including some natural killer T cells (NKT) can also produce IL-17. It has been found that type 3 innate lymphoid cells (ILC3) which produce IL-22 and IL-17 have been enriched in serum and synovium of individuals who suffer from SpA and contribute to the human enthesis. It is suggested that this RAR-related orphan receptor gamma isoform t positive (RORγt)$^+$ group of cells (ILC3) participate in enthesitis of SpA by producing IL-17 [69–71]. Besides, IL-17A$^+$ neutrophils have been found in the synovium and joints of patients with PsA and AS [72, 73].

Produced IL-17 upregulates the expansion of Th17 in a positive feedback loop in SpA patients [74]. IL-17 induces mRNA transcription or stabilization of pro-inflammatory cytokine, chemokines, and matrix metalloproteinases (MMPs) from macrophages, dendritic cells (DCs), endothelial cells, and fibroblasts and induces joints destruction [75]. Moreover, IL-17 participates in bone erosion and new bone formation processes of AS [76].

3.3.2.1 IL-17 and Enthesitis

Enthesitis is a key feature of AS and PsA. It is suggested that IL-23 and prostaglandin E2 (PGE2) initiate entheseal inflammation by vasodilation and induction of IL-17 production by resident innate and adaptive immune cells [76, 77]. Entheseal resident LC3 and gamma delta (γδ) T cells with the IL-17 production capacity have been found in humans [71]. In a study by Sherlock *et al.*, it is suggested that IL-23 induces resident RORγt$^+$ CD4$^-$ CD8$^-$ T cells to produce several inflammatory cytokines such as IL-17 and IL-22 and resulted in enthesitis, bone remodeling, and spondyloarthropathy in the mouse model [78]. Several murine models demonstrated the crucial role of the IL-23/IL-17 signaling axis in the initiation and progression of entheseal inflammation [79–81]; however, other models indicate that enthesitis can also develop independently of T cells in the T lymphocytes depleted models [82–84]. The role of IL-17 in the entheseal inflammatory responses needs more investigation; nevertheless, it seems that IL-17 reinforces entheseal inflammatory responses. IL-17 accelerates neutrophils and macrophages migration and activation directly and also induces resident mesenchymal cells to produce inflammatory cytokines including IL-6, IL-8, and granulocyte-macrophage colony-stimulating factor (GM-CSF), and recruits them indirectly. Neutrophils act as effector cells that produce and release different protease and reactive oxygen species (ROS) (Figure 3.1) [19, 77, 85–87].

3.3.2.2 IL-17 and Bone Remodeling

Prolonged entheseal inflammation may lead to significant tissue responses including bone erosion, formation, remodeling, and syndesmophyte formation. IL-17 along with IL-22 and PEG2 is one of the main factors that connect enthesitis with bone and cartilage remodeling responses [88]. Several studies demonstrated bone resorption and pro-osteoclastogenic function of IL-17 in experimental arthritis models [89–91]. It is suggested that IL-17 directly or indirectly contributes to osteoclast differentiation and survivance by inducing the transcription of macrophage colony-stimulating factor (M-CSF) and receptor activator of nuclear factor-kappa B (RANKL) [88]. M-CSF and RANKL are key factors in osteoclast differentiation from monocyte/macrophage precursors. Th17 also supports osteoclast formation by expressing RANKL and activates osteoclastogenesis [92]. It was also demonstrated that IL-17 can also promote osteoclastogenesis by instigating the production of pro-inflammatory cytokines; for instance, TNF-α, IL-6, and IL-17 from macrophages and other immune cells [93] (Fig. 3.1).

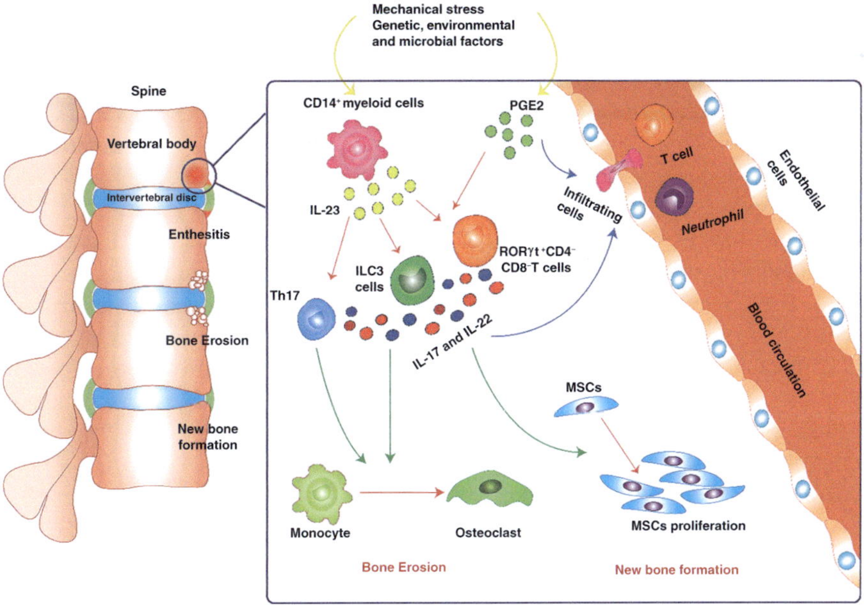

Fig. 3.1 IL-17, enthesitis, and bone remodeling in SpA disorders. Mechanical stress, genetic, environmental, and microbial factors induce the production of prostaglandin E2 (PGE2) and IL-23 in the enthesis of PsA patients. PGE2 triggers vasodilation and IL-17 production by immune cells. Produced IL-23 by CD14$^+$ myeloid cells in the enthesis causes IL-17 and IL-22 secretion by RORγt$^+$ CD4$^-$ CD8$^-$ T, type 3 innate lymphoid (ILC3), and Th17 cells. IL-17 accelerates neutrophils and macrophages migration and activation. Th17 and IL-17 support osteoclast formation, activate osteoclastogenesis, and bone erosion. Besides, IL-17 along with IL-22 can trigger proliferation and activation of residential mesenchymal stem cells (MSCs) and may contribute to the new bone formation.

Residential mesenchymal cells have the ability to differentiate into chondroblasts and osteoblasts in response to inflammatory conditions and are the main cells that correlate inflammation and bone remodeling [94]. There are contradictory results regarding the effect of IL-17 on osteoblasts. Some research have shown that IL-17 can properly activate mesenchymal cells and boost osteoblast differentiation and activate osteoblasts by JAK2/STAT3 signaling pathway [95]. Besides, it is found that the IL-17 knockout experimental models have impaired bone regeneration, and IL-17 inhibition results in a suppressed formation of new bone in HLA-B27 transgenic rats [96, 97].

However, other studies have found inhibitory effects of IL-17 on osteoblasts, and its effect on bone loss in erosive arthritis has been well known [98–100]. It is suggested that IL-17A in combination with TNF-α induces bone resorption in fetal mouse [101]. It is thought that IL-17 inhibits osteoblast activity and differentiation by stimulating RANKL expression and by inhibiting wingless protein (Wnt) signaling [102, 103].

3.3.2.3 Targeting Th17 in SpAs

Targeting Th17 responses and IL-23/IL-17 axis in SpA disorders has been considered in recent years by several clinical trial studies. The use of IL-23/IL-17 axis inhibitors has resulted in suppressed disease activity in PsA and AS patients and can reduce joint radiographic progression in patients [104–107]. Different monoclonal antibodies including Ixekizumab and Secukinumab (both target IL-17A), Ustekinumab (targets p40 subunit of IL-23), and Brodalumab (targets IL17RA) have been developed [108]. Secukinumab administration ameliorates the clinical signs and symptoms of AS and PsA patients in randomized clinical trial studies [106, 109]. Secukinumab has reduced significantly the assessment of spondyloarthritis international society criteria for improvement (ASAS20) responses in patients in comparison to control groups [109]. The effect of long-term use of Secukinumab was also assessed in a phase-III clinical trial. The results showed that Secukinumab results in sustained amelioration in the clinical symptoms, ASAS 20/40 response rates, and Bath Ankylosing Spondylitis Disease Activity Index (BASDAI) of individuals with AS [110]. The enthesitis score of PsA patients was improved by Secukinumab and Ixekizumab treatment in about 50% and 30-40% of patients, respectively [106, 111].

The efficacy and safety of Ixekizumab have been assessed in various clinical trials on different groups of SpA patients in recent years. In two phase-III randomized clinical trials, it is found that Ixekizumab significantly improved 16 week-radiographic signs and symptoms in patients who suffer from radiographic axial SpA and were not priorly receive biological disease-modifying anti-rheumatic drugs (bDMARDs) and in patients with prior intolerance or improper response to TNF inhibitors compared to the placebo group [112, 113]. It was also found that this significant efficacy maintains up to 52 weeks in both groups of patients [114]. In addition, Ixekizumab has had beneficial effects on axial SpA patients without sacroiliitis or radiographic symptoms who were nonsteroidal anti-inflammatory drug (NSAID) intolerance or had improper responses to NSAIDs [115]. In a meta-analysis by Yin et al. the ability and safety of IL-17 inhibitors (Secukinumab and Ixekizumab) have been investigated in 6 clinical trials conducted on AS patients. The results indicated that IL-17 inhibitors resulted in increased ASAS20 and ASAS40 response rate in patients. Although IL-17 inhibitors did not produce serious adverse events, the risk of non-severe infection was increased after treatment [116].

Besides, the effect of brodalumab treatment on 159 patients with axial SpA at week 16 has been investigated in a phase-III randomized trial by Cheng-Chung Wei et al. Brodalumab has significantly elevated the ASAS40 response rate in patients and it seems that it has effective and tolerable results in axSpA patients [117].

3.3.3 Th22 and IL-22 in SpAs

Th22 lymphocytes are a novel lineage of CD4^{+} effector T cells. Same as Th17 lymphocytes, these lymphocytes are one of the main sources of IL-22. They also express and produce various inflammatory cytokines containing TNF-α, IL-13, and chemokine receptors CCR4, 6, and 10. On the other hand, they do not express the markers of Th17 (IL-17, IL-23R, and CD161), Th1 (IFN-γ), and Th2 (IFN-γ) cells [118–120]. It is demonstrated that Th22 can differentiate from naïve $CD4^+$ T lymphocytes in the presence of TNF-α and IL-6 and their expansion is regulated by the aryl hydrocarbon receptor (AHR) transcription factor [121, 122].

IL-22 is one of the IL-10 superfamily members. It is produced by different immune cell populations such as Th22, Th17, Th1, NKT, ILC3, $CD8^+T$, macrophages, neutrophils, and γδT cells during infection and inflammation and binds to its heterodimeric receptor (IL-10R2/IL-22R1) on target cells [123, 124]. IL-22 by targeting resident entheseal cells including epithelial and mesenchymal cells induces osteogenesis and new bone formation and contributes to SpA disease pathogenesis [125]. In a study by Zhang et al., increased peripheral blood Th22 and IL-22 levels of AS patients have been shown compared to OA and healthy individuals [60]. Besides, an elevated level of $IL\text{-}22^+$ $CD4^+$ T cells was detected in peripheral blood of AS and PsA patients in comparison to healthy controls [52, 58]. In addition, increased IL-22 transcript level in the terminal ileum of AS individuals with gut inflammation was observed [126]. However, Ezeonyeji et al. have found a lower proportion of $CD4^+$ $IL\text{-}22^+$ T cells and Th22 ($IL\text{-}22^+$ $IL\text{-}17^-$ $CD4^+$) cells in the activated PBMCs of PsA patients than in healthy individuals [54]. In a study by Mitra et al., it has been reported that IL-22 was considerably upregulated in synovial fluid of PsA patients compared to OA controls. Their results showed that recombinant IL-22 induces PsA fibroblast-like synoviocytes (FLS) proliferation alone or in combination with TNF-α. It has also been found that PsA activated synovial T cells produce significantly elevated IL-22 compared to OA T cells [53].

3.3.4 Functional Abnormalities of Regulatory T Cells in SpAs

Regulatory T cells are also known as Tregs are a subgroup of T lymphocytes that regulate or suppress other leukocytes and play an essential role in maintaining immune tolerance and preventing autoimmunity by repressing effector cell proliferation and cytokine production [127, 128]. Treg cells are differentiated from naïve T cells and forkhead box protein P3 (FOXP3) transcription factor is a well-known feature of these groups of cells and is crucial for their gene expression, development, and function [129]. Although FOXP3 is essential for Treg cells maintenance and function, its expression is not limited to regulatory cells and is detected in a remarkable number of human activated effector T lymphocytes [127]. Currently, there is not any specified marker for characterizing human Treg cells, and human $CD4^+$ $CD25^+$ T cells that do not express α-chain of IL-7R (CD127) are considered as regulatory T cells [130].

Several phenotypically and functionally distinct types of $CD4^+$ Treg have been identified which are either derived from the thymus (natural Treg) or induced in the peripheral environment upon exposure to antigens (inducible Treg). Natural Treg cells are one of the largest subsets of Treg and constitutively express the IL-2 receptor (CD25) and FOXP3 transcription factor, IL-2 is required for the proliferation and survival of them [131, 132]. Inducible Treg that develop in the periphery are secondary suppressor T cells. Their suppressive properties are mediated mainly through inhibitory cytokines such as IL-10 produced by T regulatory 1 (Tr1) cells and TGF-β produced by T helper 3 (Th3) regulatory cells [133–135]. Dysregulated Treg numbers and function lead to abnormal immune responses and are supposed to contribute to the pathogenesis and development of many rheumatic disorders including SpA disorders [136, 137].

Some studies did not found a remarkable alteration in the number of Treg cells in AS patients. Wang et al. have reported that the percentage of Treg cells does not show a notable difference between AS and healthy individuals. However, as previously mentioned it has beenn found that the proportion of Th17 lymphocytes and the ratio of Th17/Treg cells is significantly higher in AS patients [10]. Ye et al. have analyzed the frequency of $CD4^{+}CD25^{high}CD39^{+}CD45RO^{+}$ naïve and $CD4^{+}CD25^{high}$ $CD39^{-}CD45RO^{-}$ effector Treg cells subset and their regulatory capacity in AS patients. Their results demonstrated that although the regulatory capacity of both groups significantly reduced in AS patients, there are no meaningful differences in the proportion of Treg subset groups between patients and healthy individuals [138].

On the other hand, some research found an increased frequency of Tregs in patients. In a study by Ciccia et al. the frequency of $CD4^{+}CD25^{high}$ regulatory T cells and the level of their related cytokines and transcription factors have been investigated in the gut ileum and blood of AS patients in contrast to healthy controls. A notable increase in the proportion of Treg cells in the gut ileum as well as in the peripheral circulation of AS patients has been found in comparison to controls. It was also found that TGF-β and IL-10 Treg cytokines and STAT-5 and FOXP3 Tregs transcription factors have upregulated expression in the ileum of AS patients [139]. Tzung Liao et al. have reported a higher percentage of $CD4^{+}$ $CD25^{+}$ $FOXP3^{+}$ Treg cells in PBMCs of AS patients. The level of Treg cells was directly correlated with the levels of ESR and CRP in patients. After using TNF-α inhibitor in patients, Treg numbers along with CRP and ESR levels were notably decreased over time [140]. In another study, the functional capacity and the frequency of $CD4^{+}$ $CD25^{+}$ $CD127^{-}$ $FOXP3v^{+}$ Tregs have been investigated in PBMCs from AS patients related to healthy individuals. Although the results showed that the frequency of Treg lymphocytes was slightly raised in AS patients, the level of FOXP3 mean fluorescence intensity (MFI) and suppressive capacity of Tregs ($Tim\text{-}3^{+}$ Tregs) were significantly diminished in patients. $Tim\text{-}3^{+}$ Tregs express upregulated levels of FOXP3, IL-10, and TGF-β, and exhibit more intense suppressive and inhibition capacity. Besides, the level of $Tim\text{-}3^{-}/Tim\text{-}3^{+}$ ratio was positively correlated with BASDI score, ESR, and CRP level in patients [141]. In a study by Guo et al., it has been found that peripheral Tregs from active AS patients have higher CpG island methylation in the FOXP3 gene, lower FOXP3 MFI, and STAT5 phosphorylation compared to healthy Treg cells. They reported that AS Treg cells cannot properly inhibit the proliferation of naïve T cells and have defects in IL-2 signaling [142].

In contrast, a significantly lower number of $CD4^{+}$ $CD25^{high}$ $CD127^{low}$ Treg cells have been reported in treatment-naïve AS patients in a study by Zhao et al. The number of Tregs was inversely correlated with patients' serum IgA level; however, they did not find a significant correlation between Tregs and BASDAI score of patients [143]. In a meta-analysis conducted by Lin Lai et al., no considerable difference in the proportion of peripheral Treg cells has been found between AS and controls regardless of their surface markers. Although single $CD25^+$ Tregs were remarkably increased in patients, the levels of $CD4^+$ $CD25^{high/+}$ $CD127^{low/-}$ and $CD4^+$ $CD25^+$ $FOXP3^+$ showed a significant decrease in AS individuals [144].

Data regarding Treg proportion in PsA patients are also conflicting. Wang et al. have been reported that the number of Treg cells in the peripheral blood of PsA cases was reduced and was restored by using a low dose of IL-2 treatment [50]. In contrast, Fiocco et al. reported that the proportion of both $CD4^+$ $CD25^{high}$ $CD127^{low}$ and $CD4^+$ $CD25^{high}$ $FOXP3^+$ Treg cells and their expression of FOXP3 protein were elevated in synovial fluid of PsA patients [145]. Christoforou et al. also reported reduced proportions of $CD25^{bright}FOXP3^+$ Treg cells in SpA patients with diminished suppressive activity. Their result showed an increase in the proportion of Tregs and a reduction in the proportion of Th17 lymphocytes after receiving anti-IL-17 treatment in patients [146].

Given these results, it seems that Treg status and functional capacity are more important than the proportion of them in SpA pathogenesis. Improvement in Treg mediated suppression may be a potential mechanism to design new therapeutic agents for patients. The alternations of Treg lymphocytes subsets and activity in SpA disorders have been summarized in Table 3.2.

3.3.5 Cytotoxic T Cell in SpAs

$CD8^+$ T lymphocytes mainly participate in the immune responses to the tumor cells and intracellular pathogens. However, they also play a main role in autoimmunity and participate in the pathogenesis of SpA diseases. HLA-B27 and other MHC class I molecules interact with and present different antigens to naïve $CD8^+$ T lymphocytes and may induce differentiation of self-reactive CTL. Effector cytotoxic T cells including Tc1, Tc2, Tc17, and regulatory $CD8^+$ T lymphocytes can be differentiated from naïve $CD8^+$ T cells upon antigen presentation and TCR activation based on the environmental cytokine, markers, and co-stimulatory molecules [147, 148].

Numbers of studies have investigated the role of cytotoxic T lymphocytes in the immune responses of SpAs disorders. In a study by Szanto et al. elevated IL-10 producing T lymphocytes and decreased Tc1 cells were reported in peripheral blood of AS patients rather than healthy controls. However, they have reported that the frequency of IL-10^+ Tc lymphocytes was markedly lower in AS patients in the active phase rather than patients in the inactive phase [44]. By contrast, Wang et al. have reported higher Tc1 numbers and increased Tc1/Tc2 ratio in mild and severe AS patients [10]. In another research, an elevated number of memory $CD8^+$ T cells and a diminished number of fully differentiated $CD8^+$ T lymphocytes and Tc1 cells have been found in AS patients [149].

Table 3.2 The alternations of Treg lymphocytes subsets and activity in patients with SpA disorders

Authors	Patients	Sample	Frequency	Activity	References
Wang et al.	95 PsA patients compared to healthy controls	Peripheral blood	Reduced Treg cell numbers	–	[50]
Fiocco et al.	15 PsA patients compared to healthy controls	Synovial fluid	Increased proportion of $CD4^+$ $CD25^{high}$ $CD127^{low}$ and $CD4^+$ $CD25^{high}$ $FOXP3^+$ Treg cells	Elevated level of FOXP3 MFI in Tregs	[145]
Christoforou et al.	PsA patients compared to healthy controls	–	Reduced proportions of $CD25^{bright}FoxP3^+$ Treg cell	Diminished suppressive activity	[146]
Wang et al.	55 AS patients compared to healthy controls	Lesions and the serum sample	No significant differences in the percentage of Treg cells	–	[10]
Ye et al.	29 ASv patients compared to healthy controls	Peripheral blood	No significant differences in the proportion of $CD4^+$ $CD25^{high}CD39^+CD45RO^+$ naïve and $CD4^+CD25^{high}$ $CD39^-CD45RO^-$ effector Treg cells	Reduced regulatory capacity	[138]
Ciccia et al.	18 AS patients compared to healthy controls	Gut ileum and blood	Increased proportion of $CD4^+CD25^{high}$ Treg cells	Upregulated TGF-β and IL-10 Treg cytokines	[139]
Tzung Liao et al.	69 AS patients compared to healthy controls	PBMCs	Increased proportion of $CD4^+$ $CD25^+$ $FOXP3^+$ Treg cells	–	[140]
Wang et al.	26 AS patients compared to healthy controls	PBMCs	Increased frequency of $CD4^+CD25^+$ $Foxp3^+CD127^-$ Treg cells	Reduced level of FOXP3 MFI and suppressive capacity of Tregs	[141]
Guo et al.	76 AS patients compared to healthy controls	Peripheral blood	–	Reduced level of FOXP3 MFI Defected ability to suppress proliferation of naïve T	[142]
Zhao et al.	14 AS patients compared to healthy controls	Peripheral blood	Increased frequency of $CD4^+$ $CD25^{high}$ $CD127^{low}$ Treg cells	Treg cell numbers inversely correlated with serum IgA level	[143]

PsA psoriatic arthritis, *AS* Ankylosing spondylitis, *Treg* regulatory T cell, *TGF-β* Transforming growth factor-beta, *IL* Interleukin, *SF* Synovial fluid, *PBMC* Peripheral blood mononuclear cells, *MFI* Mean fluorescence intensity

In addition, the cytotoxicity profile of $CD8^+$ T lymphocytes has been also analyzed in blood and synovial fluid of AS patients. Gracey et al. have reported increased $CD8^+$ T lymphocyte frequency in the blood and decreased frequency in synovial fluid of AS patients. They found that the expression of both granzyme and perforin 1 as cytotoxicity markers of CTL was reduced in AS blood. However, granzymes levels were upregulated in the synovial of AS patients. It seems that CTL with cytotoxicity activity is recruited to the synovial environment [150]. Moreover, in a study by Schirmer et al. it has been demonstrated that circulating $CD8^+$ $CD28^-$ T lymphocytes, which are characterized by perforin production, are expanded more in AS individuals in comparison to healthy ones. The elevated proportion of $CD8^+$ $CD28^-$ T lymphocytes were correlated to a more intense course of the disease, and severe movement restrictions in patients [151].

In another study, it has been observed that PBMCs from individuals with AS or HLA-$B27^+$ genotype have elevated frequency of IL-4^+ $CD8^+$ regulatory T lymphocytes [152]. Previously it had been reported a novel human CD8+ T cell subset with regulatory phenotype which is not cytolytic and can respond to autoreactive HLA class I by producing IL-4, IL-13, and TGF-β [153]. Therefore, it seems that elevated IL-4^+ $CD8^+$ regulatory T lymphocytes in AS patients may participate in the development of disease but it needs more investigations. These reports suggested that dysregulation in the number and cytolytic activity of CD8+ T cells are contributed to the immunopathogenesis of AS.

Regarding the role of $CD8^+$ T lymphocytes in PsA disease, it has been found that the $CD8^+$ T cells of the synovial cavity of PsA patients have various oligoclonal expansions in the β chain of TCR, and most of these expansions only found in joint fluid and not found in the blood of patients. This finding confirms the crucial role of T $CD8^+$ T cells and their clonal expansions in the development of the disease [17]. Some other studies evaluate the proportion and activity of $CD8^+$ T lymphocytes in PsA. Colombo et al. have found a significant expansion in the peripheral blood IFN-γ^+ $CD8^+$ T cells in PsA patients in contrast to controls which was related to the number of swollen joints in patients [154]. In a study by Diani et al., the role of effector memory T lymphocyte has been considered in systemic and joint manifestations of PsA patients. Increased proportion of $CD8^+$ $CCR6^+$ $CD69^+$ effector T cell in the blood enhanced number of $CXCR3^+$ $CD8^+$ T lymphocytes in synovial fluid, and elevated infiltration of $CD8^+$ effector memory T cells in synovial tissues has been reported in PsA patients [155]. Moreover, elevated expression of CD69 and HLA-DR activation agents in the $CD4^+$ and $CD8^+$ T cells subsets within the synovial tissue of ReA patients compared with paired peripheral blood has been reported [156].

These results showed an expansion and increased activity of $CD8^+$ T cells in SpA disorders especially in their involved synovial tissues and suggested a main role for the infiltrated $CD8^+$ T lymphocytes in the inflammatory response of involved joints of PsA and other uSpA patients. Therefore, targeting cytotoxic T cells in the involved joint of patients could be a probable therapeutic aim with low systemic side effects.

3.3.6 Gamma Delta T Cells and SpAs

Gamma delta (γδ) T cells are a subset of T lymphocytes that possess distinctive TCR molecules (made up of a pair gamma/delta chain) on their surface. They participate in the immune responses against infections and cancerous cells and take part in auto-inflammatory conditions and autoimmunity by producing IL-22 and IL-17 inflammatory cytokines [157–160]. Although IL-23/IL-23R is the main signaling pathway inducing IL-17 production, Guggino et al. reported that IL-9/IL-9R interaction can also trigger γδT lymphocytes of PsA patients' activation and induce IL-17 secretion [161]. γδT cells are enriched in inflamed tissue of non-autoimmune arthritis mouse models and participate in the immunopathogenesis of SpA disease in mice and humans [81, 162, 163]. Altered frequency of γδT cells in blood or synovial tissue of SpA patients has been reported in some research. Meliconi et al. for the first time investigated the number of γδT cells in the peripheral and synovial fluid of the patients with seronegative spondyloarthritides. However, they did not find significant differences [164]. Later Kenna et al. have reported the elevated proportion of IL-17 producing IL-23R$^+$ γδT cells in the periphery of AS patients compared to RA and healthy persons [165]. In another study by Chowdhury et al., it was shown that although the frequency of γδT cells was reduced in the blood of ReA and uSpA patients in comparison to the healthy group, the level of IL-17 producing γδT cells was upregulated. They have also reported that the ratio of IL-17 producing IFN-γ$^+$ γδT lymphocytes was considerably higher in the synovial fluid of patients rather than their blood [166]. Moreover, a reduced number of γδ CD4$^+$ or CD8$^+$ T lymphocytes in the blood of PsA patients concerning the control group has been reported. In a study by Spadaro et al., they have also found an association between the value of γδT cells in synovial tissue of patients and NK and NK T cells numbers. However, they did not see a significant correlation between γδT cells proportion and patients' clinical and serological manifestations [167]. Cuvelier et al. have found the increased expansion of CD3$^+$ lymphocytes in the ileal mucosa of the patients with SpA-related gut inflammation. However, they did not found remarkable differences in the level of γδT cells, and an observed increase was probably due to the expansion of αβ T lymphocytes in patients [168]. Due to the mentioned results, it seems that following an increase in the IL-23 level in the inflamed synovium of SpA disorders, IL-17 producing γδT cells may be enriched in them and participates in the auto-inflammatory responses.

3.4 B Cell Activation and Signaling

B cells play important roles in various autoimmune diseases by antibody production, antigens presentation, and inflammatory cytokines release [169]. However, their role in the pathogenesis of SpA disorders remains still undetermined. Previously SpA disease was considered as auto-inflammatory ones; however, in recent years several autoantibodies have been detected in the patients' serum [170]. B lymphocyte imbalance and hyperactivity have been shown in patients with

SpA. Increased numbers of B lymphocytes and immunoblast cells along with an elevated level of serum immunoglobulins have been also found in AS patients [171–174]. A decreased number of $CD27^+$ $CD19^+$ (memory) B cells and an elevated number of $CD27^-$ $CD19^+$ (naive) B cells have been described in peripheral blood of AS patients in comparison to controls. It was suggested that the reduction in memory B cells might be due to their differentiation to plasma cells.

Besides, an increased number of $CD86^+$ $CD19^+$ and $CD27^-$ $CD95^+$ $CD19^+$ B cells has been found in the blood of AS patients which indicates an upregulation in the activated phenotype of naïve and memory B cells in patients. It has suggested that $CD86^+$ $CD19^+$ and $CD27^-$ $CD95^+$ $CD19^+$ B lymphocytes may be potential targets in AS patients [175]. Also, in a study by Lin et al., it has been suggested that the proportion of $CD19^+$ B cells was increased in active AS patients or patients with peripheral joint involvement in comparison to patients with stable disease, and the increase was correlated with the rate of patients' BASDAI and back pain scores. The proportion of $CD19^+$ $CD27^{high}$ plasmablasts was considerably higher in AS patients with peripheral joint involvement rather than healthy individuals or patients with axial involvements [176]. Besides, an elevated proportion of $CD19^+$ B cells has been demonstrated in PBMCs from PsA patients [177]. Hence, it is suggested that naïve and memory B cells and their activated phenotypes contribute to the immune abnormalities of SpA diseases mostly in AS patients with involved peripheral joints, and the exact mechanism underlying their contribution needs more research.

Moreover, it has been shown that the expression level of α and γ globulin, IgG, IgM, and IgA immunoglobulins was remarkably increased in the serum samples of AS patients [10]. Besides, several autoantibodies including anti-beta2 microglobulin [178], anti-heat shock protein 65 (anti-HSP65) [179], anti-nuclear components (ANA) [180], anti-mutated citrullinated vimentin (MCV) [179], anti-cardiolipin (anti-phospholipid) [181], anti-14-3-3η (eta) [182], anti-protein phosphatase magnesium-dependent 1A (anti-PPM1A) [183], anti-neutrophil cytoplasmic antibody (ANCA) [184], anti-sclerostin (anti-SOST) [185], anti-microbial targets [186–188], and anti-CD74 [189] autoantibodies have been detected in SpA patients [170, 190]. Curry et al. have detected the IgG antibodies against beta2 microglobulin in 68% of studied patients. Interestingly, the rate of anti-beta2 microglobulin antibodies was higher in AS patients compared to patients with RA and lupus [191]. The prevalence of serum anti-MCV antibodies has been shown to be 13.9% and 15.2% in patients with spondyloarthropathy and PsA, respectively [192]. It has been also demonstrated that the prevalence of anti-CMV antibodies is 37% in AS patients and is remarkably higher regarding to healthy controls that have not anti-CMV antibodies in their serum [179]. Results regarding anti-HSP56 are contradictory. Although elevated anti-HSP56 antibodies have been reported in AS patients compared to healthy controls with back pain by Bondnar et al. [179], McLean et al. have not found significant differences in the level of this antibody in patients [193]. Moreover, the elevated expression level of 14-3-3η intracellular protein and increased level of anti-14-3-3η antibodies have been reported in AS patients [194, 195].

PPM1A is a phosphatase that regulates bone morphogenetic proteins (BMP) and Wnt signaling pathways and participates in bone remodeling. A significantly elevated level of PPM1A expression and anti-PPM1A autoantibodies have been detected in treatment-naïve AS patients and the level was associated with the severity of sacroiliitis [183]. Sclerostin is an inhibitor of Wnt and BMP pathways and bone formation. Lower sclerostin levels and increased levels of anti-sclerostin antibodies have been reported in AS patients [196, 197]. It has also been found that the rate of anti-SOST antibodies was notably elevated in patients with axial SpA-associated IBD compared with IBD patients and can be considered as a potential biomarker in this group of patients [185]. CD74 is a protein that participates in the MHC class-II antigen presentation. The extracellular segment of CD74 contains two domains: class II-associated invariant chain peptide (CLIP) and thyroglobulin type-1 [198, 199]. In a study by Baerlecken et al., it was found that anti-CD74 IgG antibodies were found in 67% of patients with SpA and 45% of patients with PsA, while only 0.8% of control blood donors were positive for these antibodies [200]. Anti-CLIP antibodies were also found in 85.1% of patients with axial SpA and the rate was remarkably higher than non-SpA patients [201]. Therefore, anti-CD74 antibodies might also be a potential biomarker for SpA patients. The role of autoantibodies in the inflammatory cascades of SpA disorders has not been considered enough. Autoantibodies can be used as a diagnosis, prognosis, and treatment response biomarkers in SpA disorders. Therefore, more researches on the level and type of autoantibodies in the different stages of SpA diseases are essential.

3.5 Conclusions and Future Directions

The role of adaptive immunity in the pathogenesis of SpA disorders has not received enough attention and needs more considerations. The role of different subsets of adaptive immune cells and their surface markers, their related cytokines, and their activity status in the different stages of the disease need special investigations. Due to the discussed role of Th17, Th22, regulatory T cells, and γδT in the immunopathogenesis of these groups of disorders especially in the inflamed tissues, it seems that T cell-targeted therapy especially Treg cells immunotherapy can be a possible therapeutic target. Considering the enrichment of various subsets of pathogenic lymphocytes in the inflamed tissue of patients, it appears that synovial or inflamed tissue specified therapy may have a more beneficial outcome in patients.

References

1. Hoebe K, Janssen E, Beutler B. The interface between innate and adaptive immunity. Nat Immunol. 2004;5(10):971–4. https://doi.org/10.1038/ni1004-971.
2. Blanco P, Palucka AK, Pascual V, Banchereau J. Dendritic cells and cytokines in human inflammatory and autoimmune diseases. Cytokine Growth Factor Rev. 2008;19(1):41–52. https://doi.org/10.1016/j.cytogfr.2007.10.004.
3. Scherer HU, Burmester GR. Adaptive immunity in rheumatic diseases: bystander or pathogenic player? Best Pract Res Clin Rheumatol. 2011;25(6):785–800. https://doi.org/10.1016/j.berh.2011.11.005.

4. Weissert R. Adaptive immunity is the key to the understanding of autoimmune and paraneoplastic inflammatory central nervous system disorders. Front Immunol. 2017;8:336. https://doi.org/10.3389/fimmu.2017.00336.
5. Goldfarb Y, Peligero-Cruz C, Abramson J. Chapter 5 – Immunological tolerance—T cells. In: Rose NR, Mackay IR, editors. The autoimmune diseases. 6th ed. St. Louis, MO: Academic Press; 2020. p. 65–90.
6. Norman MU, Hickey MJ. Mechanisms of lymphocyte migration in autoimmune disease. Tissue Antigens. 2005;66(3):163–72. https://doi.org/10.1111/j.1399-0039.2005.00434.x.
7. McGonagle D, Savic S, McDermott MF. The NLR network and the immunological disease continuum of adaptive and innate immune-mediated inflammation against self. Semin Immunopathol. 2007;29(3):303–13. https://doi.org/10.1007/s00281-007-0084-1.
8. Sibley CH. Autoinflammation and HLA-B27: Beyond Antigen Presentation. Ocul Immunol Inflamm. 2016;24(4):460–9. https://doi.org/10.1080/09273948.2016.1175641.
9. Stoll ML. Interactions of the innate and adaptive arms of the immune system in the pathogenesis of spondyloarthritis. Clin Exp Rheumatol. 2011;29(2):322–30.
10. Wang C, Liao Q, Hu Y, Zhong D. T lymphocyte subset imbalances in patients contribute to ankylosing spondylitis. Exp Ther Med. 2015;9(1):250–6. https://doi.org/10.3892/etm.2014.2046.
11. Tam LS, Gu J, Yu D. Pathogenesis of ankylosing spondylitis. Nat Rev Rheumatol. 2010;6(7):399–405. https://doi.org/10.1038/nrrheum.2010.79.
12. Ranganathan V, Gracey E, Brown MA, Inman RD, Haroon N. Pathogenesis of ankylosing spondylitis – recent advances and future directions. Nat Rev Rheumatol. 2017;13(6):359–67. https://doi.org/10.1038/nrrheum.2017.56.
13. Sherlock JP, Joyce-Shaikh B, Turner SP, Chao C-C, Sathe M, Grein J, et al. IL-23 induces spondyloarthropathy by acting on ROR-γt+ CD3+CD4−CD8− entheseal resident T cells. Nat Med. 2012;18(7):1069–76. https://doi.org/10.1038/nm.2817.
14. Ebihara S, Date F, Dong Y, Ono M. Interleukin-17 is a critical target for the treatment of ankylosing enthesitis and psoriasis-like dermatitis in mice. Autoimmunity. 2015;48(4):259–66. https://doi.org/10.3109/08916934.2014.976630.
15. Wedderburn LR, Patel A, Varsani H, Woo P. Divergence in the degree of clonal expansions in inflammatory T cell subpopulations mirrors HLA-associated risk alleles in genetically and clinically distinct subtypes of childhood arthritis. Int Immunol. 2001;13(12):1541–50. https://doi.org/10.1093/intimm/13.12.1541.
16. Treviño MA, Teixeiro E, Bragado R. CD8+ T cells oligoclonally expanded in synovial fluid at onset of spondyloarthropathy selectively proliferate in response to self-antigens: characterization of cell specificities in nonclonal populations. J Rheumatol. 2004;31(10):1962–72.
17. Costello PJ, Winchester RJ, Curran SA, Peterson KS, Kane DJ, Bresnihan B, et al. Psoriatic arthritis joint fluids are characterized by CD8 and CD4 T cell clonal expansions appear antigen driven. J Immunol. 2001;166(4):2878–86. https://doi.org/10.4049/jimmunol.166.4.2878.
18. Braun J, Bollow M, Neure L, Seipelt E, Seyrekbasan F, Herbst H, et al. Use of immunohistologic and in situ hybridization techniques in the examination of sacroiliac joint biopsy specimens from patients with ankylosing spondylitis. Arthritis Rheum. 1995;38(4):499–505. https://doi.org/10.1002/art.1780380407.
19. McGonagle D, Marzo-Ortega H, O'Connor P, Gibbon W, Hawkey P, Henshaw K, et al. Histological assessment of the early enthesitis lesion in spondyloarthropathy. Ann Rheum Dis. 2002;61(6):534–7. https://doi.org/10.1136/ard.61.6.534.
20. Appel H, Kuhne M, Spiekermann S, Ebhardt H, Grozdanovic Z, Köhler D, et al. Immunohistologic analysis of zygapophyseal joints in patients with ankylosing spondylitis. Arthritis Rheum. 2006;54(9):2845–51. https://doi.org/10.1002/art.22060.
21. Kinsella TD, Espinoza L, Vasey FB. Serum complement and immunoglobulin levels in sporadic and familial ankylosing spondylitis. J Rheumatol. 1975;2(3):308–13.
22. Cowling P, Ebringer R, Ebringer A. Association of inflammation with raised serum IgA in ankylosing spondylitis. Ann Rheum Dis. 1980;39(6):545–9. https://doi.org/10.1136/ard.39.6.545.

23. Veys EM, van Leare M. Serum IgG, IgM, and IgA levels in ankylosing spondylitis. Ann Rheum Dis. 1973;32(6):493–6. https://doi.org/10.1136/ard.32.6.493.
24. Szalay B, Mészáros G, Cseh Á, Ács L, Deák M, Kovács L, et al. Adaptive immunity in ankylosing spondylitis: phenotype and functional alterations of T-cells before and during infliximab therapy. Clin Dev Immunol. 2012;2012:808724. https://doi.org/10.1155/2012/808724.
25. Hammer RE, Maika SD, Richardson JA, Tang JP, Taurog JD. Spontaneous inflammatory disease in transgenic rats expressing HLA-B27 and human beta 2m: an animal model of HLA-B27-associated human disorders. Cell. 1990;63(5):1099–112. https://doi.org/10.1016/0092-8674(90)90512-d.
26. Taurog JD, Maika SD, Satumtira N, Dorris ML, McLean IL, Yanagisawa H, et al. Inflammatory disease in HLA-B27 transgenic rats. Immunol Rev. 1999;169:209–23. https://doi.org/10.1111/j.1600-065x.1999.tb01317.x.
27. Breban M, Fernández-Sueiro JL, Richardson JA, Hadavand RR, Maika SD, Hammer RE, et al. T cells, but not thymic exposure to HLA-B27, are required for the inflammatory disease of HLA-B27 transgenic rats. J Immunol. 1996;156(2):794–803.
28. Breban M, Hammer RE, Richardson JA, Taurog JD. Transfer of the inflammatory disease of HLA-B27 transgenic rats by bone marrow engraftment. J Exp Med. 1993;178(5):1607–16. https://doi.org/10.1084/jem.178.5.1607.
29. Skapenko A, Leipe J, Lipsky PE, Schulze-Koops H. The role of the T cell in autoimmune inflammation. Arthritis Res Ther. 2005;7(2):S4. https://doi.org/10.1186/ar1703.
30. Sallusto F, Lenig D, Förster R, Lipp M, Lanzavecchia A. Two subsets of memory T lymphocytes with distinct homing potentials and effector functions. Nature. 1999;401(6754):708–12. https://doi.org/10.1038/44385.
31. Lucey DR, Clerici M, Shearer GM. Type 1 and type 2 cytokine dysregulation in human infectious, neoplastic, and inflammatory diseases. Clin Microbiol Rev. 1996;9(4):532–62. https://doi.org/10.1128/cmr.9.4.532-562.1996.
32. May E, Dorris ML, Satumtira N, Iqbal I, Rehman MI, Lightfoot E, et al. CD8αβ T cells are not essential to the pathogenesis of arthritis or colitis in HLA-B27 transgenic rats. J Immunol. 2003;170(2):1099–105. https://doi.org/10.4049/jimmunol.170.2.1099.
33. Duftner C, Goldberger C, Falkenbach A, Würzner R, Falkensammer B, Pfeiffer KP, et al. Prevalence, clinical relevance and characterization of circulating cytotoxic CD4+CD28- T cells in ankylosing spondylitis. Arthritis Res Ther. 2003;5(5):R292–300. https://doi.org/10.1186/ar793.
34. Roberts AR, Vecellio M, Chen L, Ridley A, Cortes A, Knight JC, et al. An ankylosing spondylitis-associated genetic variant in the IL23R-IL12RB2 intergenic region modulates enhancer activity and is associated with increased Th1-cell differentiation. Ann Rheum Dis. 2016;75(12):2150–6. https://doi.org/10.1136/annrheumdis-2015-208640.
35. Berger A. Th1 and Th2 responses: what are they? BMJ (Clinical research ed). 2000;321(7258):424. https://doi.org/10.1136/bmj.321.7258.424.
36. Cortés A, Muñoz-Antoli C, Esteban JG, Toledo R. Th2 and Th1 responses: clear and hidden sides of immunity against intestinal helminths. Trends Parasitol. 2017;33(9):678–93. https://doi.org/10.1016/j.pt.2017.05.004.
37. Wen JT, Zhang DH, Fang PF, Li MH, Wang RJ, Li SH. Role of Th1/Th2 cytokines in the diagnosis and prognostic evaluation of ankylosing spondylitis. Genet Mol Res: GMR. 2017;16(1) https://doi.org/10.4238/gmr16019322.
38. Bautista-Herrera LA, De la Cruz-Mosso U, Morales-Zambrano R, Villanueva-Quintero GD, Hernández-Bello J, Ramírez-Dueñas MG, et al. Expression of MIF and TNFA in psoriatic arthritis: relationship with Th1/Th2/Th17 cytokine profiles and clinical variables. Clin Exp Med. 2018;18(2):229–35. https://doi.org/10.1007/s10238-017-0475-0.
39. Singh R, Aggarwal A, Misra R. Th1/Th17 cytokine profiles in patients with reactive arthritis/undifferentiated spondyloarthropathy. J Rheumatol. 2007;34(11):2285–90.
40. Yin Z, Braun J, Neure L, Wu P, Liu L, Eggens U, et al. Crucial role of interleukin-10/interleukin-12 balance in the regulation of the type 2 T helper cytokine response in reactive arthritis. Arthritis Rheum. 1997;40(10):1788–97. https://doi.org/10.1002/art.1780401010.

41. Braun J, Yin Z, Spiller I, Siegert S, Rudwaleit M, Liu L, et al. Low secretion of tumor necrosis factor alpha, but no other Th1 or Th2 cytokines, by peripheral blood mononuclear cells correlates with chronicity in reactive arthritis. Arthritis Rheum. 1999;42(10):2039–44. https://doi.org/10.1002/1529-0131(199910)42:10<2039::aid-anr3>3.0.co;2-6.
42. Simon AK, Seipelt E, Sieper J. Divergent T-cell cytokine patterns in inflammatory arthritis. Proc Natl Acad Sci U S A. 1994;91(18):8562–6. https://doi.org/10.1073/pnas.91.18.8562.
43. Cañete JD, Martínez SE, Farrés J, Sanmartí R, Blay M, Gómez A, et al. Differential Th1/Th2 cytokine patterns in chronic arthritis: interferon gamma is highly expressed in synovium of rheumatoid arthritis compared with seronegative spondyloarthropathies. Ann Rheum Dis. 2000;59(4):263–8. https://doi.org/10.1136/ard.59.4.263.
44. Szántó S, Aleksza M, Mihály E, Lakos G, Szabó Z, Végvári A, et al. Intracytoplasmic cytokine expression and T cell subset distribution in the peripheral blood of patients with ankylosing spondylitis. J Rheumatol. 2008;35(12):2372–5. https://doi.org/10.3899/jrheum.070839.
45. Limón-Camacho L, Vargas-Rojas MI, Vázquez-Mellado J, Casasola-Vargas J, Moctezuma JF, Burgos-Vargas R, et al. *In Vivo* peripheral blood proinflammatory T cells in patients with ankylosing spondylitis. J Rheumatol. 2012;39(4):830–5. https://doi.org/10.3899/jrheum.110862.
46. Brandt J, Haibel H, Cornely D, Golder W, Gonzalez J, Reddig J, et al. Successful treatment of active ankylosing spondylitis with the anti-tumor necrosis factor alpha monoclonal antibody infliximab. Arthritis Rheum. 2000;43(6):1346–52. https://doi.org/10.1002/1529-0131(200006)43:6<1346::aid-anr18>3.0.co;2-e.
47. Yang PT, Kasai H, Zhao LJ, Xiao WG, Tanabe F, Ito M. Increased CCR4 expression on circulating CD4(+) T cells in ankylosing spondylitis, rheumatoid arthritis and systemic lupus erythematosus. Clin Exp Immunol. 2004;138(2):342–7. https://doi.org/10.1111/j.1365-2249.2004.02617.x.
48. Rudwaleit M, Siegert S, Yin Z, Eick J, Thiel A, Radbruch A, et al. Low T cell production of TNFalpha and IFNgamma in ankylosing spondylitis: its relation to HLA-B27 and influence of the TNF-308 gene polymorphism. Ann Rheum Dis. 2001;60(1):36–42. https://doi.org/10.1136/ard.60.1.36.
49. Wang J, Zhao Q, Wang G, Yang C, Xu Y, Li Y, et al. Circulating levels of Th1 and Th2 chemokines in patients with ankylosing spondylitis. Cytokine. 2016;81:10–4. https://doi.org/10.1016/j.cyto.2016.01.012.
50. Wang J, Zhang SX, Hao YF, Qiu MT, Luo J, Li YY, et al. The numbers of peripheral regulatory T cells are reduced in patients with psoriatic arthritis and are restored by low-dose interleukin-2. Ther Adv Chronic Dis. 2020;11:2040622320916014. https://doi.org/10.1177/2040622320916014.
51. Menon B, Gullick NJ, Walter GJ, Rajasekhar M, Garrood T, Evans HG, et al. Interleukin-17+CD8+ T cells are enriched in the joints of patients with psoriatic arthritis and correlate with disease activity and joint damage progression. Arthritis Rheumatol (Hoboken, NJ). 2014;66(5):1272–81. https://doi.org/10.1002/art.38376.
52. Benham H, Norris P, Goodall J, Wechalekar MD, FitzGerald O, Szentpetery A, et al. Th17 and Th22 cells in psoriatic arthritis and psoriasis. Arthritis Res Ther. 2013;15(5):R136-R. https://doi.org/10.1186/ar4317.
53. Mitra A, Raychaudhuri SK, Raychaudhuri SP. Functional role of IL-22 in psoriatic arthritis. Arthritis Res Ther. 2012;14(2):R65-R. https://doi.org/10.1186/ar3781.
54. Ezeonyeji A, Baldwin H, Vukmanovic-Stejic M, Ehrenstein MR. CD4 T-Cell dysregulation in psoriatic arthritis reveals a regulatory role for IL-22. Front Immunol. 2017;8:1403. https://doi.org/10.3389/fimmu.2017.01403.
55. Shen H, Goodall JC, Gaston JS. Frequency and phenotype of T helper 17 cells in peripheral blood and synovial fluid of patients with reactive arthritis. J Rheumatol. 2010;37(10):2096–9. https://doi.org/10.3899/jrheum.100146.
56. Singh AK, Misra R, Aggarwal A. Th-17 associated cytokines in patients with reactive arthritis/undifferentiated spondyloarthropathy. Clin Rheumatol. 2011;30(6):771–6. https://doi.org/10.1007/s10067-010-1646-5.

57. Jandus C, Bioley G, Rivals JP, Dudler J, Speiser D, Romero P. Increased numbers of circulating polyfunctional Th17 memory cells in patients with seronegative spondylarthritides. Arthritis Rheum. 2008;58(8):2307–17. https://doi.org/10.1002/art.23655.
58. Shen H, Goodall JC, Hill Gaston JS. Frequency and phenotype of peripheral blood Th17 cells in ankylosing spondylitis and rheumatoid arthritis. Arthritis Rheum. 2009;60(6):1647–56. https://doi.org/10.1002/art.24568.
59. Wang X, Lin Z, Wei Q, Jiang Y, Gu J. Expression of IL-23 and IL-17 and effect of IL-23 on IL-17 production in ankylosing spondylitis. Rheumatol Int. 2009;29(11):1343–7. https://doi.org/10.1007/s00296-009-0883-x.
60. Zhang L, Li YG, Li YH, Qi L, Liu XG, Yuan CZ, et al. Increased frequencies of Th22 cells as well as Th17 cells in the peripheral blood of patients with ankylosing spondylitis and rheumatoid arthritis. PLoS One. 2012;7(4):e31000. https://doi.org/10.1371/journal.pone.0031000.
61. Taams LS, Steel KJA, Srenathan U, Burns LA, Kirkham BW. IL-17 in the immunopathogenesis of spondyloarthritis. Nat Rev Rheumatol. 2018;14(8):453–66. https://doi.org/10.1038/s41584-018-0044-2.
62. Ruyssen-Witrand A, Luxembourger C, Cantagrel A, Nigon D, Claudepierre P, Degboe Y, et al. Association between IL23R and ERAP1 polymorphisms and sacroiliac or spinal MRI inflammation in spondyloarthritis: DESIR cohort data. Arthritis Res Ther. 2019;21(1):22. https://doi.org/10.1186/s13075-018-1807-5.
63. Rueda B, Orozco G, Raya E, Fernandez-Sueiro JL, Mulero J, Blanco FJ, et al. The IL23R Arg381Gln non-synonymous polymorphism confers susceptibility to ankylosing spondylitis. Ann Rheum Dis. 2008;67(10):1451–4. https://doi.org/10.1136/ard.2007.080283.
64. Zhong L, Wang W, Song H. Complex role of IL-23R polymorphisms on ankylosing spondylitis: a meta-analysis. Expert Rev Clin Immunol. 2018;14(7):635–43. https://doi.org/10.1080/1744666x.2018.1491308.
65. Li X, Bechara R, Zhao J, McGeachy MJ, Gaffen SL. IL-17 receptor–based signaling and implications for disease. Nat Immunol. 2019;20(12):1594–602. https://doi.org/10.1038/s41590-019-0514-y.
66. Gu C, Wu L, Li X. IL-17 family: cytokines, receptors and signaling. Cytokine. 2013;64(2):477–85. https://doi.org/10.1016/j.cyto.2013.07.022.
67. Menon B, Gullick NJ, Walter GJ, Rajasekhar M, Garrood T, Evans HG, et al. Interleukin-17+CD8+ T cells are enriched in the joints of patients with psoriatic arthritis and correlate with disease activity and joint damage progression. Arthritis Rheum. 2014;66(5):1272–81. https://doi.org/10.1002/art.38376.
68. Xueyi L, Lina C, Zhenbiao W, Qing H, Qiang L, Zhu P. Levels of circulating Th17 cells and regulatory T cells in ankylosing spondylitis patients with an inadequate response to anti-TNF-α therapy. J Clin Immunol. 2013;33(1):151–61. https://doi.org/10.1007/s10875-012-9774-0.
69. Soare A, Weber S, Maul L, Rauber S, Gheorghiu AM, Luber M, et al. Cutting edge: homeostasis of innate lymphoid cells is imbalanced in psoriatic arthritis. J Immunol. 2018;200(4):1249–54. https://doi.org/10.4049/jimmunol.1700596.
70. Leijten EF, van Kempen TS, Boes M, Michels-van Amelsfort JM, Hijnen D, Hartgring SA, et al. Brief report: enrichment of activated group 3 innate lymphoid cells in psoriatic arthritis synovial fluid. Arthritis Rheum. 2015;67(10):2673–8. https://doi.org/10.1002/art.39261.
71. Cuthbert RJ, Fragkakis EM, Dunsmuir R, Li Z, Coles M, Marzo-Ortega H, et al. Brief Report: Group 3 Innate Lymphoid Cells in Human Enthesis. Arthritis Rheum. 2017;69(9):1816–22. https://doi.org/10.1002/art.40150.
72. Moran EM, Heydrich R, Ng CT, Saber TP, McCormick J, Sieper J, et al. IL-17A expression is localised to both mononuclear and polymorphonuclear synovial cell infiltrates. PLoS One. 2011;6(8):e24048. https://doi.org/10.1371/journal.pone.0024048.
73. Appel H, Maier R, Wu P, Scheer R, Hempfing A, Kayser R, et al. Analysis of IL-17(+) cells in facet joints of patients with spondyloarthritis suggests that the innate immune pathway might be of greater relevance than the Th17-mediated adaptive immune response. Arthritis Res Ther. 2011;13(3):R95. https://doi.org/10.1186/ar3370.

74. Benedetti G, Miossec P. Interleukin 17 contributes to the chronicity of inflammatory diseases such as rheumatoid arthritis. Eur J Immunol. 2014;44(2):339–47. https://doi.org/10.1002/eji.201344184.
75. Amatya N, Garg AV, Gaffen SL. IL-17 Signaling: The Yin and the Yang. Trends Immunol. 2017;38(5):310–22. https://doi.org/10.1016/j.it.2017.01.006.
76. McGonagle DG, McInnes IB, Kirkham BW, Sherlock J, Moots R. The role of IL-17A in axial spondyloarthritis and psoriatic arthritis: recent advances and controversies. Ann Rheum Dis. 2019;78(9):1167–78. https://doi.org/10.1136/annrheumdis-2019-215356.
77. Schett G, Lories RJ, D'Agostino MA, Elewaut D, Kirkham B, Soriano ER, et al. Enthesitis: from pathophysiology to treatment. Nat Rev Rheumatol. 2017;13(12):731–41. https://doi.org/10.1038/nrrheum.2017.188.
78. Sherlock JP, Joyce-Shaikh B, Turner SP, Chao CC, Sathe M, Grein J, et al. IL-23 induces spondyloarthropathy by acting on ROR-γt+ CD3+CD4-CD8- entheseal resident T cells. Nat Med. 2012;18(7):1069–76. https://doi.org/10.1038/nm.2817.
79. Benham H, Rehaume LM, Hasnain SZ, Velasco J, Baillet AC, Ruutu M, et al. Interleukin-23 mediates the intestinal response to microbial β-1,3-glucan and the development of spondyloarthritis pathology in SKG mice. Arthritis Rheum. 2014;66(7):1755–67. https://doi.org/10.1002/art.38638.
80. Ebihara S, Date F, Dong Y, Ono M. Interleukin-17 is a critical target for the treatment of ankylosing enthesitis and psoriasis-like dermatitis in mice. Autoimmunity. 2015;48(4):259–66. https://doi.org/10.3109/08916934.2014.976630.
81. Khmaladze I, Kelkka T, Guerard S, Wing K, Pizzolla A, Saxena A, et al. Mannan induces ROS-regulated, IL-17A-dependent psoriasis arthritis-like disease in mice. Proc Natl Acad Sci U S A. 2014;111(35):E3669–78. https://doi.org/10.1073/pnas.1405798111.
82. Cambré I, Gaublomme D, Burssens A, Jacques P, Schryvers N, De Muynck A, et al. Mechanical strain determines the site-specific localization of inflammation and tissue damage in arthritis. Nat Commun. 2018;9(1):4613. https://doi.org/10.1038/s41467-018-06933-4.
83. De Wilde K, Martens A, Lambrecht S, Jacques P, Drennan MB, Debusschere K, et al. A20 inhibition of STAT1 expression in myeloid cells: a novel endogenous regulatory mechanism preventing development of enthesitis. Ann Rheum Dis. 2017;76(3):585–92. https://doi.org/10.1136/annrheumdis-2016-209454.
84. Jacques P, Lambrecht S, Verheugen E, Pauwels E, Kollias G, Armaka M, et al. Proof of concept: enthesitis and new bone formation in spondyloarthritis are driven by mechanical strain and stromal cells. Ann Rheum Dis. 2014;73(2):437–45. https://doi.org/10.1136/annrheumdis-2013-203643.
85. Yu JJ, Ruddy MJ, Wong GC, Sfintescu C, Baker PJ, Smith JB, et al. An essential role for IL-17 in preventing pathogen-initiated bone destruction: recruitment of neutrophils to inflamed bone requires IL-17 receptor-dependent signals. Blood. 2007;109(9):3794–802. https://doi.org/10.1182/blood-2005-09-010116.
86. Ye P, Rodriguez FH, Kanaly S, Stocking KL, Schurr J, Schwarzenberger P, et al. Requirement of interleukin 17 receptor signaling for lung CXC chemokine and granulocyte colony-stimulating factor expression, neutrophil recruitment, and host defense. J Exp Med. 2001;194(4):519–27. https://doi.org/10.1084/jem.194.4.519.
87. Adamopoulos IE, Tessmer M, Chao CC, Adda S, Gorman D, Petro M, et al. IL-23 is critical for induction of arthritis, osteoclast formation, and maintenance of bone mass. J Immunol. 2011;187(2):951–9. https://doi.org/10.4049/jimmunol.1003986.
88. Lee Y. The role of interleukin-17 in bone metabolism and inflammatory skeletal diseases. BMB Rep. 2013;46(10):479–83. https://doi.org/10.5483/bmbrep.2013.46.10.141.
89. Chabaud M, Lubberts E, Joosten L, van Den Berg W, Miossec P. IL-17 derived from juxta-articular bone and synovium contributes to joint degradation in rheumatoid arthritis. Arthritis Res. 2001;3(3):168–77. https://doi.org/10.1186/ar294.
90. Chabaud M, Miossec P. The combination of tumor necrosis factor alpha blockade with interleukin-1 and interleukin-17 blockade is more effective for controlling synovial inflam-

mation and bone resorption in an ex vivo model. Arthritis Rheum. 2001;44(6):1293–303. https://doi.org/10.1002/1529-0131(200106)44:6<1293::aid-art221>3.0.co;2-t.

91. Lubberts E, van den Bersselaar L, Oppers-Walgreen B, Schwarzenberger P, Coenen-de Roo CJ, Kolls JK, et al. IL-17 promotes bone erosion in murine collagen-induced arthritis through loss of the receptor activator of NF-kappa B ligand/osteoprotegerin balance. J Immunol. 2003;170(5):2655–62. https://doi.org/10.4049/jimmunol.170.5.2655.
92. Kikuta J, Wada Y, Kowada T, Wang Z, Sun-Wada GH, Nishiyama I, et al. Dynamic visualization of RANKL and Th17-mediated osteoclast function. J Clin Invest. 2013;123(2):866–73. https://doi.org/10.1172/jci65054.
93. Huang H, Kim HJ, Chang EJ, Lee ZH, Hwang SJ, Kim HM, et al. IL-17 stimulates the proliferation and differentiation of human mesenchymal stem cells: implications for bone remodeling. Cell Death Differ. 2009;16(10):1332–43. https://doi.org/10.1038/cdd.2009.74.
94. Loi F, Córdova LA, Pajarinen J, Lin TH, Yao Z, Goodman SB. Inflammation, fracture and bone repair. Bone. 2016;86:119–30. https://doi.org/10.1016/j.bone.2016.02.020.
95. Jo S, Wang SE, Lee YL, Kang S, Lee B, Han J, et al. IL-17A induces osteoblast differentiation by activating JAK2/STAT3 in ankylosing spondylitis. Arthritis Res Ther. 2018;20(1):115. https://doi.org/10.1186/s13075-018-1582-3.
96. Ono T, Okamoto K, Nakashima T, Nitta T, Hori S, Iwakura Y, et al. IL-17-producing γδ T cells enhance bone regeneration. Nat Commun. 2016;7:10928. https://doi.org/10.1038/ncomms10928.
97. van Tok MN, van Duivenvoorde LM, Kramer I, Ingold P, Pfister S, Roth L, et al. Interleukin-17A inhibition diminishes inflammation and new bone formation in experimental spondyloarthritis. Arthritis Rheum. 2019;71(4):612–25. https://doi.org/10.1002/art.40770.
98. Kotake S, Udagawa N, Takahashi N, Matsuzaki K, Itoh K, Ishiyama S, et al. IL-17 in synovial fluids from patients with rheumatoid arthritis is a potent stimulator of osteoclastogenesis. J Clin Invest. 1999;103(9):1345–52. https://doi.org/10.1172/jci5703.
99. Sato K, Suematsu A, Okamoto K, Yamaguchi A, Morishita Y, Kadono Y, et al. Th17 functions as an osteoclastogenic helper T cell subset that links T cell activation and bone destruction. J Exp Med. 2006;203(12):2673–82. https://doi.org/10.1084/jem.20061775.
100. Komatsu N, Okamoto K, Sawa S, Nakashima T, Oh-hora M, Kodama T, et al. Pathogenic conversion of Foxp3+ T cells into TH17 cells in autoimmune arthritis. Nat Med. 2014;20(1):62–8. https://doi.org/10.1038/nm.3432.
101. Van Bezooijen RL, Farih-Sips HC, Papapoulos SE, Löwik CW. Interleukin-17: A new bone acting cytokine in vitro. J Bone Mineral Res: The Official Journal of the American Society for Bone and Mineral Research. 1999;14(9):1513–21. https://doi.org/10.1359/jbmr.1999.14.9.1513.
102. Ke D, Fu X, Xue Y, Wu H, Zhang Y, Chen X, et al. IL-17A regulates the autophagic activity of osteoclast precursors through RANKL-JNK1 signaling during osteoclastogenesis in vitro. Biochem Biophys Res Commun. 2018;497(3):890–6. https://doi.org/10.1016/j.bbrc.2018.02.164.
103. Wang Z, Jia Y, Du F, Chen M, Dong X, Chen Y, et al. IL-17A inhibits osteogenic differentiation of bone mesenchymal stem cells via wnt signaling pathway. Med Sci Monitor: International Medical Journal of Experimental and Clinical Research. 2017;23:4095–101. https://doi.org/10.12659/msm.903027.
104. Mease P, van der Heijde D, Landewé R, Mpofu S, Rahman P, Tahir H, et al. Secukinumab improves active psoriatic arthritis symptoms and inhibits radiographic progression: primary results from the randomised, double-blind, phase III FUTURE 5 study. Ann Rheum Dis. 2018;77(6):890–7. https://doi.org/10.1136/annrheumdis-2017-212687.
105. Mease PJ, McInnes IB, Kirkham B, Kavanaugh A, Rahman P, van der Heijde D, et al. Secukinumab inhibition of interleukin-17A in patients with psoriatic arthritis. N Engl J Med. 2015;373(14):1329–39. https://doi.org/10.1056/NEJMoa1412679.
106. McInnes IB, Mease PJ, Kirkham B, Kavanaugh A, Ritchlin CT, Rahman P, et al. Secukinumab, a human anti-interleukin-17A monoclonal antibody, in patients with psoriatic

arthritis (FUTURE 2): a randomised, double-blind, placebo-controlled, phase 3 trial. Lancet. 2015;386(9999):1137–46. https://doi.org/10.1016/S0140-6736(15)61134-5.

107. Baeten D, Sieper J, Braun J, Baraliakos X, Dougados M, Emery P, et al. Secukinumab, an Interleukin-17A Inhibitor, in Ankylosing Spondylitis. N Engl J Med. 2015;373(26):2534–48. https://doi.org/10.1056/NEJMoa1505066.
108. Jeon C, Sekhon S, Yan D, Afifi L, Nakamura M, Bhutani T. Monoclonal antibodies inhibiting IL-12, -23, and -17 for the treatment of psoriasis. Hum Vaccin Immunother. 2017;13(10):2247–59. https://doi.org/10.1080/21645515.2017.1356498.
109. Baeten D, Baraliakos X, Braun J, Sieper J, Emery P, van der Heijde D, et al. Anti-interleukin-17A monoclonal antibody secukinumab in treatment of ankylosing spondylitis: a randomised, double-blind, placebo-controlled trial. Lancet (London, England). 2013;382(9906):1705–13. https://doi.org/10.1016/s0140-6736(13)61134-4.
110. Marzo-Ortega H, Sieper J, Kivitz A, Blanco R, Cohen M, Delicha EM, et al. Secukinumab provides sustained improvements in the signs and symptoms of active ankylosing spondylitis with high retention rate: 3-year results from the phase III trial, MEASURE 2. RMD open. 2017;3(2):e000592. https://doi.org/10.1136/rmdopen-2017-000592.
111. Mease PJ, van der Heijde D, Ritchlin CT, Okada M, Cuchacovich RS, Shuler CL, et al. Ixekizumab, an interleukin-17A specific monoclonal antibody, for the treatment of biologic-naive patients with active psoriatic arthritis: results from the 24-week randomised, double-blind, placebo-controlled and active (adalimumab)-controlled period of the phase III trial SPIRIT-P1. Ann Rheum Dis. 2017;76(1):79–87. https://doi.org/10.1136/annrheumdis-2016-209709.
112. van der Heijde D, Cheng-Chung Wei J, Dougados M, Mease P, Deodhar A, Maksymowych WP, et al. Ixekizumab, an interleukin-17A antagonist in the treatment of ankylosing spondylitis or radiographic axial spondyloarthritis in patients previously untreated with biological disease-modifying anti-rheumatic drugs (COAST-V): 16 week results of a phase 3 randomised, double-blind, active-controlled and placebo-controlled trial. Lancet. 2018;392(10163):2441–51. https://doi.org/10.1016/s0140-6736(18)31946-9.
113. Deodhar A, Poddubnyy D, Pacheco-Tena C, Salvarani C, Lespessailles E, Rahman P, et al. Efficacy and safety of ixekizumab in the treatment of radiographic axial spondyloarthritis: sixteen-week results from a phase III randomized, double-blind, placebo-controlled trial in patients with prior inadequate response to or intolerance of tumor necrosis factor inhibitors. Arthritis Rheum. 2019;71(4):599–611. https://doi.org/10.1002/art.40753.
114. Correction: Efficacy and safety of ixekizumab through 52 weeks in two phase 3, randomised, controlled clinical trials in patients with active radiographic axial spondyloarthritis (COAST-V and COAST-W). Ann Rheum Dis. 2020;79(6):e75. https://doi.org/10.1136/annrheumdis-2019-216118corr1.
115. Deodhar A, van der Heijde D, Gensler LS, Kim T-H, Maksymowych WP, Østergaard M, et al. Ixekizumab for patients with non-radiographic axial spondyloarthritis (COAST-X): a randomised, placebo-controlled trial. Lancet. 2020;395(10217):53–64. https://doi.org/10.1016/S0140-6736(19)32971-X.
116. Yin Y, Wang M, Liu M, Zhou E, Ren T, Chang X, et al. Efficacy and safety of IL-17 inhibitors for the treatment of ankylosing spondylitis: a systematic review and meta-analysis. Arthritis Res Ther. 2020;22(1):111. https://doi.org/10.1186/s13075-020-02208-w.
117. Wei JC-C, Kim T-H, Kishimoto M, Morishige T, Ogusu N, Kobayashi S. OP0234 efficacy and safety of brodalumab, an anti-interleukin-17 receptor a monoclonal antibody, in patients with axial spondyloarthritis: a 16 week results of a phase 3, multicenter, randomized, double-blind, placebo-controlled study. Ann Rheum Dis. 2019;78(Suppl 2):195. https://doi.org/10.1136/annrheumdis-2019-eular.6888.
118. Larsen M, Arnaud L, Hié M, Parizot C, Dorgham K, Shoukry M, et al. Multiparameter grouping delineates heterogeneous populations of human IL-17 and/or IL-22 T-cell producers that share antigen specificities with other T-cell subsets. Eur J Immunol. 2011;41(9):2596–605. https://doi.org/10.1002/eji.201041131.

119. Trifari S, Kaplan CD, Tran EH, Crellin NK, Spits H. Identification of a human helper T cell population that has abundant production of interleukin 22 and is distinct from T(H)-17, T(H)1 and T(H)2 cells. Nat Immunol. 2009;10(8):864–71. https://doi.org/10.1038/ni.1770.
120. Jia L, Wu C. The biology and functions of Th22 cells. Adv Exp Med Biol. 2014;841:209–30. https://doi.org/10.1007/978-94-017-9487-9_8.
121. Gholamreza A, Anita S, Nadia MMER, Abbas M. Th22 cells contribution in immunopathogenesis of rheumatic diseases. Iranian J Allergy, Asthma Immunol. 2015;14(3):246–54.
122. Baba N, Rubio M, Kenins L, Regairaz C, Woisetschlager M, Carballido JM, et al. The aryl hydrocarbon receptor (AhR) ligand VAF347 selectively acts on monocytes and naïve CD4(+) Th cells to promote the development of IL-22-secreting Th cells. Hum Immunol. 2012;73(8):795–800. https://doi.org/10.1016/j.humimm.2012.05.002.
123. Jones BC, Logsdon NJ, Walter MR. Structure of IL-22 bound to its high-affinity IL-22R1 chain. Structure. 2008;16(9):1333–44. https://doi.org/10.1016/j.str.2008.06.005.
124. Dudakov JA, Hanash AM, van den Brink MRM. Interleukin-22: immunobiology and pathology. Annu Rev Immunol. 2015;33:747–85. https://doi.org/10.1146/annurev-immunol-032414-112123.
125. El-Zayadi AA, Jones EA, Churchman SM, Baboolal TG, Cuthbert RJ, El-Jawhari JJ, et al. Interleukin-22 drives the proliferation, migration and osteogenic differentiation of mesenchymal stem cells: a novel cytokine that could contribute to new bone formation in spondyloarthropathies. Rheumatology. 2017;56(3):488–93. https://doi.org/10.1093/rheumatology/kew384.
126. Ciccia F, Accardo-Palumbo A, Alessandro R, Rizzo A, Principe S, Peralta S, et al. Interleukin-22 and interleukin-22-producing NKp44+ natural killer cells in subclinical gut inflammation in ankylosing spondylitis. Arthritis Rheum. 2012;64(6):1869–78. https://doi.org/10.1002/art.34355.
127. Vignali DAA, Collison LW, Workman CJ. How regulatory T cells work. Nat Rev Immunol. 2008;8(7):523–32. https://doi.org/10.1038/nri2343.
128. Haque M, Fino K, Lei F, Xiong X, Song J. Utilizing regulatory T cells against rheumatoid arthritis. Front Oncol. 2014;4:209. https://doi.org/10.3389/fonc.2014.00209.
129. Lu L, Barbi J, Pan F. The regulation of immune tolerance by FOXP3. Nat Rev Immunol. 2017;17(11):703–17. https://doi.org/10.1038/nri.2017.75.
130. Liu W, Putnam AL, Xu-Yu Z, Szot GL, Lee MR, Zhu S, et al. CD127 expression inversely correlates with FoxP3 and suppressive function of human CD4+ T reg cells. J Exp Med. 2006;203(7):1701–11. https://doi.org/10.1084/jem.20060772.
131. Sakaguchi S. Naturally arising Foxp3-expressing CD25+CD4+ regulatory T cells in immunological tolerance to self and non-self. Nat Immunol. 2005;6(4):345–52. https://doi.org/10.1038/ni1178.
132. Sakaguchi S, Sakaguchi N, Asano M, Itoh M, Toda M. Immunologic self-tolerance maintained by activated T cells expressing IL-2 receptor alpha-chains (CD25). Breakdown of a single mechanism of self-tolerance causes various autoimmune diseases. J Immunol. 1995;155(3):1151–64.
133. Wehrens EJ, van Wijk F, Roord ST, Albani S, Prakken BJ. Treating arthritis by immunomodulation: is there a role for regulatory T cells? Rheumatology. 2010;49(9):1632–44. https://doi.org/10.1093/rheumatology/keq130.
134. Jonuleit H, Schmitt E. The regulatory T cell family: distinct subsets and their interrelations. J Immunol. 2003;171(12):6323–7. https://doi.org/10.4049/jimmunol.171.12.6323.
135. Zhang H, Kong H, Zeng X, Guo L, Sun X, He S. Subsets of regulatory T cells and their roles in allergy. J Transl Med. 2014;12:125. https://doi.org/10.1186/1479-5876-12-125.
136. Wing K, Sakaguchi S. Regulatory T cells exert checks and balances on self tolerance and autoimmunity. Nat Immunol. 2010;11(1):7–13. https://doi.org/10.1038/ni.1818.
137. Miao J, Zhu P. Functional defects of treg cells: new targets in rheumatic diseases, including ankylosing spondylitis. Curr Rheumatol Rep. 2018;20(5):30. https://doi.org/10.1007/s11926-018-0729-1.

138. Ye L, Goodall JC, Zhang L, Putintseva EV, Lam B, Jiang L, et al. TCR usage, gene expression and function of two distinct FOXP3+Treg subsets within CD4+CD25hi T cells identified by expression of CD39 and CD45RO. Immunol Cell Biol. 2016;94(3):293–305. https://doi.org/10.1038/icb.2015.90.
139. Ciccia F, Accardo-Palumbo A, Giardina A, Di Maggio P, Principato A, Bombardieri M, et al. Expansion of intestinal CD4+CD25(high) Treg cells in patients with ankylosing spondylitis: a putative role for interleukin-10 in preventing intestinal Th17 response. Arthritis Rheum. 2010;62(12):3625–34. https://doi.org/10.1002/art.27699.
140. Liao HT, Lin YF, Tsai CY, Chou CT. Regulatory T cells in ankylosing spondylitis and the response after adalimumab treatment. Joint, Bone, Spine: revue du rhumatisme. 2015;82(6):423–7. https://doi.org/10.1016/j.jbspin.2015.03.003.
141. Wang M, Liu C, Bond A, Yang J, Zhou X, Wang J, et al. Dysfunction of regulatory T cells in patients with ankylosing spondylitis is associated with a loss of Tim-3. Int Immunopharmacol. 2018;59:53–60. https://doi.org/10.1016/j.intimp.2018.03.032.
142. Guo H, Zheng M, Zhang K, Yang F, Zhang X, Han Q, et al. Functional defects in CD4+ CD25high FoxP3+ regulatory cells in ankylosing spondylitis. Sci Rep. 2016;6(1):37559. https://doi.org/10.1038/srep37559.
143. Zhao SS, Hu JW, Wang J, Lou XJ, Zhou LL. Inverse correlation between CD4+ CD25high CD127low/- regulatory T-cells and serum immunoglobulin A in patients with new-onset ankylosing spondylitis. J Int Med Res. 2011;39(5):1968–74. https://doi.org/10.1177/147323001103900543.
144. Lai NL, Zhang SX, Wang J, Zhang JQ, Wang CH, Gao C, et al. The proportion of regulatory T cells in patients with ankylosing spondylitis: a meta-analysis. J Immunol Res. 2019;2019:1058738. https://doi.org/10.1155/2019/1058738.
145. Fiocco U, Martini V, Accordi B, Caso F, Costa L, Oliviero F, et al. Transcriptional network profile on synovial fluid T cells in psoriatic arthritis. Clin Rheumatol. 2015;34(9):1571–80. https://doi.org/10.1007/s10067-015-3002-2.
146. Christoforou T, Prelog M, Almanzar G, Feuchtenberger M, Schmalzing M, Tony H-P et al. Proportions of regulatory T cells (Treg) and suppressive Treg function in patients with psoriasis arthritis (PsA) or spondyloarthritis (SpA) after switching to anti-IL-17 treatment. 2020.
147. Mittrücker HW, Visekruna A, Huber M. Heterogeneity in the differentiation and function of $CD8^{+}$ T cells. Arch Immunol Ther Exp. 2014;62(6):449–58. https://doi.org/10.1007/s00005-014-0293-y.
148. Narjes S, Ali AA, Mahdi M, Ali AP, Esfandiar A, Ahmad RJ, Nima R, Mohammad TT, Katayoon B, Behrouz N, Mohammad HN. Study of Programmed Cell Death 1 (PDCD1) Gene Polymorphims in Iranian Patients with Ankylosing Spondylitis. Inflammation. 2011;34(6):707–12.
149. Yang M, Lv Q, Wei Q, Jiang Y, Qi J, Xiao M, et al. TNF-α inhibitor therapy can improve the immune imbalance of CD4+ T cells and negative regulatory cells but not CD8+ T cells in ankylosing spondylitis. Arthritis Res ther. 2020;22(1):149. https://doi.org/10.1186/s13075-020-02226-8.
150. Gracey E, Yao Y, Qaiyum Z, Lim M, Tang M, Inman RD. Altered cytotoxicity profile of CD8+ T cells in ankylosing spondylitis. Arthritis Rheum. 2020;72(3):428–34. https://doi.org/10.1002/art.41129.
151. Schirmer M, Goldberger C, Würzner R, Duftner C, Pfeiffer K-P, Clausen J, et al. Circulating cytotoxic CD8(+) CD28(-) T cells in ankylosing spondylitis. Arthritis Res. 2002;4(1):71–6. https://doi.org/10.1186/ar386.
152. Zhang L, Jarvis LB, Baek HJ, Gaston JS. Regulatory IL4+CD8+ T cells in patients with ankylosing spondylitis and healthy controls. Ann Rheum Dis. 2009;68(8):1345–51. https://doi.org/10.1136/ard.2008.088120.
153. Jarvis LB, Matyszak MK, Duggleby RC, Goodall JC, Hall FC, Gaston JS. Autoreactive human peripheral blood CD8+ T cells with a regulatory phenotype and function. Eur J Immunol. 2005;35(10):2896–908. https://doi.org/10.1002/eji.200526162.

154. Colombo E, Galleri G, Erre GL, Piras C, Biondi G, Taras L, et al. Peripheral blood CD8+ T-cell profiles in patients with psoriatic arthritis: a cross-sectional case-control study. Eur Rev Med Pharmacol Sci. 2017;21(22):5166–71. https://doi.org/10.26355/eurrev_201711_13834.
155. Diani M, Casciano F, Marongiu L, Longhi M, Altomare A, Pigatto PD, et al. Increased frequency of activated CD8+ T cell effectors in patients with psoriatic arthritis. Sci Rep. 2019;9(1):10870. https://doi.org/10.1038/s41598-019-47310-5.
156. Beacock-Sharp H, Young JL, Gaston JS. Analysis of T cell subsets present in the peripheral blood and synovial fluid of reactive arthritis patients. Ann Rheum Dis. 1998;57(2):100–6. https://doi.org/10.1136/ard.57.2.100.
157. Reinhardt A, Prinz I. Whodunit? The contribution of interleukin (IL)-17/IL-22-producing γδ T cells, αβ T cells, and innate lymphoid cells to the pathogenesis of spondyloarthritis. Front Immunol. 2018;9:885. https://doi.org/10.3389/fimmu.2018.00885.
158. Sutton CE, Mielke LA, Mills KHG. IL-17-producing γδ T cells and innate lymphoid cells. Eur J Immunol. 2012;42(9):2221–31. https://doi.org/10.1002/eji.201242569.
159. Prinz I, Silva-Santos B, Pennington DJ. Functional development of γδ T cells. Eur J Immunol. 2013;43(8):1988–94. https://doi.org/10.1002/eji.201343759.
160. Papotto PH, Reinhardt A, Prinz I, Silva-Santos B. Innately versatile: γδ17 T cells in inflammatory and autoimmune diseases. J Autoimmun. 2018;87:26–37. https://doi.org/10.1016/j.jaut.2017.11.006.
161. Guggino G, Ciccia F, Di Liberto D, Lo Pizzo M, Ruscitti P, Cipriani P, et al. Interleukin (IL)-9/IL-9R axis drives γδ T cells activation in psoriatic arthritis patients. Clin Exp Immunol. 2016;186(3):277–83. https://doi.org/10.1111/cei.12853.
162. Cornelissen F, Mus AM, Asmawidjaja PS, van Hamburg JP, Tocker J, Lubberts E. Interleukin-23 is critical for full-blown expression of a non-autoimmune destructive arthritis and regulates interleukin-17A and RORgammat in gammadelta T cells. Arthritis Res Ther. 2009;11(6):R194. https://doi.org/10.1186/ar2893.
163. Avau A, Mitera T, Put S, Put K, Brisse E, Filtjens J, et al. Systemic juvenile idiopathic arthritis-like syndrome in mice following stimulation of the immune system with Freund's complete adjuvant: regulation by interferon-γ. Arthritis Rheum. 2014;66(5):1340–51. https://doi.org/10.1002/art.38359.
164. Meliconi R, Pitzalis C, Kingsley GH, Panayi GS. Gamma/delta T cells and their subpopulations in blood and synovial fluid from rheumatoid arthritis and spondyloarthritis. Clin Immunol Immunopathol. 1991;59(1):165–72. https://doi.org/10.1016/0090-1229(91)90090-w.
165. Kenna TJ, Davidson SI, Duan R, Bradbury LA, McFarlane J, Smith M, et al. Enrichment of circulating interleukin-17-secreting interleukin-23 receptor-positive γ/δ T cells in patients with active ankylosing spondylitis. Arthritis Rheum. 2012;64(5):1420–9. https://doi.org/10.1002/art.33507.
166. Chowdhury AC, Chaurasia S, Mishra SK, Aggarwal A, Misra R. IL-17 and IFN-γ producing NK and γδ-T cells are preferentially expanded in synovial fluid of patients with reactive arthritis and undifferentiated spondyloarthritis. Clin Immunol. 2017;183:207–12. https://doi.org/10.1016/j.clim.2017.03.016.
167. SpAdaro A, Scrivo R, Moretti T, Bernardini G, Riccieri V, Taccari E, et al. Natural killer cells and gamma/delta T cells in synovial fluid and in peripheral blood of patients with psoriatic arthritis. Clin Exp Rheumatol. 2004;22(4):389–94.
168. Cuvelier CA, De Wever N, Mielants H, De Vos M, Veys EM, Roels H. Expression of T cell receptors alpha beta and gamma delta in the ileal mucosa of patients with Crohn's disease and with spondylarthropathy. Clin Exp Immunol. 1992;90(2):275–9. https://doi.org/10.1111/j.1365-2249.1992.tb07942.x.
169. Yoshizaki A, Sato S. Abnormal B lymphocyte activation and function in systemic sclerosis. Ann Dermatol. 2015;27(1):1–9. https://doi.org/10.5021/ad.2015.27.1.1.
170. Liu Y, Liao X, Shi G. Autoantibodies in Spondyloarthritis, focusing on Anti-CD74 antibodies. Front Immunol. 2019;10:5. https://doi.org/10.3389/fimmu.2019.00005.

171. Hickling P, Turnbull L, Dixon JS. The relationship between disease activity, immunoglobulins and lymphocyte sub-populations in ankylosing spondylitis. Rheumatology. 1982;21(3):145–50. https://doi.org/10.1093/rheumatology/21.3.145.
172. Eghtedari AA, Davis P, Bacon PA. Immunological reactivity in ankylosing spondylitis. Circulating immunoblasts, autoantibodies, and immunoglobulins. Ann Rheum Dis. 1976;35(2):155–7. https://doi.org/10.1136/ard.35.2.155.
173. Howell FA, Chamberlain MA, Perry RA, Torrigiani G, Roitt IM. IgG antiglobulin levels in patients with psoriatic arthropathy, ankylosing spondylitis, and gout. Ann Rheum Dis. 1972;31(2):129–31. https://doi.org/10.1136/ard.31.2.129.
174. Wendling D, Didier JM, Seilles E. Serum secretory immunoglobulins in ankylosing spondylitis. Clin Rheumatol. 1996;15(6):590–3. https://doi.org/10.1007/bf02238549.
175. Niu XY, Zhang HY, Liu YJ, Zhao D, Shan YX, Jiang YF. Peripheral B-cell activation and exhaustion markers in patients with ankylosing spondylitis. Life Sci. 2013;93(18-19):687–92. https://doi.org/10.1016/j.lfs.2013.09.003.
176. Lin Q, Gu JR, Li TW, Zhang FC, Lin ZM, Liao ZT, et al. Value of the peripheral blood B-cells subsets in patients with ankylosing spondylitis. Chin Med J. 2009;122(15):1784–9.
177. Lu J, Ding Y, Yi X, Zheng J. CD19+ B cell subsets in the peripheral blood and skin lesions of psoriasis patients and their correlations with disease severity. Braz J Med Biol Res= Revista brasileira de pesquisas medicas e biologicas. 2016;49(9):e5374. https://doi.org/10.1590/1414-431x20165374.
178. Curry R, Thoen J, Shelborne C, Gaudernack G, Messner R. Antibodies to and elevations of beta 2 microglobulin in the serum of ankylosing spondylitis patients. Arthritis Rheum. 1982;25(4):375–80. https://doi.org/10.1002/art.1780250403.
179. Bodnár N, Szekanecz Z, Prohászka Z, Kemény-Beke A, Némethné-Gyurcsik Z, Gulyás K, et al. Anti-mutated citrullinated vimentin (anti-MCV) and anti-65 kDa heat shock protein (anti-hsp65): new biomarkers in ankylosing spondylitis. Joint Bone, Spine: revue du rhumatisme. 2012;79(1):63–6. https://doi.org/10.1016/j.jbspin.2011.03.010.
180. Vasey FB, Kinsella TD. Increased frequency of leukocyte-reactive antinuclear antibody in patients with ankylosing spondylitis. J Rheumatol. 1977;4(2):158–64.
181. Juanola X, Mateo L, Domenech P, Bas J, Contreras N, Nolla JM, et al. Prevalence of antiphospholipid antibodies in patients with ankylosing spondylitis. J Rheumatol. 1995;22(10):1891–3.
182. Maksymowych WP, Boire G, van Schaardenburg D, Wichuk S, Turk S, Boers M, et al. 14-3-3η Autoantibodies: Diagnostic Use in Early Rheumatoid Arthritis. J Rheumatol. 2015;42(9):1587–94. https://doi.org/10.3899/jrheum.141385.
183. Kim YG, Sohn DH, Zhao X, Sokolove J, Lindstrom TM, Yoo B, et al. Role of protein phosphatase magnesium-dependent 1A and anti-protein phosphatase magnesium-dependent 1A autoantibodies in ankylosing spondylitis. Arthritis Rheum. 2014;66(10):2793–803. https://doi.org/10.1002/art.38763.
184. Locht H, Skogh T, Kihlström E. Anti-lactoferrin antibodies and other types of anti-neutrophil cytoplasmic antibodies (ANCA) in reactive arthritis and ankylosing spondylitis. Clin Exp Immunol. 1999;117(3):568–73. https://doi.org/10.1046/j.1365-2249.1999.01008.x.
185. Luchetti MM, Ciccia F, Avellini C, Benfaremo D, Guggino G, Farinelli A, et al. Sclerostin and Antisclerostin Antibody Serum Levels Predict the Presence of Axial Spondyloarthritis in Patients with Inflammatory Bowel Disease. J Rheumatol. 2018;45(5):630–7. https://doi.org/10.3899/jrheum.170833.
186. Tani Y, Sato H, Tanaka N, Hukuda S. Antibodies against bacterial lipopolysaccharides in Japanese patients with ankylosing spondylitis. Br J Rheumatol. 1997;36(4):491–3. https://doi.org/10.1093/rheumatology/36.4.491.
187. Andretta MA, Vieira TD, Nishiara R, Skare TL. Anti-Saccharomyces cerevisiae (ASCA) and anti-endomysial antibodies in spondyloarthritis. Rheumatol Int. 2012;32(2):551–4. https://doi.org/10.1007/s00296-010-1722-9.
188. Wallis D, Asaduzzaman A, Weisman M, Haroon N, Anton A, McGovern D, et al. Elevated serum anti-flagellin antibodies implicate subclinical bowel inflammation in ankylosing

spondylitis: an observational study. Arthritis Res Ther. 2013;15(5):R166. https://doi.org/10.1186/ar4350.

189. Riechers E, Baerlecken N, Baraliakos X, Achilles-Mehr Bakhsh K, Aries P, Bannert B, et al. Sensitivity and Specificity of Autoantibodies Against CD74 in Nonradiographic Axial Spondyloarthritis. Arthritis Rheum. 2019;71(5):729–35. https://doi.org/10.1002/art.40777.
190. Quaden DHF, De Winter LM, Somers V. Detection of novel diagnostic antibodies in ankylosing spondylitis: An overview. Autoimmun Rev. 2016;15(8):820–32. https://doi.org/10.1016/j.autrev.2016.06.001.
191. Curry R, Thoen J, Shelborne C, Gaudernack G, Messner R. Antibodies to and elevations of beta 2 microglobulin in the serum of ankylosing spondylitis patients. Arthritis Rheum. 1982;25(4):375–80. https://doi.org/10.1002/art.1780250403.
192. Damjanovska L, Thabet MM, Levarth EW, Stoeken-Rijsbergen G, van der Voort EI, Toes RE, et al. Diagnostic value of anti-MCV antibodies in differentiating early inflammatory arthritis. Ann Rheum Dis. 2010;69(4):730–2. https://doi.org/10.1136/ard.2009.108456.
193. McLean IL, Archer JR, Cawley MI, Pegley FS, Kidd BL, Thompson PW. Specific antibody response to the mycobacterial 65 kDa stress protein in ankylosing spondylitis and rheumatoid arthritis. Br J Rheumatol. 1990;29(6):426–9. https://doi.org/10.1093/rheumatology/29.6.426.
194. Maksymowych WP, Naides SJ, Bykerk V, Siminovitch KA, van Schaardenburg D, Boers M, et al. Serum 14-3-3η is a novel marker that complements current serological measurements to enhance detection of patients with rheumatoid arthritis. J Rheumatol. 2014;41(11):2104–13. https://doi.org/10.3899/jrheum.131446.
195. Kalyoncu U, Karadag O, Kilic L, Ertenli I, Bilgen SA, Akdogan A, et al. THU0104 risk factors of advanced spinal disease and/or bamboo disease in patients with ankylosing sponylitis during TNFI treatments: HÜR-BİO REAL life results. Ann Rheum Dis. 2014;73(Suppl 2):213. https://doi.org/10.1136/annrheumdis-2014-eular.4041.
196. Appel H, Ruiz-Heiland G, Listing J, Zwerina J, Herrmann M, Mueller R, et al. Altered skeletal expression of sclerostin and its link to radiographic progression in ankylosing spondylitis. Arthritis Rheum. 2009;60(11):3257–62. https://doi.org/10.1002/art.24888.
197. Tsui FW, Tsui HW, Las Heras F, Pritzker KP, Inman RD. Serum levels of novel noggin and sclerostin-immune complexes are elevated in ankylosing spondylitis. Ann Rheum Dis. 2014;73(10):1873–9. https://doi.org/10.1136/annrheumdis-2013-203630.
198. Lotteau V, Teyton L, Peleraux A, Nilsson T, Karlsson L, Schmid SL, et al. Intracellular transport of class II MHC molecules directed by invariant chain. Nature. 1990;348(6302):600–5. https://doi.org/10.1038/348600a0.
199. Matza D, Wolstein O, Dikstein R, Shachar I. Invariant chain induces B cell maturation by activating a TAF(II)105-NF-kappaB-dependent transcription program. J Biol Chem. 2001;276(29):27203–6. https://doi.org/10.1074/jbc.M104684200.
200. Baerlecken NT, Nothdorft S, Stummvoll GH, Sieper J, Rudwaleit M, Reuter S, et al. Autoantibodies against CD74 in spondyloarthritis. Ann Rheum Dis. 2014;73(6):1211–4. https://doi.org/10.1136/annrheumdis-2012-202208.
201. Baraliakos X, Baerlecken N, Witte T, Heldmann F, Braun J. High prevalence of anti-CD74 antibodies specific for the HLA class II-associated invariant chain peptide (CLIP) in patients with axial spondyloarthritis. Ann Rheum Dis. 2014;73(6):1079–82. https://doi.org/10.1136/annrheumdis-2012-202177.

Part III

Genes

4 Association of HLA and HLA-Related Genes with Ankylosing Spondylitis

Mazdak Ganjalikhani Hakemi

4.1 Biology of HLA Expression and Functions

In contrary to B cells, T lymphocytes have to recognize their specific antigens in the context of MHC molecules. MHC genes are the most polymorphic ones among the others. In humans, MHC is called Human Leukocyte Antigen (HLA) and is inherited as a co-dominant trait across the generations. As HLA alleles are inherited as haplotypes, therefore, each person has one maternal and one paternal HLA haplotype in his/her genome.

4.1.1 Genomic Organization

HLA alleles which are located on the short arm of chromosome 6, occupied a place approaches 3500 base pair length. There are two different classes of HLA named HLA-class I and HLA-class II. Class I HLA is responsible for presenting cytosolic (endogenous) peptides to CD8+ T cells and HLA-class II is dedicated to present endocytosed (exogenous) antigens to CD4+ T cells. Class I is located on the telomeric end of the chromosome and, from this end, consists of HLA-A, -C, and -B loci, respectively. Inside this area, there are some other genes that encode non-classical HLA class I or MHC class IB molecules, like HLA-G, -E, and -HEF, as well as MICA and MICB. These are structurally related to HLA-class I molecules but are not so polymorph and do not present antigenic peptides. On the centromeric site, HLA-class II area is located where the loci of HLA-DP, -DQ, and -DR are placed in order from the centromeric end. Throughout the HLA class II area, there

M. Ganjalikhani Hakemi (✉)
Department of Immunology, Faculty of Medicine, Isfahan University of Medical Sciences, Isfahan, Iran
e-mail: mghakemi@med.mui.ac.ir

M. H. Nicknam (ed.), *Ankylosing Spondylitis - Axial Spondyloarthritis*,
https://doi.org/10.1007/978-981-16-4733-8_4

are genes that encode necessary molecules in the process of antigen presentation by HLA-class I, such as Transporter in Antigen-Presenting (TAP) 1, TAP2, and Tapasin (Fig. 4.1).

4.1.1.1 HLA Nomenclature

The accepted nomination of HLA genes and their encoded proteins is based on similarities among their sequences and their molecular structure. As is depicted in Fig. 4.1, only one allele is present per each HLA-class I locus while for class II, every single locus consists of at least two different alleles. These alleles encode different HLA chains. For this, there are some differences in the way of HLA class I and II nomination.

Each locus for HLA-class I is named by a letter in capital format, like HLA-B while for class two, there are two capital letters indicating a locus, such as DR. To determine an allele (allelic group) for HLA class I, a number is added after the letter, like HLA-B27. For the nomination of an allele of HLA-class II, one letter and one number are added after the two-letter code for locus. This latte letter defines the type of HLA-class II chain. For example, HLA-DRB1 stands for the chain β1 from HLA-DR locus. In order to define a specific allelic subtype, after the capital letter determining an HLA-class I locus, an asterisk and a four-digit number are written. For example, HLA-B*2705 means that this is the fifth subtype of allele B27 from HLA-class I locus. Defining an HLA-class II allelic subtype is similar to what is used for class one. After the three letters and one number, an asterisk and a

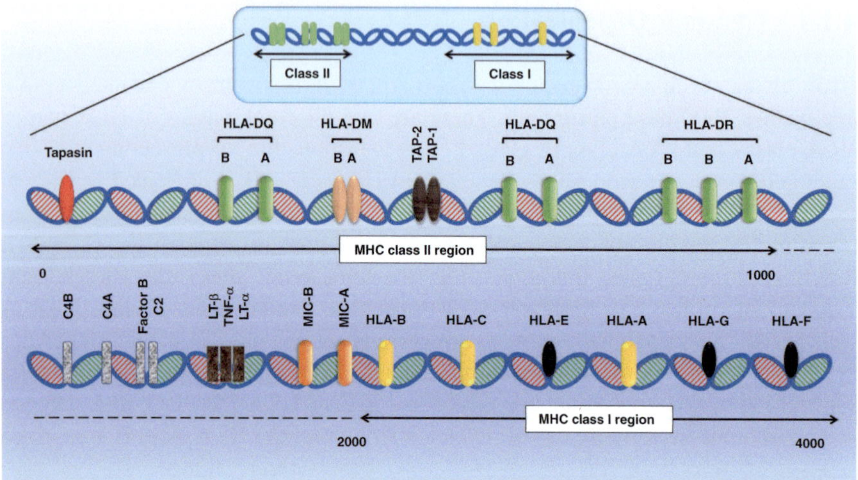

Fig. 4.1 Organization of HLA genes on chromosome 6p. Class I HLA loci are located on the telomeric side of the chromosome while on the centromeric side is the area for HLA class-II. Distributed among HLA class-I, there are several non-classical HLA-I genes (HLA class-Ib). On the other hand, genes encoding for effector molecules in antigen presentation are found in HLA class-II area. The area between class-I and class-II loci is the region of the genes encoding some cytokines, hormones, and complement proteins

four-digit number are written. In this way, HLA-DRB1*1502 indicates for the second subtype of the allele 15 from the chain β1 in the HLA-DR locus.

4.1.2 Molecular Structure

MHC molecules are heterodimeric transmembrane proteins with a peptide-binding cleft that encompass polymorphic residues. As different HLAs bind to and present different peptides, the kind of immune response against the same antigen in distinct individuals is different. HLA molecules also have a non-polymorph region for binding to T cells co-receptors.

4.1.2.1 Molecular Structure of HLA-Class I

MHC-I molecules are expressed on all nucleated cells except sperm and trophoblast. Class I HLA consists of two different chains named α and β2-microglobulin (β2m). The light chain, β2m, is encoded in chromosome 15 which is out of the MHC locus. This chain has only one extracellular domain with no activity for antigen binding. Its role is to stabilize the structure of HLA-class I. In contrast, α chain is encoded inside the HLA locus and consists of three extracellular, transmembrane, and intra-cytoplasmic parts. The extracellular part includes three domains which numbered from N-terminal side as α1, α2, and α3, respectively. The peptide binding cleft (PBC) is formed between the α1 and α2 domains. Domain α3 is a non-polymorphic member of the Ig super-family which binds to the CD8 co-receptor of T lymphocytes (Fig. 4.2a).

4.1.2.2 Molecular Structure of HLA-Class II

This molecule has a limited distribution and is expressed only by B lymphocytes, macrophages, and dendritic cells (professional APCs) as well as thymic epithelial cells. MHC-II molecules consist of two nearly similar chains, α and β, that both of them are encoded in the HLA locus. Both chains have three intracellular, transmembrane, and extracellular areas. The extracellular part includes two domains which are numbered from the N-terminal end of the chains as α1 and α2 as well as β1 and β2. The peptide binding cleft is made of α1 and β1 domains where the most polymorphic residues are located, especially in β1. The CD4 binding site of HLA-class II is the invariant β2 domain (Fig. 4.2b).

4.1.3 Pathways of Antigen Presentation

MHC molecules bind to peptide antigens in order to present them to a relevant T cell receptor (TCR) on specific T cells. The role of discrimination between self and foreign peptides is played by TCR as MHC molecules do not have such ability. For binding to MHC, the peptide must have specific structural properties like a defined size. Peptides with 8–11 amino acid length and hydrophobic or basic residues in their C-terminal end bind to MHC-I while those with 10–30 amino acid residues

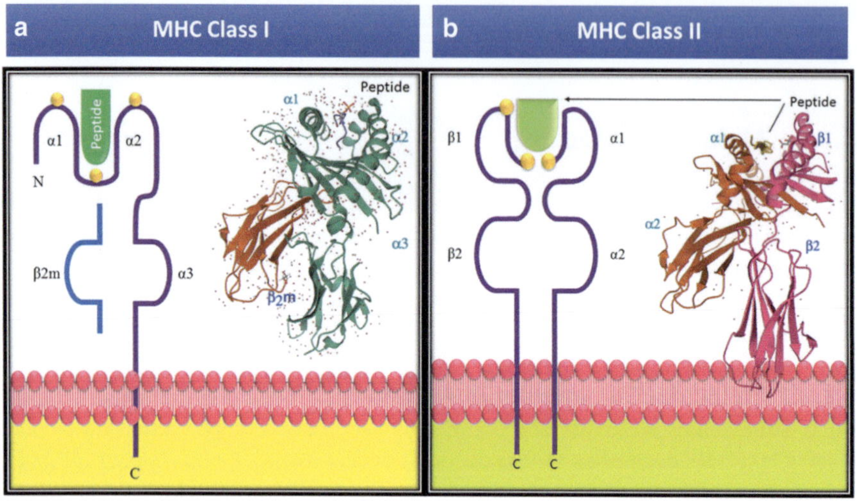

Fig. 4.2 Molecular structure of MHC. (**a**) Class-I MHC consists of one heavy chain named α and one light chain called β2-microglobulin (β2m). The α chain is comprised of three, extracellular, transmembrane, and intracellular, parts. The extracellular part consists of three domains which are numbered in order from the N-terminal end as α1, α2, and α3. The area between domains α1 and α2 is the peptide binding cleft. The α3 is the site of interaction with CD8 marker on T cells. (**b**) Class-II MHC is comprised of two almost similar chains named α and β. Both chains include extracellular, transmembrane, and intracellular, parts. The extracellular part of both chains is comprised of two domains which are numbered in order from N-terminal end as α1 and α2 for α chain, and β1 and β2 for β chain. The peptide binding cleft is formed by α1 and β1. The β2 domain is the site of interaction with CD4 marker on T cells

present with MHC-II. Some amino acid residues may have branched chains through them can be linked to the PBC packets via hydrophobic interactions. These branched-chain amino acids are named "anchor residues." However, the overall affinity of MHC molecules for their relevant peptide is low (kd = 10^{-6} M) and their connection is made by non-covalent forces.

The residues which are recognized by TCR are different from those linked to MHC. In fact, TCR recognizes both antigenic peptide and MHC molecules and hence, possesses two specificities while having just one capacity. Positively selected T cells have been instructed to recognize peptides presented by self MHC molecules. Simultaneously, the non-polymorphic domains of MHC molecules are identified by CD4 or CD8 co-receptors.

4.1.3.1 Processing and Presentation of Endocytosed Antigens

On one hand, when an exogenous protein is engulfed by an antigen-presenting cell (APC), enters the cell in a vesicle called a phagosome. This phagosome then fuses to lysosomes in cytosol and forms phagolysosome in which, acidic pH and proteolytic enzymes disintegrate the protein antigen. Through this process, so-called "antigen processing," different antigenic peptides are produced. On the other hand, synthesis of MHC-II chains is done in the endoplasmic reticulum (ER) linked ribosomes and newly formed chains enter the ER. In order to fold in the right way and assembling together, Calnexin, a chaperon, binds to them in ER. When the process of forming a two-chain MHC-II molecule is completed, an invariant protein called "Ii" binds to its PBC and prevents it from binding to endogenous peptides. After transferring to the Golgi complex, this three-peptide complex enters into secretary vesicles which then fuse to phagolysosomes containing the peptide antigens and forms the MHC-II compartment (MIIC). Here in MIIC, the "Ii" is proteolytically broken, and then, HLA-DM, a non-classical MHC class II, replaces its remnant with a specific peptide antigen. Finally, the vesicle goes out and the peptide: MHC-II complex emerges on the cell surface to be recognized by a specific CD4+ T cell.

4.1.3.2 Processing and Presentation of Cytosolic Antigens

Every single endogenous protein that enters the cytosol will be ubiquitinated after a while. In this way, they are marked to be trapped by a cylinder form organelle named "proteasome" where they are converted to small peptides via proteolytic degradation. These small peptides will then enter the ER through a heterodimer gate-operating protein called transporters in antigen presenting (TAP). Thereafter, longer peptides will be further cleaved by ER aminopeptidase (ERAP) 1 and ERAP2 to approach the length which is appropriate for antigen presentation. ERAP1/2 efficiently cleaves these newly entered peptides to oligopeptides with 8 or 9 residues in length, which is optimal for binding to HLA class I. Simultaneously, newly synthesized chains of MHC-I come into the ER, fold and join together by Calnexin, and link to Tapasin by Calreticulin. As Tapasin is also connected to TAP, brings the new MHC-I molecule into the vicinity of the TAP. Now, small peptides which come into ER are trapped by these MHC-I molecules. Then, these peptides: MHC-I complexes exit the ER and will be transported from the Golgi apparatus to the plasma membrane of the cell. Here, these complexes are ready to be recognized by specific CD8+ T cells.

4.2 Association of HLA loci with Ankylosing Spondylitis

4.2.1 HLA-B27

Ankylosing spondylitis (AS) is a chronic inflammatory rheumatic disease from the category of seronegative spondyloarthritis (SpA). AS is inherited as an intricate genetic trait in which 4–10 predisposing genes have been estimated [1, 2]. Genetic studies have prepared invaluable knowledge to our perception of AS etiology. Familial aggregation studies have clarified a substantial heritability of AS susceptibility as the occurrence risk of AS in monozygotic twins is 63% and in first-degree relatives is 8.2% in comparison with 0.1% in the general population. In addition, the risk of AS is appraised as 16 times higher in the HLA-B27 positive relatives in comparison with isolated HLA-B27 positive individuals in general population. Unlike most complex genetic diseases, a significant genetic predisposition has been established by the discovery of one of the strongest associations among HLA alleles and diseases between AS and HLA-B27 in 1973. The correlation between HLA-B27 and AS is one of the most significant associations between a disease and an HLA molecule, as though its contribution is approaching 50% of genetic susceptibility to AS [2–7]. Among the populations with a high frequency of HLA-B27, the prevalence of AS and other SpAs is raised up. For instance, in the Haida Native Americans, the HLA-B27 frequency in the population is 50%, and the frequency of AS is 6.1%, while in the Japanese, HLA-B27 frequency is less than 1%, and the AS prevalence is only 0.0065% [8]. Not only has the HLA-B27 been shown as a predisposing factor, a lot of studies have suggested that HLA-B27 positive patients with AS show more severe clinical and radiological manifestations than those who do not express HLA-B27. It means that HLA-B27 may affect many features of AS, such as the age of onset, sex, and family history. For example, several studies have shown a younger age of onset in HLA-B27 positive patients. Moreover, several studies have shown that the presence of HLA-B27 is associated with increased occurrence of uveitis, cardiac involvement, worse sacroiliitis, hip joint involvement, peripheral arthritis, and significantly more symptoms of involvement of spinal column such as increased dorsal kyphosis, and decreased cervical slope, in AS patients. In fact, HLA-B27 expressing AS patients have significantly extended disease duration and shows worse Bath Ankylosing Spondylitis Disease Activity Index (BASDAI), Bath Ankylosing Spondylitis Functional Index (BASFI), and Ankylosing Spondylitis Quality of Life (ASQoL) in comparison with HLA-B27 negative AS patients. Although AS is an intricated genetic disease and a proportion of HLA-B27 negative AS patients have been reported, B27 is still considered as the main factor in the development of AS [2, 3, 6].

About 80–98% of white patients with AS are HLA-B27 positive, while the prevalence of this gene is less than 8% in the general population. However, in different races and ethnic groups, the degree of this association is different. For example, only 50% of American blacks with AS are HLA-B27 positive and in Iran, HLA-B27 has been reported in 70% of AS patients [2, 5–7, 9, 10]. Differences in the distribution of HLA-B27 subtypes among distinct populations and ethnic groups might be the main reason for such a different amount of association with AS.

The genome-wide association studies and technological advances in high throughput genotyping of single nucleotide polymorphisms (SNPs) have enabled us to identify many risk alleles predisposing to AS. Based on what is reported by the Anthony Nolan Trust database (http://hla.alleles.org/alleles/class1.html) and IMGT (https://www.ebi.ac.uk/ipd/imgt/hla/) there are 187 distinct HLA-B27 subtypes (designated HLA-B*27:01 to-B*27:188; the subtype B27:22 has been withdrawn), making B27 one of the most polymorphic alleles among HLA-B alleles. The difference among these subtypes is the occurrence of one or more mutations, generally affecting the peptide-binding cleft which is the polymorphic part of the molecule [2, 4, 11].

The geographic and ethnic distribution of the HLA-B27 alleles is considerably different. The most prevalent subtype which is found in all populations around the world is B*27:05 and accounts for about 90–96% of HLA-B27 positive individuals in the Euro-Caucasian (Aryan) tribes (odds ratio = 62.41, CI = 95%) [5, 6, 12]. Although HLA-B*27:05 has been found to be associated with AS virtually in all populations studied, it does not appear to abdicate risk in West Africa and American blocks. The predominant subtype in these populations is B*27:03 which is less strongly associated with the disease than B*27:05 [6, 9, 11]. The relatively common subtypes including B*27:05, B*27:08 (Caucasians), B*27:02 (Mediterranean), B*27:07 and B*27:04 (Asians) are present in multiple populations have been associated with AS. In contrast to B*27:05 which is over-represented in circumpolar and sub artic regions of Eurasia, B*27:02 is the predominant subtype among the Middle East and the Jewish populations. This allele is the second most AS-associated subtype among European-descent subjects (odds ratio = 43.41, CI = 95%). Based on studies on Asian populations, it has been suggested that B*27:04 might be more strongly associated with AS than B*27:05 in areas where both alleles coexist, such as in Taiwan, China or India. The two alleles, B*27:06 and B*27:09, appear to be unassociated or perhaps weakly associated with the disease and have been reported to have a possible protective role in Thais and Sardinians, respectively [4, 5, 9, 11, 12]. However, reports of B*27:06 and B*27:09 presence in patients with AS are emerging [3, 6, 9]. These cases confirm that B*27:09 and B*27:06 have a weaker association with AS, and are not absolutely protective for the disease [11]. In Caucasians, the AS-related subtype B*27:01 is the less frequent allele of HLA-B27. In China and Singapore, only B*27:04, B*27:05, and B*27:06 have been found which is completely different from those in Caucasians [9]. An uncommon European allele that was first observed in Britain is B*27:08. Its association with AS in a large family from the Azores Islands of Portugal has been reported. In Brazilians and Western Indians, B*27:13 and B*27:14 have been found to be associated with AS, respectively. More recently, B*27:10, B*27:12, B*27:15, B*27:17, B*27:19, B*27:24, B*27:27, B*27:30 and B*27:49 have also been reported to be predisposing factors for AS. However, the epidemiologic evidence for their association has remained unreliable [4, 5, 11].

Apart from these pieces of information, the molecular basis for such an association has not yet been convincingly explained. Currently, there are three main hypotheses presented to explain the mechanism of the association between HLA-B27 alleles and AS:

- The arthritogenic peptide hypothesis: based on this theory, it is assumed that the presence of a similarity (molecular mimicry) between pathogens and self-derived peptides could lead to T cells cross-reactivity, resulting in AS.
- The HLA-B27 misfolding hypothesis: it is proposed that the accumulation of unusually folded HLA-B27 chains or β2m accumulation and deposition in the endoplasmic reticulum (ER) provoke intracellular signaling, ends up to a stress in ER and unfolded protein response (UPR).
- The HLA-B27 dimer hypothesis: the generation of HLA-B27 homodimers on the cell surface could lead to an unusual immune response. These dimers could be recognized by an activating type of a group of natural killer (NK) and CD4+ T cells receptors named killer immunoglobulin-like receptor (KIR) [2–4].

4.2.1.1 Arthritogenic Peptide Hypothesis

From the date that the association between HLA B27 and AS has firstly been described, great attempts have been done to elucidate the molecular biology of HLA-B27 molecules and their role in the presentation of antigenic peptides to T cells. When the molecular structure of HLA B27 was clarified, it was revealed that peptides composed of nine amino acids in length with a highly conserved binding motif, including the existence of an arginine at position 2 and another basic residue located at position 9 were typically presented by this molecule. However, the precise mechanism of the association between AS and HLA B27 remains obscure [13].

The "molecular mimicry" theory recommends that a microbial pathogen-derived cross-reactive peptide provokes T cells responses. Consequently, the T cells could respond to a "self-peptide" which is associated with HLA-B27, or to peptides directly derived from HLA-B27 per se. Based on this, a great deal of self and foreign antigen peptides has been interrogated and sequenced to find candidate peptides. However, no convincing evidence indicating that any of these peptides are self-peptides or cross-reactive has been found [3].

It appeared that few residues in the α1 and α2 domains of the very first HLA-B27 alleles, forming the peptide-binding cleft (PBC) of the molecule, are different from other HLA-B alleles. These include His-9, Glu-45, Cys-67, Lys-70, and Ala-71. Interestingly, all of these unique disease-specific residues are located around the B-pocket of the PBC, where the second anchor residue of the peptide antigen accommodates [4]. Following this observation, the "arthritogenic" peptide hypothesis on the role of HLA-B27 in AS predisposition emerged.

The "arthritogenic" peptide theory, proposed by Benjamin and Parham, suggests that the pathogenicity of HLA-B27 may be due to its unique capability to present a particular repertoire of peptides to pathogenic CD8+ T cells [4, 6]. As is argued in this hypothesis, the apparently unique peptide binding specificity of HLA-B27 could be, in large part, due to its unusual B pocket. This might be responsible for selecting self-peptides that are similar to pathogen-derived peptides that might induce an autoreactive T cell response [6]. In comparison with most of the alleles, it seems that the HLA-B27 heavy chain is unusually slow to fold. In order to correct the problem, a hybrid HLA-B27 molecule consists of an HLA-A2-like B pocket transplant (referred to as B27.A2B) is formed and causes the heavy chain of HLA-B27 (B27.A2B) to fold, bind β2m, and then, exit the ER faster than the "wild type" B27 allele, more similar to other A and B alleles. This hybrid class I molecule can select and present a unique set of antigenic peptides. The B27.A2B molecule does not present peptides that are naturally restricted to HLA-B27 unless they are modified at position 2 in a way that the side chain of amino acid could fit appropriately into an HLA-A2-like B pocket [6].

Nevertheless, there are several problems with this theory. The first one is the failure to recognize any peptide specially presented by disease-associated HLA-B27 subtypes. The second problem is that apparently CD8+ T cells are not necessary for disease development in the HLA-B27 transgenic rat model of spondyloarthropathies (SpA) [4].

4.2.1.2 HLA-B27 Misfolding Hypothesis

In recent years, a considerable body of researches has focused on uncommon features of HLA-B27, including a tendency to misfold in HLA-B27 heavy chain and stable BiP binding in the ER before its assembly with peptide and β2m and to make disulfide-linked homodimers after arriving at the cell surface [6]. As mentioned before, there are a few residues such as Glu-45, Cys-67, and Lys-70 which are virtually unique to HLA-B27 (www.anthonynolan.com/HIG/). Mutagenesis experiments have defined that Glu-45 and Cys-67 in B pocket are necessary for HLA-B27 misfolding. Thus, it could be assumed that misfolding is extremely uncommon in other HLA-B alleles if not unique to HLA-B27. Moreover, it has been shown that, HLA-B27 needs about 30-fold higher concentration of antigen peptide to attain the same half-maximal binding capacity as B27.A2B and other class I alleles. This lower binding capacity of wild-type B27 allele suggests that B27 folding abnormality may affect its peptide-binding ability [1].

A reduced rate of folding in the majority of the disease-related forms of HLA-B27 subtypes (HLA-B*2705, HLA-B*2704, and HLA-B*2702) has been demonstrated compared with HLA-B*2706 and HLA-B*2709 and most of other non-AS related MHC class-I molecules. Increased duration for assembly of the disease-associated HLA-B27 subtypes appears to cause the accumulation of misfolded HLA-B27 molecules in the ER. The accumulation of unfolded and/or misfolded proteins may disturb ER function and lead to ER stress and activation of the unfolded protein response (UPR), in order to rescue from the burden of misfolded proteins [3]. ER stress and activation of UPR in the result of HLA-B27 misfolding might be involved in AS pathogenesis. Cells exhibiting UPR activation has altered response to innate immune stimuli which in turn alters the cytokine production pattern. In fact, the UPR activation or its subsequent outcomes such as autophagy may work as additional signals that promote the production of particular pro-inflammatory cytokines by macrophages in response to TLR agonists such as LPS and other bacterial products. In this way, innate immune stimuli polarize macrophages toward increased production of IFN-β, IL-23, and IL-6. As has been demonstrated before, IL-23 and IL-6 are important for the differentiation of Th17 cells. This recommends a novel mechanism that may describe, at least in part, the pathologic role of HLA-B27, as the IL-23/IL17 axis could be important as an upstream factor in AS pathogenesis. In addition, implications of HLA-B27 misfolding during the response to other inflammatory cytokines such as TNFα and IFNγ may play a more highlighted downstream role which contributes to the AS phenotype. It has been indicated that IFNγ upregulates several components of the MHC class I assembly pathway such as TAP1 and 2, Tapasin, ERAP1, β2m, and proteasome subunits LMP2 and LMP7. This, in turn, exacerbates HLA-B27 misfolding and UPR activation [1, 14, 15].

4.2.1.3 HLA-B27 Dimer Hypothesis

As is mentioned before, three main features of HLA-B27 that are known to distinguish it from other class I HLA molecules are proposed to describe how it may contribute to AS development. We have discussed in detail about arthritogenic peptide presentation and the predilection of HLA-B27 to misfold in the ER which triggers ER stress and provokes the UPR. The third hypothesis that try to describe the role of B27 in the pathogenesis of AS is a tendency for forming HLA-B27 heavy chain homodimers during cell surface recycling [14]. Usually, misfolded proteins may activate ER-associated degradation while, misfolded HLA-B27 heavy chains tend to form dimers or multimers [3]. Peptide-binding studies have revealed that newly synthesized B27 heavy chains oligomerize in disulfide-linked structures whose formation depends on the presence of unpaired cysteine at position 67 (Cys67) [14]. Cell surface expression of HLA-B27 dimers may be important in the pathogenesis of AS, because of their role in binding to immune cells receptors.

It has been shown that HLA-B27 homodimers could bind to immunoreceptors expressed on NK cells and other leukocytes and hence might be important in the immunopathogenesis of autoimmune diseases like AS [3]. These receptors include killer cell immunoglobulin-like receptors (KIR) and leucocyte immunoglobulin-like receptors (LILR). Enhanced survival and proliferation of KIR3DL2+ IL-17-producing CD4+ T cells and increased IL-23 receptor expression and the production of IL-17, TNF-α and IFN-γ have been observed in patients with AS following stimulation with HLA-B27 homodimers expressing antigen-presenting cells (APCs). Differential association of B27 alleles with AS might be due to the formation of these dimers from different HLA-B27 subtypes. For instance, it has been demonstrated that HLA-B*2705, which is significantly associated with AS, forms a higher number of B27 heavy chain dimers for KIR3DL2 in comparison with HLA-B*2709 that is almost not associated with AS [3].

Another proposed mechanism by which B27 dimers can be involved in AS pathogenesis is the "β2m over-expression" hypothesis. Based on this, following B27 dimers dissociation, β2m may accumulate and become trapped in the synovia, where they may bind to collagen and make deposits of amyloid or interact with synovial fibroblasts. In this manner, they can stimulate the production and secretion of proteins involved in tissue destruction, which in turn lead to AS development [3].

Apart from what was discussed in the above-mentioned theories, there are evidences of the role of other possible mechanisms which associate HLA-B27 to AS development. One of them is that the ER chaperone BiP transiently binds to many newly synthesized MHC class I heavy chains to fold them properly. Nevertheless, HLA-B27 heavy chains show a prolonged association with BiP in ER. It has been shown that BiP has a predilection to bind oligomers of HLA-B27 in cells. This prolonged association might be a consequence of oligomerization of HLA-B27 heavy chains. The biochemical details of this BiP/HLA-B27 association have not yet been explicated but it is considered as a potential factor for developing AS. As has been reported, expression of BiP protein in peripheral joints macrophages of subjects with ankylosing spondylitis is greater than in osteoarthritis. Moreover, a correlation between synovial fluid inflammatory cytokines, TNFα and IL-6, and expression of BiP in macrophages, as well as between serum level of IL-6, disease activity, and macrophage BiP level has also been found [14].

In addition, it has been demonstrated that the macrophages of individuals who are HLA-B27-positive have altered intracellular killing in particular infections. It has been observed that transfected cell lines with HLA-B27 but no other HLA allele show enhanced intracellular bacterial survival and replication. This could be important for the pathogenesis of SpAs as the p38 MAP kinase pathway may be disrupted in these cells. This evidence presumably represents an intracellular or at least a non-antigen presenting effect of HLA-B27 in the pathogenesis of AS [1]. This suggests that infection or altered immune response may work as a trigger of SpA in B27 expressing individuals [8]. Based on this, another proposed mechanism is the modified serological recognition of B27 by oxidation of the free sulfhydryl group of its Cys67. This might be attained by the interaction of HLA-B27 with a bacterial product, homocysteine. There are certain factors recognized to be able to alter the serological properties of HLA-B27, which in people could result in recognition of B27 as a non-self-antigen [6, 16].

Despite extensive studies being done to clarify the mechanism of function of HLA-B27 in AS development, the problem remains open and not fully answered [2]. In human, only as few as 1–5% of HLA-B27 positive individuals develop AS, and there are increasing evidences to support that susceptibility to AS is complicated and B27 is only one of several genes that are involved in predisposition and phenotype of the disease [6, 11]. One of the main non-HLA-B27 contributions to susceptibility to AS is proposed by the higher concordance rate of monozygotic twins (60–75%) in comparison with B27-positive dizygotic twin pairs (24%) [11, 17]. Thus, an attractive subject is to explain why only a proportion of individuals with HLA B27 develop AS [13]. Today, whole-genome association studies (GWAS) are applied to identify other human predisposing genes [1]. The GWAS has enabled us to identify non-MHC associations of AS with more velocity. GWAS findings have underlined a number of important pathways involved in the pathogenesis of AS including aminopeptidases and peptide presentation, the IL-23 pathway, stimulation of innate immune responses, and the interaction and homeostasis of normal microbial flora [17].

4.2.2 HLA Genes Other Than HLA-B27

Although HLA-B27 is evidently the main AS-associated MHC gene, is clearly not the only one and several studies have indicated that there are several other HLA-B and non-HLA-B alleles that are important in the risk of AS development [11]. In this way, both linkage and association of other class I and II HLA loci with AS have been demonstrated [8]. Possibly HLA-B40, specifically with B*40:01 (a DNA-defined allele that is serologically defined as HLA-B60) subtype, has the second most characterized and validated association after HLA-B27. This association was defined for the first time in HLA-B27-positive patients with AS from Europe and the USA in 1989 [8]. Thereafter, several studies demonstrated that the strong epistatic interaction between B27 and B40 multiplies the predisposition to AS in B27 positive Caucasians by 3.6 to 4.7-fold [2, 13]. However, further studies by many research groups confirmed the association of AS with HLA-B*40:01 as well as B*40:02 (serologically defined as B61) alleles in both B27-positive and B27-negative AS patients in European and East Asian populations (odds ratio = 1.22 and

1.59, respectively, CI = 95%). However, the power of association of HLA-B40 with AS is much weaker than the association with HLA-B27, having an odds ratio of 3.6 [4, 11, 12, 18].

HLA-B14 is another HLA-B allele described to be associated with AS in French families with SpA. In addition, recent studies have shown a remarkable association of AS with HLA-B*14:03 in several sub-Saharan African populations (Burkina Faso, Zambia, and Togo). This is a very low frequent allele that has been detected in 32% of SpA patients in those areas but in none of the healthy controls. Both SpA and HLA-B27 are rare in West Africa [4, 8].

In Tunisia, in Belgian patients with undifferentiated SpA as well as in Mexican patients with peripheral spondyloarthritis, an association has been reported with HLA-B15. An association between HLA-B39 and HLA-B27-negative AS patients has also been described [8, 18].

In addition to HLA-B alleles, using single-nucleotide polymorphisms (SNPs) studies to ascribe other HLA alleles, a significant association between HLA-A*02:01 (rs2394250) and AS susceptibility with odds ratios of 1.21 in B27 positive and 1.36 in B27 negative samples has been revealed. Thus, the association of the HLA-A*02:01 allele is independent of the HLA-B*27 genotype and no linkage disequilibrium with HLA-B27 has been explained [8, 18].

After controlling for the associated haplotypes in HLA class-I, independent associations with the class-II HLA alleles have also been observed [18]. Initial studies from the United Kingdom had implicated HLA-DRB1*01:01. Nevertheless, this was then attributed to its linkage disequilibrium with HLA-B*27:05-bearing haplotypes. Further studies have shown a significant association with HLA-DRB1 irrespective of whether the haplotype includes HLA-B27. These reports evidenced a predisposing role for HLA-DR4 (DRB1*04:04) in a French family-based study and subsequently, in a North American case–control study. The impact of these associations is considerable, as the attributable risk of these haplotypes is 34% [8, 11].

In a large case–control study performed in an HLA-B27+ Spanish population, a region placed around the HLA-DPA1 and HLA-DPB1 loci has been described as weakly but significantly associated with susceptibility to AS. This association is with the DPA1*01:03, DPA1*02:01, and DPB1*13:01 subtypes. Interestingly, the HLA-DPA1 and -DPB1 molecules make a heterodimer implicated in the presentation of extracellular antigens (e.g., microbial) to CD4+ T cells Afterward, the association of AS with HLA-DPA1*01:03 was found again in the Portuguese population, supporting its validity [4].

On the short arm of chromosome 6, the closest gene to the HLA-B locus is major histocompatibility complex class I chain A related (MICA). The MICA gene encodes a cell stress-inducible glycoprotein as a ligand for natural killer group 2D receptor (NKG2D) activation associated with the proinflammatory pathway. NKG2D is an activating receptor from the C-type lectin-like family which is expressed on natural killer (NK) cells, CD8+ T cells, and NK T cells [19]. In addition to HLA genes, there is strong evidence for the association of MICA alleles with susceptibility to SpA. A triplet repeat polymorphism in the transmembrane section of the MICA-A4 gene closely linked to the HLA-B locus has been reported to be associated with AS. In fact, a high frequency of MICA-A4 allele in HLA-B27 negative AS patients from Sardinia has marked this allele as a susceptibility factor albeit weaker than B27 for AS. Other data have proposed that MICA is a strong predisposing factor for AS in the US white population [8]. It is well established that the two MICA alleles reported as positively associated with SpA are MICA*007:01 (in Caucasian and Han Chinese populations) and MICA*019 (in Chinese patients). Interestingly, these associations have been found both in B27-negative and B27-positive patients that indicate them as independent of HLA-B27 [4].

It has been evidenced that MICA 129 Val/Val constitutes a negative genetic association with SpA and indeed, protects against PsA. This polymorphism in exon 3 results in the replacement of methionine by valine which can influence NKG2D signaling. In fact, the presence of methionine instead of valine at position 129 of the α2-heavy chain domain of MICA results in strong binding to the NKG2D receptor, while MICA-129 Val/Val leads to a weak binding affinity. Therefore, SpA patients with MICA129 Val/Val polymorphism show lower levels of inflammation close to their sacroiliac joint and hence suffer less injury from sacroiliitis. Present studies have shown that MICA129 val/val, MICA A5.1 and NKC3 C/C polymorphisms (the latter is related to low level of NK cell cytotoxic activity) protect against SpA. On contrary, MICA129 met/met, NKC3 G/G, and G/C polymorphisms (related to an increased level of cytotoxic activity) are considered as risk factors for SpA. NKC3 G/G polymorphism could be used to improve the diagnosis of SpA, especially when the patient is HLA-B27 negative [19].

4.3 Association of HLA-Related Genes with Ankylosing Spondylitis

Genome-Wide Association Studies (GWAS) have identified 31 non-HLA genetic loci In AS patients with European ancestry [20]. However, as is estimated, all of these non-HLA predisposing loci account only for 4.3% of heritability in AS, while HLA-B27 alleles contribute more than 20%, indicating that a majority of predisposing loci have still been undefined [21].

4.3.1 Transporters in Antigen Presenting (TAP)

It has been proposed that differences in susceptibility to AS among different B27-positive individuals may be due to the differences in the peptides presented by HLA-B27. Interestingly, there are evidences that some B27-positive persons fail to present viral epitopes which are restricted to B27 in other individuals. One possible elucidation for this could be the involvement of the well-defined polymorphisms of a group of genes encoding components of the pathway by which peptide fragments are produced as the result of breaking down of the complex antigens and transported to the ER. TAP 1 and TAP 2 are two examples of these genes [13]. The TAP1 and TAP2 genes code for subunits of the functional TAP gate, which transport proteasome processed cytosolic derived peptides into the ER. Mutations in TAP1 or TAP2 genes entail to structural alterations that inhibit TAP heterodimer formation and affect antigen recognition and presentation [22]. It is hypothesized that there is a linkage disequilibrium between particular alleles at the TAP loci and HLA B27 in both the HLA-B27 positive healthy controls and AS patients. Finding an association with specific TAP alleles, TAP1B, TAP1C, and TAP2E have been shown to be rare in the general population, while they are increased in B27 positive individuals, either healthy or patient. Thus, this may not have a profound effect and is not of primary importance in AS susceptibility [8, 13].

Although the importance of TAP in the pathogenesis of autoimmune disorders like AS is almost unknown, many studies have demonstrated its direct or indirect participation in the development of AS. It is possible that TAP alleles may affect the selection of epitopes that play a role in the pathogenesis of AS and other autoimmune inflammatory diseases [22].

Polymorphism in the TAP1 gene was first identified in the early 1990s. The main polymorphic positions in TAP1 are 333 (Val) and 637 (Asp) which corresponds to cDNA positions 1069 and 1982. In TAP2, the main polymorphic site is 565 (Thr) which corresponds to cDNA position 1693. Interestingly, strong associations have been detected between the TAP1-333, -637, and TAP2-565 and AS compared with total and HLA-B27 negative, but not with HLA-B27 positive controls. It has been demonstrated that TAP1-333Val, TAP1-637Gly, and TAP2-565Thr are potential risk factors for AS in HLA-B27 negative cases. In the British population, the frequency of allele TAPIC (333 Val-637 Asp) has been shown to be significantly increased in the AS patients compared with normal controls. In addition, it has been reported that the frequency of the TAP1B allele is significantly elevated in AS patients with the extra-spinal disease compared with AS patients without extra-spinal disease or normal controls. In a Chinese population, TAP1-637 and TAP2-565 have been demonstrated to be associated with AS in comparison with HLA-B27 negative control. Nevertheless, no significant association has been identified between TAP1 and TAP2 alleles in Japanese, Spanish, and Caucasian populations [22].

In the genotype analyses, allele G and genotype A/G at TAP1 site 1910 have been described as possible risk factors for AS in HLA-B27 negative controls. Interestingly, this position has also been described to be associated with infection with hepatitis B virus, dengue virus, allergic rhinitis, and hypersensitivity pneumonitis. Both TAP1 position 1910 SNP A/G and TAP2 position 1693 G/A led to Asp637Gly and Ala565Thr replacements, respectively. The presence of both Asp and Gly at the position of amino acid 637 for TAP1 may influence peptide transport to ER and contribute to AS susceptibility, while being homozygous for either Gly or Asp does not. With regard to TAP2 SNP 1693, only the presence of Thr and not Ala at the position of amino acid 565 may play a role in AS development [23].

4.3.2 M1 zinc-Aminopeptidases

Antigenic peptides are obligatory for oligomerization and expression of HLA-B27. Thus, it could be logical to assume that occurrence of polymorphisms in intracellular peptidases can affect the quality and quantity of antigenic peptides available for presentation with MHC class I molecules and influence the susceptibility to AS [14]. In this way, aminopeptidases play an essential role in peptide trimming which is a required step for the generation of suitable peptides for HLA class I-binding [20]. In mammals, the M1 zinc-aminopeptidase family contains 5 integral transmembrane proteins and 4 non-transmembrane enzymes. From these, the endoplasmic reticulum aminopeptidase (ERAP)-1, ERAP2, and insulin-regulated aminopeptidase (IRAP or LNPEP) belong to the oxytocinase subfamily and are encoded in human chromosome 5p15 locus. This enzyme family is recognized by the HEXXH(X18) E Zn-binding and GAMEN motifs which are necessary for their activity. NPEPPS gene which encodes puromycin-sensitive aminopeptidase is located on the chromosome 17q21 locus. ERAP1 is a type II integral membrane enzyme, while ERAP2 and NPEPPS are non-transmembrane enzymes [17, 24]. ERAP1 and ERAP2 have been reported as important components of the final processing of antigenic peptides for MHC-I in the ER. In particular, they are recognized to trim peptides that are going to be presented by MHC class I molecules [24, 25]. Alterations within several aminopeptidases, such as ERAP1, ERAP2, LNPEP, and NPEPPS, have been identified.

4.3.2.1 Endoplasmic Reticulum Aminopeptidase (ERAP)-1

Studies done on patients with HLAB27 negative AS patients prepared a wider view of non-HLA-B27 genetic predisposition factors associated with AS. However, a number of these genes have been shown to have a significant relationship with HLA-B27 [2]. Abnormal peptide processing and presentation might be involved in the pathogenesis of AS owing to the interaction between ERAP1 and HLA-B27 [3]. Both susceptible and protective variants of ERAP1 associated with AS have been recognized by genome-wide association studies (GWAS). The relative attributable risk of ERAP1 for AS is around 25%, while that of HLA-B27 is around 50%. These two genes are the two strongest disease risk factors for AS development. Interestingly, the association of ERAP1 is limited to HLA-B27 positive AS patients [21]. The relationship between HLA-B27 and ERAP1 supports the hypothesis that asserts the mechanism of action of B27 in AS development involves abnormal processing and presentation of antigenic peptides. The discovery of the mechanism of the contribution of ERAP1 and HLA-B27 interaction in the pathogenesis of AS will open a door to better understanding and management of AS [2]. However, the exact fundamental molecular mechanisms of this process have not been fully clarified [25].

The protein ERAP1 has four domains (I to IV). Domain II includes the catalytic site. On the top of domain II, domain I is located and contains binding residues for the N-termini of the substrate. The Gln181 and Glu183 are such binding residues whose mutations influence the enzyme's specificity and activity. Domain III is a small one with a β-sandwich structure that connects the catalytic domain II with the large C-terminal domain IV. Domain IV is a big α-helical domain that extends away from the catalytic part and makes a large cavity between domains II and IV which is probably a substrate-binding site accommodating different length peptides for catalysis [24, 25].

Preliminary studies have shown that the association of AS with ERAP1 occurs only among HLA-B27 positive cases as shown in Caucasians and Taiwanese populations [25]. In fact, those data demonstrating genetic interaction between ERAP1 and HLA-B27 as well as the involvement of ERAP1 mutations in protein changes propose that abnormal peptide presentation might be influential in AS susceptibility. Genetic variants associated with diminished function of ERAP1, and loss of ERAP2 expression, are protective for AS. Presumably, these genes work in AS by influencing the quantity of MHC class I peptide presentation or by a qualitative impact on the peptide repertoire presented. It has also been shown that down-regulation of ERAP1 and ERAP2 expression declines the cell-surface expression of class-I MHC molecules [8, 25].

HLA class-I molecules enforce strict limitations to peptide length, binding mainly 9 or 10-mers peptides. Thus, the N-terminal peptides entering the ER must be trimmed to achieve optimized length for HLA class-I binding. This is done by ERAP1, presumably in concert with the action of ERAP2. Apparently, a unique property of ERAP1, called the "molecular ruler" mechanism, is to cleave substrates longer than 9-mers efficiently, while doing that with less efficiency for 9-mers and almost is unable to cleave 8-mers or shorter peptides. This feature makes ERAP1 ideal for generating optimal HLA class-I ligands [25]. It is also recognized to cleave substrates with a hydrophobic C-terminal residue, more efficiently [24]. In fact, positively charged and nonpolar residues, except Trp and Val, are preferred over polar, basic, and acidic residues. Anywhere in the peptide sequence, Glu, Gly, or Pro disfavored cleavage [25].

Variants of ERAP1 have been widely reported by GWA studies in East Asians and in populations of white European ancestry. ERAP1 is known as a highly polymorphic molecule and certain ERAP1 haplotypes, or combinations of particular SNPs, are predisposing for AS susceptibility. However, very tight linkage disequilibrium between ERAP1 variants complicates the assignment of a given SNP as a predisposing factor for AS [25]. Fine-mapping studies on ERAP1 have indicated that the SNP rs30187 (R528 or Lys528Arg), as the major allele, and the minor allele of rs10050860/rs17482078 (N575/Q725 or Asp575Asn/ Arg725Gln) are significantly associated with AS [17]. In addition, another AS-associated SNP (rs27434) in ERAP1 has been reported in the Chines population [26]. The risk of AS in B27-positive homozygous carriers of ERAP1 protective variants in combination is three- to fourfold lower [24]. Haplotype evolution studies have evidenced that among the most strongly associated haplotypes with AS, the haplotype of rs30187-rs10050860-rs27044 (AGG) is predisposing, while the haplotype of rs26653-rs26618-rs30187 (CAG) is protecting against AS [18]. Apart from a very strong linkage disequilibrium between rs10050860 and rs17482078, in vitro studies of peptidase activity of ERAP1 variants have indicated that the protective variants of rs17482078 and rs30187 are associated with a 40% decrease in peptidase function, while rs10050860 has no impact [17, 24]. Indeed, the polymorphisms associated with protection from AS are related to decreasing ERAP1 activity. It has also been suggested that a main mechanism of the functional ERAP1 and HLA-B27 interaction is the variations induced in the balance between epitope generation and degradation by ERAP1 polymorphisms [25]. In this way, ERAP1 may degrade some antigenic peptides and hence, prevent their presentation [17]. The SNP rs30187 of ERAP1 has been shown to change a highly conserved residue (Arg528Lys, located near the entrance of the substrate pocket) which entails to a dramatic decrease of the enzyme catalytic activity. The SNP rs17482078 (Arg725Gln), on the other hand, reduces enzyme activity by influencing the substrate sequence specificity as it is exposed on the inner surface of the C-terminal cavity. Therefore, ERAP1 variants could affect AS susceptibility through both the amount of antigenic peptide presented by HLA-B27, as well as the length and sequence of the presented peptides [24]. More recently, the interaction between the rs30187 SNP and HLA-B40 (B*40:01) which is another AS-associated HLA-B allele has been demonstrated. This has been confirmed by the observation of rs30187 association with AS among HLA-B27 negative/HLA-B40 positive patients, but not among HLA-B27 negative/HLA-B40 negative patients [18, 24].

AS-associated variants of ERAP1 alter the amount, length, and stability of peptides presented by the MHC molecule. The high level of alterations in the cell's peptidome induced by polymorphism of ERAP1 may affect other aspects of HLA-B27 related ERAP1 pathogenetic roles in AS, such as stability, folding, and generation of heavy chain homodimers at the cell surface [17, 25]. For instance, if the presence of an ERAP1 variant with diminished activity disrupts the optimization of the HLA-B27 peptidome, this could result in retention of HLA-B27 in the endoplasmic reticulum and increased misfolding level in an AS-protective context. This is in contrary to the misfolding hypothesis of the pathogenesis of AS which was mentioned earlier. Nevertheless, this prediction has not been yet established experimentally. In addition, the expression of heavy chain homodimers at the cell surface might also happen as the result of decreased HLA-B27 stability. This means that, in the presence of less functional ERAP1 variants, higher amounts of suboptimal HLA-B27/peptide complexes could be exported to the cell surface and dissociate under the acidic situation of the endosome which favors homodimer formation. Again, it seems that the effect of AS-associated polymorphism of ERAP1 which leads to a decrease of surface expression of HLA-B27 homodimers contradicts their above-mentioned pathogenetic role [25]. Some studies have demonstrated that ERAP1 suppression as the result of genetic polymorphism could lead to a B27-subtype-specific effect ending up to increased intracellular free B27 heavy chain which influences the cells expressing HLA-B*27:04 or B*27:05 but not B*27:06 and B*27:09. These observations confirm that alterations in the ERAP1/HLA-B27 interactions entail variable peptide presentation and provide a possible explanation for the absence of, or at least weak, the association of the HLA-B27 subtypes B*27:06 and B*27:09 with ankylosing spondylitis (AS) [12, 24].

In addition to its function to trim peptides before loading into newly synthesized class-I HLA molecules, ERAP1 may affect disease susceptibility through its role in cleaving receptors of pro-inflammatory cytokine from the cell surface, such as IL-1 receptor 2, TNF receptor 1, and IL-6 receptor. The effect of cytokine receptor cleavage has been argued but there are no in vivo evidences to support this function as of yet [11]. Altogether, these suggest that inhibition of ERAP1 could potentially be applied as a promising therapeutic target both in Ankylosing Spondylitis and in other HLA/ERAP1 associated diseases [24].

4.3.2.2 ERAP2

ERAP2 is another zinc-dependent M1 aminopeptidases member in ER which is structurally related to ERAP1 and other members of this family. ERAP1 and ERAP2 share around 50% identity in amino acid sequence with many similarities in their three-dimensional structure. ERAP1 and 2 are an integral part of the class-I MHC presentation pathway in ER and it is evident that ERAP1 and ERAP2 can form heterodimers more efficient trimming activity in comparison with ERAP1 or ERAP2 homodimers [17, 24, 27]. In this manner, ERAP1 and ERAP2 together are responsible for trimming peptides to optimize their length for presenting by HLA class-I. Therefore, they have a central role in the regulation of immune responses. It has been evidenced that there is a strong association of ERAP2 with AS, inflammatory bowel disease (IBD), and psoriasis [12, 24].

The most recent GWAS outcomes have shown an association of AS in HLA-B27-negative cases with two functionally important variants of ERAP2 [21]. The most important variant is the synonymous SNP rs2248374 G allele which alters the stability of the exon 10 splice site, leading to a larger exon 10 transcript with 2 stop codons [18]. This leads to transcription of a truncated mRNA that undergoes nonsense-mediated decay causing the loss of ERAP2 protein production. This loss-of-enzyme variant phenomenon is associated with decreased HLA class I surface expression and is protective of AS, in a similar manner to the loss-of-function variants in ERAP1 which is also protective of AS [17]. Another variant of ERAP2 is rs2549782 (Asn392Lys) which alters both the speed of action and specificity of ERAP2 trimming activity. This variant is also associated with AS, IBD, and psoriasis and is in significant linkage disequilibrium (LD) with rs2248374 [17, 18, 20, 24]. It has been demonstrated that an ERAP1/ERAP2 haplotype (rs27044[G] rs30187[T] rs2549782[T]) is in association with familial AS. As mentioned before, ERAP1 variants rs27044 and rs30187 affect the peptide-trimming activity and ERAP2 SNP rs2549782 changes its specificity and activity of ERAP2 [21]. Regarding the strong LD between ERAP1 and HLA-B27, as well as between ERAP1 and ERAP2, it is almost impossible to determine whether ERAP2 is associated with AS in HLA-B27 positive samples. However, as mentioned earlier, its association with AS is evident in HLA-B27 negative cases [17].

4.3.2.3 NPEPPS

NPEPPS, also known as puromycin-sensitive aminopeptidase or cytosol alanyl aminopeptidase, is the only cytosolic aminopeptidase that cleaves polyQ sequences and hydrolyzes N-terminal amino acids from its peptide substrates. NPEPPS prefers hydrophobic and basic residues in the peptide substrate. There is rarely a knowledge on the impact of mutations on NPEPPS functional activity and its functional variants. Genome-wide association studies demonstrated a significant association at synonymous SNP rs9901869 of NPEPPS at chromosome 17q21 with AS [24]. Whether NPEPPS operates in AS through influencing autophagy or via alternate effects on intracellular peptide handling needs further explorations [17, 20].

4.3.2.4 Ubiquitinases

Ubiquitination is another factor that plays an important role in determining what antigenic peptides are presented to the immune system. GWA studies have revealed two ubiquitinases, UBE2E3 and UBE2L3, in association with AS. UBE2E3 and UBE2L3 encode the UbcH9 and UbcH7 enzymes, respectively. UbcH9 cannot form bonds with ubiquitin but is able to do that with a similar protein SUMO. In contrary to ubiquitination, when a protein undergoes sumoylation it will not be degraded and instead, it may increase the protein's stability, change its position, or direct involvement in other cellular processes such as signal transduction. On the other hand, UBE2L3 variants are involved in the regulation of NF-κB and it has been associated with a number of other inflammatory disorders [17, 18]. Collectively, these findings further emphasize the importance of antigen presentation in AS pathogenesis [20].

4.3.2.5 LMP2

It has been demonstrated that the large multifunctional protease (LMP) 2 and LMP7 subunits which are coded in the HLA class-II region act to amplify specific endopeptidase functions of the proteasome. IFNγ and the expression of the *LMP2* and *LMP7* genes could favor the generation of peptides almost exclusively with hydrophobic or basic residues by proteasomes [28, 29]. It has previously been shown that LMP2 is associated with both AS and uveitis in patients with AS. Based on its association with uveitis, LMP2 could be considered as a marker representing a more aggressive form of AS which may result in more structural damage. In addition, the proteasome breaks down the β-catenin, and hence, aberrations in LMP2 may lead to excess Wnt/β-catenin signaling and osteoblastic activity [21, 30].

4.4 Role of Epigenetics in Ankylosing Spondylitis Pathogenesis

Epigenetics is typically recognized as potentially reversible but heritable changes in gene expression without aberration in nucleotide sequence. Therefore, this phenomenon is largely responsible for controlling the profile of the cell-specific expression of genes during the cell cycle, development, and in response to biological or environmental conditions. This explains that how a limited number of genes can result in the differentiation of a cell into several different cell types. Epigenetic modifications involved in regulating the gene expression include modification of histones proteins by acetylation, DNA methylation, and microRNAs functions. Environmental factors can affect some epigenetic processes like acetylation and methylation, while other epigenetic factors are inherited [20]. Histone acetylation facilitates gene expression by converting a heterochromatin structure to euchromatin form and therefore, promotes the accessibility of DNA regulatory regions to the transcriptional factors or to other DNA binding proteins, while methylation of DNA in the promoter region of genes hampers gene transcription activity. Considering several surveys, it has been established that epigenetics is involved in the etiopathogenesis of AS [18, 31].

4.4.1 DNA Methylation

The most extensively studied epigenetic mechanism is DNA methylation which is mediated by two DNA methyltransferase (DNMT) enzymes, with S adenosylmethionine (SAM) as the methyl donor. There are five members of DNMT enzymes categorized into two main classes: de novo DNA methyltransferases (DNMT3a, DNMT3b, and DNMT3L) and maintenance methyltransferases (DNMT1, DNMT2). Methyltransferases transfer the methyl group (CH3) onto the C5 position of cytosines to generate the 5-methylcytosine (5mC). Regulation of genomic imprinting, gene expression, genome defense, and X-chromosome inactivation are done by DNA methylation. Cytosine–guanine dinucleotides (CpG) are the regions of DNA where methylation frequently occurs and are termed CpG islands (CGIs). Four general types of DNA methylation based on the target sites are the methylation of CpG islands clustered within gene promoter regions, the methylation of the edge of CpG islands (CpG island shores), the methylation throughout the whole gene, and the methylation of repetitive sequences. DNA methylation is a highly stable marker so that is maintained throughout mitotic cell division [32]. DNA Methyltransferases have dual activities as are involved in the addition of methyl groups to DNA and also its removal. By the addition of methyl groups to DNA, transcription is blocked through diminished binding of transcription factors and enhanced binding of methyl-CpG-binding domain (MBD) proteins. In such a situation, the chromatin structure is affected and a co-repressor complex is generated. By contrast, removal of methyl groups from DNA leads to the euchromatin structure formation and allows binding of transcription factors to the correct regions [18].

It has been evidenced that abnormal DNA methylation can play an important role in several diseases in humans [33]. However, little has been explored with regard to the association of DNA methylation with AS, so far [18]. Whole-blood transcriptional profiling studies on AS have demonstrated that the expression level of DNMT1 is down-regulated and CpG islands at the promoter of DNMT1 are highly methylated in the PBMCs from patients with AS in comparison with the healthy controls. Based on the role of the DNMT1 enzyme in preserving the methylation pattern of DNA, it is expected that a decrease of DNMT1 can influence the level of DNA methylation of downstream genes that could probably contribute to the development of AS [34, 35].

DNMT3A and DNM3TB are de novo methyltransferases that have been shown to be involved in genomic imprinting and inactivation of X-chromosome, to impress development of hematopoietic stem cells, and activation of UBE2 ubiquitin ligases, which are also known to be associated with AS. The functions of these genes have led to the suggestion that they might be responsible for the male gender bias in AS [12].

Methylation in other genes has been reported as associated with AS. It has been shown that the methylation of SOCS-1 can only be found in the serum of HLA-B27-positive patients with AS but not in any of B27-positive healthy controls. Interestingly, the amount of methylated SOCS-1 has been shown to be significantly correlated with the degree of inflammation as measured through sacroiliitis, acute phase reactant, erythrocyte sedimentation rate (ESR) and C-reactive protein (CRP), as well as cytokine level of IL-6 and TNF-α in AS patients [18, 20, 33]. In addition, down-regulation of BCL11B expression as well as its CpG island hyper-methylation in PBMCs from AS patients compared with healthy subjects has been observed. More detailed studies would be advantageous to explain the exact mechanisms by which both DNMT1 and BCL11B hyper-methylation are involved in the AS etiopathogenesis [18, 35]. One important finding of a study is that the HLA-DQB1 gene is involved in AS development. Interestingly, a significant level of hyper-methylation of the HLA-DQB1 gene in AS PBMCs has been identified [36].

4.4.2 Histone Modifications

Histones are conserved proteins involved in packaging and organizing DNA to form nucleosome structure. Histones are classified into two main groups of cores (H2A, H2B, H3, and H4) and linker (H1 and H5) proteins. Histone proteins can undergo a series of post-translational modifications such as acetylation, phosphorylation, sumoylation, ubiquitination, and methylation. These mechanisms regulate the transcription of the genes in two major ways. On one hand, histone modification changes chromatin conformation and hence makes the gene promoters accessible for transcription factors. On the other hand, histone modification may affect the binding of chromatin-associated factors. Histone methylation does not change the charge of histone proteins while acetylation does. Histone acetylation is necessary for the regulatory factors access to the transcription factors and for the following gene expression [32]. Histone acetylation is mediated by two enzymes named histone acetyltransferases (HATs) and histone deacetylases (HDACs). Histone acetyltransferases transfer an acetyl group to the amino group of lysine side chains from acetyl CoA. This alteration neutralizes the positive charge of lysine and diminishes the interaction between the DNA strand and the histone and hence, entails a less integrated and accessible chromatin structure, which rises the gene expression. By contrast, histone deacetylases remove an acetyl group from the acetylated lysine side chain, adding a positive charge and leading to an intense chromatin configuration, which reduces the gene expression

[18]. It has been reported that in AS, HAT and HDAC activities are significantly decreased and HDAC inhibitors are capable of down-regulating TNF production by PBMC in patients with AS [20].

4.4.3 MicroRNAs

Another element of the epigenetic machinery is microRNA (miRNA). MicroRNAs are endogenous short non-coding RNAs that contain 18–23 nucleotides that play important roles in regulating gene expression at the post-transcriptional level. Their genes are located throughout the genome and are transcribed from intronic regions of protein-coding genes, within intronic or exonic sequences of noncoding RNAs, and approximately 30% in intergenic regions [32]. The miRNAs are generated in the nucleus and then moves to the cytoplasm. Primary miRNAs (pri-miRNAs), as long primary transcripts, are transcribed by RNA polymerase II from mono- or polycistronic miRNA genes in the nucleus. These pri-miRNAs fold into hairpin structures and then, processed by a multiprotein complex, which comprises an identifier component named RNA-binding protein DiGeorge syndrome critical region 8 (DGCR8), and a catalyzer component named RNase III type endonuclease Drosha (or RN3). The Drosha catalyzes the conversion of pri-miRNA to precursor miRNA (pre-miRNA), which subsequently will be transported to the cytoplasm via Exportin 5. In the cytoplasm, another RNase III type endonuclease, called Dicer, processes the pre-miRNA into a mature miRNA duplex. Finally, at the core of a multiprotein RNA-induced silencing complex (RISC), the guide (antisense) strand is selectively separated to bind to the 3′UTR of complementary mRNA sequences, which leads to degradation or translational suppression. The passenger (sense) strand is generally released and rapidly degraded (Fig. 4.3) [37]. Silencing of gene expression by miRNAs is mediated by two pathways. First, induction of degradation of target mRNA when a part of its 3'UTR sequence is completely matched with the miRNA. Second, steric hindrance which prevents translation when miRNA strand is matched incompletely with target mRNA 3'UTR. In addition, miRNAs can influence the gene expression either positively or negatively by the means of modulating promoter DNA methylation as well as histone modifications [18].

As fine-tuning regulators of gene expression, microRNAs target numerous mRNAs participating in different physiological processes of cells, including proliferation, development and differentiation, cell metabolism, and apoptosis. Therefore, any abnormality in their expression profile can lead to dysregulation of the normal functions of the cell. MiRNAs are also important players in regulating the development of the immune system, normal immune function, autoimmunity, and osteoblast differentiation [15, 20]. Therefore, their deregulation can be associated with the pathogenesis of many human diseases [15, 18]. The pathological role of miRNAs has recently been studied most intensively in malignant diseases and also in autoimmune disorders. In recent years, some researchers have been engrossed in the potential role of miRNAs in autoimmune disorders and several unusual expression profiles have been defined as biomarkers of certain autoimmune disorders [37].

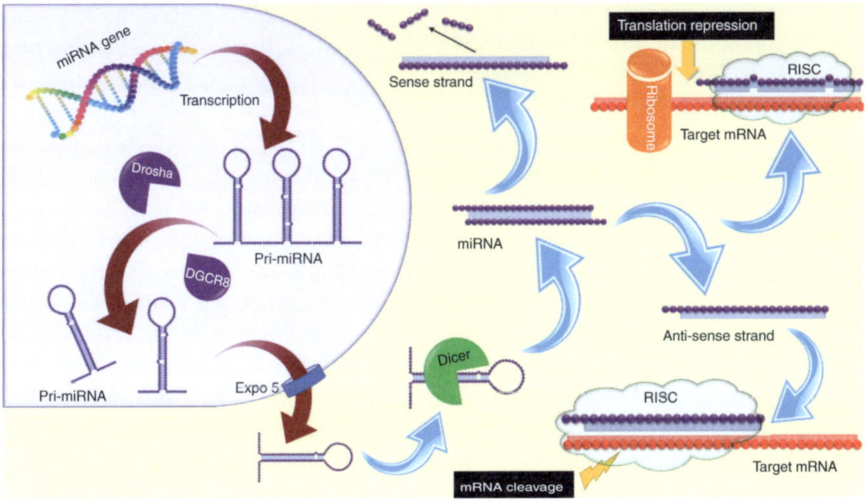

Fig. 4.3 The microRNA biogenesis pathway. Pri-miRNA is the first product of transcription of miRNA genes in the nucleus. This is then processed by Drosha and DGCR8 to generate pre-miRNAs. Pre-miRNAs exit from the nucleus toward cytosol via exportin 5 (Expo 5). Inside the cytosol, pre-miRNA is further processed by Dicer and a double-stranded RNA with about 21–23 nt length is generated. Then, miRNA is incorporated into a multicomponent enzyme complex named RNA Induced Silencing Complex (RISC). The RISC complex, using the antisense strand of the miRNA as a guide, searches for the mRNA target and degrades it. In the case of incomplete matching between miRNA and target mRNA, steric hindrance prevents the translation of the target mRNA. If the antisense strand is completely matched with complementary mRNA, antisense hybridizes to the target mRNA and induces its degradation by the intracellular enzyme RNase H

There are many studies evaluating the role of different miRNAs in AS. Expression profile studies of miRNAs in AS patients has revealed upregulation of several miRNAs including miR-16, miR-17-5p, miR-31, miR-32, miR-34a, miR-99b, miR-130a, miR-146a, miR-150, miR-221, miR-342-5p, let-7b, let-7i, miR-155-5p, miR-210-3p, and miR-513-5p, while down-regulation of miR-10b, miR-27b-3p, miR-29a, miR-30a, miR-30e, miR-126-3p, miR-154, miR-199a-5p, miR-215, miR-218, and miR-409-3p compared with healthy controls. On the contrary, the down-regulation of miR-16 and miR-150 has been shown in AS patients in one study [37–40]. Among the overexpressed microRNAs, miR-221 and let-7i have been confirmed to be correlated positively with the Bath Ankylosing Spondylitis Radiology Index (BASRI) of the lumbar spine. The contribution of the elevated expression of let-7i in T cells AS patients in the immunopathogenesis of AS via increasing the IFNγ production and Th1 inflammatory response has been indicated [18, 20, 37].

A remarkable higher level of miR-21 in AS patients, positively correlated with programmed cell death 4 (PDCD4) and C-telopeptide (CTX) mRNAs in patients with AS who are taking sulfasalazine has been demonstrated. By contrast, the high expression level of miR-21 has been seen to be negatively correlated with PDCD4 mRNA expression in AS patients who are taking neither NSAID nor DMARD. Positive correlations of miR-21 and CTX expression level have also been observed in AS patients with less than 7 years of disease duration and in active disease. The binding of miR-21 to PDCD4 can suppress the expression of PDCD4 and further induce the osteoclasts activation. It seems that the expression of miR-21 might be important in the AS development [18, 20].

A significant upregulated expression of miR-29a in PBMCs of AS patients compared with RA patients and healthy controls has been reported. The miR-29a regulates TNF-α mediated bone resorption mainly by targeting Dickkopf homolog 1 (Dkk-1) and GSK3b, and hence, activates the Wnt signaling pathway. Negative regulation of Dkk-1 in Wnt signaling may contribute to new bone formation in AS. However, no correlation between miR-29a expression and level of CRP and ESR, as well as Bath Ankylosing Spondylitis Disease Activity Index (BASDAI), and Bath Ankylosing Spondylitis Functional Index (BASFI) score of patients has been reported [18, 20]. Although a specific miRNA expression profile has not yet been established for AS, miR-29a could be considered as a helpful marker for diagnosis and monitoring the new bone formation in AS and might be a potential therapeutic approach in the future. Nevertheless, miR-29a is not specific for AS and could be involved in other disorders [18].

It has been evidenced that ANTXR2 is down-regulated and miR-124 expression is upregulated in AS patients. Given that ANTXR2 suppression by miR-124 promotes JNK activation and induces autophagy, it has been suggested that miR-124 may stimulate autophagy to participate in AS pathogenesis [20, 37].

Diminished miRNA-130a and elevated TNF-α and HDAC3 expression levels have been observed in PBMCs from AS patients. Down-regulation of TNF-α mRNA in PBMCs has been shown in overexpression of miRNA-130a, while inhibition of miR-130a led to an overexpression of TNF-α. On the other hand, knockdown or silencing of HDAC3 has been shown to be associated with both overexpression of miR-130a and down-regulation of TNF-α. These findings conclude that HDAC3 through establishing a negative feedback loop with miR-130a and promotion of TNF-α expression plays an important role in the molecular etiopathology of Ankylosing Spondylitis [18].

A remarkable higher frequency of the G and GG alleles in the miR-146a rs2910164G > C SNP has been demonstrated in the AS patients compared to the healthy controls in a Han Chinese population but not in other Chinese populations [37, 39]. In Chinese Han people, down-regulation of miR-143, miR-146a, miR-9-3, miR-205, and overexpression of miR-301a and miR-23a has been shown to be associated with susceptibility to acute anterior uveitis (AAU) in AS patients but not in AS negative cases [37, 41].

References

1. Colbert RA, et al. HLA-B27 misfolding and spondyloarthropathies. Prion. 2009;3(1):15–26.
2. Akassou A, Bakri Y. Does HLA-B27 status influence ankylosing spondylitis phenotype? Clin Med Insights: Arthritis and Musculoskeletal Disorders. 2018;11:1179544117751627.
3. Chen B, et al. Role of HLA-B27 in the pathogenesis of ankylosing spondylitis. Mol Med Rep. 2017;15(4):1943–51.

4. Breban M, et al. Revisiting MHC genes in spondyloarthritis. Curr Rheumatol Rep. 2015;17(6):40.
5. Nicknam MH, et al. Determination of HLA-B27 subtypes in Iranian patients with ankylosing spondylitis. Iran J Allergy Asthma Immunol. 2008;7(1):19–24.
6. Colbert RA, et al. From HLA-B27 to spondyloarthritis: a journey through the ER. Immunol Rev. 2010;233(1):181–202.
7. Gran JT, Husby G. HLA-B27 and spondyloarthropathy: value for early diagnosis? J Med Genet. 1995;32(7):497.
8. Reveille JD. An update on the contribution of the MHC to as susceptibility. Clin Rheumatol. 2014;33(6):749–57.
9. Nicknam M, et al. Association between HLA-B27 antigen and ankylosing spondylitis in Iranian patients. Hakim. 2005;8(1):29–34.
10. Nicknam M, et al. Comparison of val idity of microlymphocytotoxicity and flowcytometry methods with PCR for HLA-B27 antigen typing. Med J Islamic Republic Iran (MJIRI). 2003;17(1):75–9.
11. Brown M. Progress in studies of the genetics of ankylosing spondylitis. in clinical and experimental rheumatology. In: Clinical & exper rheumatology via santa maria, vol. 31. Italy: PISA; 2010. p. 56126.
12. Hanson A, Brown MA. Genetics and the causes of ankylosing spondylitis. Rheum Dis Clin. 2017;43(3):401–14.
13. Burney R, et al. Analysis of the MHC class II encoded components of the HLA class I antigen processing pathway in ankylosing spondylitis. Ann Rheum Dis. 1994;53(1):58–60.
14. Colbert RA, Tran TM, Layh-Schmitt G. HLA-B27 misfolding and ankylosing spondylitis. Mol Immunol. 2014;57(1):44–51.
15. Ganjalikhani Hakemi M, et al. Optimization of human Th17 cell differentiation in vitro: evaluating different polarizing factors. In Vitro Cell Dev Biol Animal. 2011;47(8):581.
16. Ringrose J. HLA-B27 associated spondyloarthropathy, an autoimmune disease based on cross-reactivity between bacteria and HLA-B27? Ann Rheum Dis. 1999;58(10):598–610.
17. Robinson PC, Brown MA. Genetics of ankylosing spondylitis. Mol Immunol. 2014;57(1):2–11.
18. Mahmoudi M, et al. New insights toward the pathogenesis of ankylosing spondylitis; genetic variations and epigenetic modifications. Mod Rheumatol. 2017;27(2):198–209.
19. Fechtenbaum M, et al. MICA and NKG2D variants as risk factors in spondyloarthritis: a case–control study. Genes Immun. 2019;20:599–605.
20. O'rielly DD, Uddin M, Rahman P. Ankylosing spondylitis: beyond genome-wide association studies. Curr Opin Rheumatol. 2016;28(4):337–45.
21. Tsui FW, et al. The genetic basis of ankylosing spondylitis: new insights into disease pathogenesis. Appl Clin Genet. 2014;7:105.
22. Qian Y, et al. Genetic association between TAP1 and TAP2 polymorphisms and ankylosing spondylitis: a systematic review and meta-analysis. Inflamm Res. 2017;66(8):653–61.
23. Feng M, et al. TAP1 and TAP2 polymorphisms associated with ankylosing spondylitis in genetically homogenous Chinese Han population. Hum Immunol. 2009;70(4):257–61.
24. Agrawal N, Brown M. Genetic associations and functional characterization of M1 aminopeptidases and immune-mediated diseases. Genes Immun. 2014;15(8):521.
25. Alvarez-Navarro C, de Castro JAL. ERAP1 structure, function and pathogenetic role in ankylosing spondylitis and other MHC-associated diseases. Mol Immunol. 2014;57(1):12–21.
26. Zhai J, et al. Immunogenetic study in Chinese population with ankylosing spondylitis: are there specific genes recently disclosed? Clin Dev Immunol. 2013;2013:419357.
27. de Castro JAL. How ERAP1 and ERAP2 shape the peptidomes of disease-associated MHC-I proteins. Front Immunol. 2018;9:2463.
28. Driscoll J, et al. MHC-linked LMP gene products specifically alter peptidase activities of the proteasome. Nature. 1993;365(6443):262.
29. Gaczynska M, Rock KL, Goldberg AL. γ-Interferon and expression of MHC genes regulate peptide hydrolysis by proteasomes. Nature. 1993;365(6443):264.

30. Westman P, et al. TAP1 and TAP2 polymorphism in HLA-B27-positive subpopulations: no allelic differences in ankylosing spondylitis and reactive arthritis. Hum Immunol. 1995;44(4):236–42.
31. Soleimanifar N, et al. Effect of food intake and ambient air pollution exposure on ankylosing spondylitis disease activity. Adv Rheumatol. 2019;59(1):9.
32. Roberts S, et al. Epigenetics of osteoarticular diseases: recent developments. Rheumatol Int. 2015;35(8):1293–305.
33. Lai N-S, et al. Association between cytokines and methylation of SOCS-1 in serum of patients with ankylosing spondylitis. Mol Biol Rep. 2014;41(6):3773–80.
34. Aslani S, et al. Evaluation of DNMT1 gene expression profile and methylation of its promoter region in patients with ankylosing spondylitis. Clin Rheumatol. 2016;35(11):2723–31.
35. Karami J, et al. Promoter hypermethylation of BCL11B gene correlates with downregulation of gene transcription in ankylosing spondylitis patients. Genes Immun. 2017;18(3):170.
36. Hao J, et al. Genome-wide DNA methylation profile analysis identifies differentially methylated loci associated with ankylosis spondylitis. Arthritis Res Ther. 2017;19(1):177.
37. Mohammadi H, et al. MicroRNA implications in the etiopathogenesis of ankylosing spondylitis. J Cell Physiol. 2018;233(8):5564–73.
38. Perez-Sanchez C, et al. Circulating microRNAs as potential biomarkers of disease activity and structural damage in ankylosing spondylitis patients. Hum Mol Genet. 2018;27(5):875–90.
39. Li Z, et al. The role of MicroRNAS in ankylosing spondylitis. Medicine. 2016;95(14):e3325.
40. Wang M, et al. Overexpression of miR-31 in peripheral blood mononuclear cells (PBMC) from patients with ankylosing spondylitis. Medical Science Monitor: International Medical Journal of Experimental and Clinical Research. 2017;23:5488.
41. Yang L, et al. miRNA copy number variants confer susceptibility to acute anterior uveitis with or without ankylosing spondylitis. Invest Ophthalmol Vis Sci. 2017;58(4):1991–2001.

5 Association of Non-HLA Genes with Ankylosing Spondylitis

Mahshid Rahmati and Mazdak Ganjalikhani Hakemi

5.1 Cytokines and Cytokine-Receptors

Cytokines are small secretory glycoproteins that interact with their receptors in controlling the proliferation and function of many immune and non-immune cells. In fact, cytokines, by telecommunication between different parts of the immune system or, creation of a bridge between intrinsic and adaptive immunity, make coordination in the system to encounter the infections. Moreover, they participate in tissue healing by recruiting other proteins and immune cells, as well as help them to move and penetrate into the tissues. Given the cytokines' importance in the function of the immune system, it is not far-fetched that they are involved in the various autoimmune diseases pathogenesis and hence, the study of them for describing the pathogenesis of diseases and their treatment has attracted a lot of attention. However, the study of these proteins with such an abundance (over 100 known types) and functional diversity is quite difficult. Cytokines exert their functions through cytokine receptors classified as type I & II cytokine receptor family, TNF receptor family, IL-1 receptor family and the related Toll-like receptors, receptor tyrosine kinases, TGF-β receptor family and IL-17 receptor, based on Vilcek J classification (Table 5.1).

Cytokines had initially been called lymphokine because it was generally believed that they were only secreted by lymphocytes. However, as its secretion was observed in other cell types, the term of cytokine was replaced. Subsequently, interleukin was also used for them because of their function, which was a link between leukocytes. It is the base of the new nomenclature of cytokines in which, an "IL" and a number

M. Rahmati · M. Ganjalikhani Hakemi (✉)
Department of Immunology, Faculty of Medicine, Isfahan University of Medical Sciences, Isfahan, Iran
e-mail: mghakemi@med.mui.ac.ir

M. H. Nicknam (ed.), *Ankylosing Spondylitis - Axial Spondyloarthritis*,
https://doi.org/10.1007/978-981-16-4733-8_5

Table 5.1 Cytokines receptor families and their related cytokines

Receptor family	cytokine
Type I cytokine receptor family	IL-2, IL-3, IL-4, IL-5, IL-6, IL-7, IL-9,IL-11, IL-13, IL-15, IL-21, IL-23, IL-27, IL-31, IL-35, GM-CSF, G-CSF
Type II cytokine receptor family	IFN-α/β, IFN-γ, IL-10, IL-19, IL-20, IL-22, IL-24, IL-26, IL-28, IL-29, IL-30
TNF receptor family	TNF-α, TNF-β,
IL-1 receptor family	IL-1α/β, IL-1F/G, IL-18, IL-33, IL-37
Receptor tyrosine kinases	IL-32, IL-16, IL-3, M-CSF, stem cell factor, FLT-3 ligand
TGF-β receptor family	TGF-β,
IL-17 receptor	IL-17A, IL-17B, IL-17C, IL-17D. IL-17E, IL-17F, IL-25

are applied to name a given cytokine. However, there is still a descriptive naming for some cytokines, such as Tumor Necrosis Factor (TNF) or Colony Stimulating Factors (CSFs) [1].

5.1.1 IL-1RN Gene

The gene of the IL-1 family, located in the chromosome 2 long arm, encodes IL-1A, IL-1B, and IL-1RN (IL-1 receptor antagonist). *IL1A* and *IL1B* genes code for IL-1α and IL-1β protein, respectively. These are inflammatory cytokines, and in coordination with IL-6, contribute to the development of systemic acute phase response. Given the key role of these cytokines in inflammation, their significance was reported in the pathogenesis of AS disease before genome-wide associated studies (GWAS). However, in the GWA studies, no association was found between the genes of these cytokines and the AS. In contrast, the association of AS with *IL1RN* on 2q14 region that encodes an antagonist receptor for IL-1α has been reported in GWA studies. This receptor, which operates competitively with IL-1R1, has an anti-inflammatory property and prevents IL-1α from sending the signal to the cells [2].

There is a difference between the type of mutations in IL-1RN and the onset of the disease in distinct races. The rs2310173 SNP of IL-1RN in the European population is strongly associated with AS, whereas this association does not exist in the Asian and middle-east populations, including China, Korea, and Iran [3, 4]. In these populations, the presence of rs30735 (C vs G allele or C carrier), rs31017 (G vs C allele), and rs315952(C carrier) SNP in the *IL1RN* gene has been evidenced to be associated with AS susceptibility. The rs31017 and rs30735 mutations, in addition to the Asian population, are also involved in the occurrence of AS in the Caucasian descent [2]. Despite the discovery of the IL-1RN gene's association with the risk of AS, the use of an antagonist for IL-1 receptor, Anakinra, has not been effective in AS treatment [5].

5.1.2 IL-6 Receptor Gene

Interleukin-6 is an inflammatory cytokine which similar to IL-1β is effective in inducing inflammation in both immune defense and autoimmune conditions. This cytokine is secreted by different cells like macrophage, epithelial and mesenchymal cells, and damages the joints and bones by osteoclast activation. Besides, IL-6, in coordination with TGF-β, acts as a mediator for Th17 differentiation. As the serum level of IL-6 has been shown to be increased in patients with AS, and considering its function, this cytokine can be a major player in the pathogenesis of the AS. IL-6 exerts its function through the IL-6 receptor (IL-6R) which is encoded on chromosome 1q21. The presence of rs4129267 SNP in *IL6R* has been demonstrated to be associated with increased soluble IL-6R and susceptibility to AS diseases in both Asian and European populations [6, 7]. Despite the discovery of IL-6R association with the risk of AS, using of Tocilizumab and Sarilumab (antibodies against IL-6R) has not been successful in the treatment of this disease in clinical trials except in few cases who were refractory to Anti-TNF therapy [6–11].

5.1.3 IL-12B Gene

Cytokine IL-12, via its heterodimer receptor, causes the naive T cells to T helper1 differentiation and also provokes the IFNγ production by NK cells. Despite the slight role of this cytokine in AS disease, the *IL12β* gene has received a great deal of attention in immunogenic studies. This gene encodes a protein called P40 which is a mutual subunit between IL-12 and IL-23 [12]. Knocking out of this gene in mice disrupts the Th1 and Th17 cells development [13]. The *IL12β* gene and its variants contribute to the risk of AS development, directly and indirectly by affecting the IL-23/IL-17 pathway and Th17 cell differentiation [14]. The *IL12β* gene is located on the long arm of chromosome 5, and the incidence of rs3212227 in its 3′ region and the occurrence of the AC/CC genotypes is associated with the AS risk in Taiwanese patients [15], although this association has not been observed in AS patients from China and Bulgaria [14–16]. In the Bulgarian population with AS, the presence of rs17860508 in the gene′s promoter has been confirmed [14]. In the European population, after proving the importance of this gene and its product in the pathogenesis of the AS disease, the rs10045431 and rs6871626 SNPs have been recognized as effective variants in the risk of AS [6]. The importance of rs6871626 SNP in susceptibility and severity of the AS disease has also been proved in Chinese patients with AS [9]. Despite the difference in IL-12β gene variants and the presence of AS in different ethnic groups, the treatment of AS patients by Ab against P40 has been effective in improving their symptoms and quality of their life.

5.1.4 IL-17 Gene

IL-17 is an unconventional cytokine, because neither cytokine nor receptor is similar to other known cytokines and receptors. The family of IL-17 contains 6 proteins, among them, IL-17A and IL-17F are inflammatory cytokines [17]. The main producer of IL-17A is the Th17 lymphocyte. This cytokine binds to its heterodimer receptor expressed on variant cell types and triggers signaling, induces inflammatory cytokines production such as TNF, IL-1, and IL-6, recruits inflammatory cells such as neutrophils and also induces the production of various antimicrobial proteins to fight against fungal and bacterial infections [18]. Despite the useful role of this cytokine in controlling infection, its aberrant production could lead to various autoimmune and auto-inflammatory diseases. IL-17A, in addition to its role in inflammation, induces the destruction of joints by up-regulating the matrix metalloproteinases (MMPs) and inhibiting the production of the matrix, and also by increasing the RANKL (Receptor activator of nuclear factor-kappa-B ligand) expression on osteoblastic cells, leads to bone destruction [19]. Thus, IL-17A can contribute to AS pathogenesis through these mechanisms. The defect in the *IL17* gene in the small arm of chromosome 6 (6p12) and its receptor in the arthritis mouse model, reduces the inflammation of the joints and prevents its degradation [20]. The HLA-B27 expressed in AS patients binds to KIR3DL2 on Th17 cells and CD15+ neutrophils and activates them [21]. In this manner, HLA-B27 is involved in inflammation caused by IL-17 in patients with AS. Regarding the approved role of this cytokine, application of anti-IL-17 and anti-IL-17 receptor monoclonal antibodies (mAb), such as Ixekizumab, Secukinumab, and Bordalumab, has been successfully investigated for controlling AS disease in clinical trials [22, 23].

5.1.5 IL-23 and IL-23 Receptor

IL-23 is another heterodimer cytokine that contains two subunits, P19 and P40. This cytokine is mainly secreted from macrophages and DC cells. IL-23, by binding to its heterodimer receptor on T cells, particularly Th17, acts as an activator for these cells. IL-23 cytokine is a head factor in the maintenance of Th17 phenotype; therefore, it is thought to be involved in extracellular bacteria defense and, also in the autoimmune and inflammatory diseases pathogenesis. IL-23 and IL-23 receptors are the essential parts in Th17 regulation. Given the importance of Th17 and its cytokines in the AS disease, the IL-23 and its receptor have attracted much attention in the pathogenesis and therapy of the disease.

In patients with AS, IL-23 serum levels and *P19* gene expression rising, as well as the presence of various IL-23R variants, have been observed [24]. The *IL23R* gene is an important predisposing factor for AS, as it is responsible for 9% of the genetic load of AS susceptibility [25]. This gene is located on chromosome 1p31, which by recruiting the β1 receptor of the IL-12β receptor, creates a heterodimer receptor. The rs11209026 SNP in the *IL23R* gene by altering the Arg381 to Gln381 affects IL-23R interaction with its signaling unit inside the cell, JAK2, and hampers the signaling in response to IL-23 [26]. In other words, this variant is protective against AS diseases. The difference in the incidence of this variant among healthy and AS individuals in the European and American populations has been strongly proven (OR: 0.6, CI = 95%) [27]. Nevertheless, this relation has been rejected in the Iranian and Chinese populations [28, 29]. The rs10889677 variant in which the A is replaced with C nucleotide in the *IL23R* gene has been shown as a risk factor for autoimmune diseases, such as Crohn's and rheumatoid arthritis disease. The arisen risk of AS disease by OR: 1.19 and OR: 1.26, CI = 95% has been reported in the European and American populations, respectively [4]. While in Asians there is no association between the rs10889677 variant and this disease [30]. The above-mentioned SNP, when is coincident with rs3212227 in the IL-12β gene, increases the severity of pain and ulcers in AS patients [15].

The rs1004819 SNP of the *IL23R* gene in an Iranian race, similar to the European and American descents, has been reported to be correlated with increased susceptibility to AS, while in other Asians, this relationship has not been demonstrated. Most of the AS-associated IL-23R SNPs including rs11465804, rs10489629, rs1343151, rs10489629, rs7517847 SNPs, and other above-mentioned variants in different races, have shown not to be associated or even not be polymorphic in the East Asian region. Only in one study on AS Chinese, rs17375018 has been introduced as a risky SNP in the *IL23R* gene [31]. Generally, IL-23R Polymorphisms are thought to be unaffiliated with the East Asian race, and in this descent, the associated polymorphisms of other factors in the IL-23R/IL-17 pathway might be effective in AS incidence. Despite the difference in the role of polymorphisms with the onset of AS disease in different races, the relation of the *IL23R* gene with AS disease has been confirmed and repeated in several studies.

5.1.6 TNF and TNF Receptor

Tumor necrosis factor (TNF) mediates an acute inflammatory response to microbes at the onset of infection. This cytokine is produced and secreted by stimulating the innate immune receptors of macrophages, monocytes, and other immune cells by foreign antigens. TNF by applying fever and recruiting inflammatory cells to the place of infection and incitement of protein secretion prepares the body for rapid combat with infection. By engagement its receptors, TNFR1 and TNFR2, TNF triggers the signal transduction in cells to induce some genes expression in order to induce proliferation, differentiation, and apoptosis. Although acute inflammation contributes to immune system resistance against the presence of infections, in autoimmune diseases, however, causes tissue damage and accumulation of immune cells for autoantigens.

In AS disease, an increase in the expression of TNF and TNF receptor genes and its destructive effects on the bones and joints has been informed. Therefore, Anti-TNF agents have recently been used to treat these patients in their short periods of high inflammatory situation; however, as noted earlier, a percentage of AS patients are not responsive to this treatment [8]. The gene of this cytokine is located on the small arm of chromosome 6. Increasing the expression of this gene directly affects the risk of AS, so that GWA studies have shown that the incidence of rs1800629 or TNF-308 G/A polymorphisms in the TNF promoter, which reduces the expression of this gene, is less in AS individuals than in control subjects. Also, the incidence of this SNP along with rs361525 or TNF-238 G/A as a haplotype has been shown protective for AS [32]. In contrast, an increased incidence of TNF-α 857 C/T SNP in people with AS in Asian populations has been demonstrated [4].

The function TNF in AS disease is practiced by binding to the TNFR on the mesenchymal cells surface. The gene of this receptor, TNFRSFA1, is located on chromosome 12p13. The incidence of rs4149570, rs4149577, and rs1800693 SNPs in the *TNFRSFA1* gene results in increased expression of TNFR in AS patients [32, 33]. Concurrence of rs1800693 and rs4149577 SNPs increases the risk of AS more than when just one of them is existed [34].

One of the effective epigenetic factors for TNF inhibition is mir130a which reduces TNF expression and secretion, and hence, participates in AS improvement [35]. Despite the relative improvement of AS with the Anti-TNF treatments, the difference in the study of the TNF gene indicates that this gene should be studied in more detail.

5.1.7 IL-10 Gene

IL-10 is a member of the heterodimer cytokines family that is involved in intrinsic and adaptive immune responses controlling. The production of this cytokine is accrued by macrophages, dendritic cells, Treg cells, and T-helpers 1 and 2 cells, and as a negative feedback regulator, acts to inhibit the costimulatory receptors' expression on macrophages and dendritic cells, as well as their functions. Despite the ability of this cytokine to control immunologic reactions and inflammation, and the general idea of diminished level or function of this cytokine in autoimmune diseases, the level of this cytokine increases in AS disease [36]. The *IL10* gene is located on chromosome 1q31 and there are many associated SNPs with this gene. GWAS studies on the populations of China and Taiwan have shown that −819 C/T SNP in the promoter of the IL-10 gene with an increscent effect on IL-10 expression, increases the AS risks [36, 37]. Enhancement in AS susceptibility has also been observed for -1082 G allele in Chinese patients. Despite the mentioned SNPs in the *IL10* gene which rise the risk of AS in Chinese patients by increasing IL-10 levels, the presence of rs4937362 in long noncoding RNA namely RP11-264E20 is a protective variant in AS diseases by increasing the level of anti-inflammatory cytokine IL-10 [38]. The use of this cytokine for therapeutic aspects requires more detailed studies in different populations for the transparency of IL-10 function in AS disease.

5.2 Overview on Signal Transduction

All immune responses from immune cells, cytokines, and chemokines require the effect of these factors on specific receptors to trigger intracellular signals for expressing genes to induced cellular differentiation, cells recruitment, and cytokine secretion for fighting against infections and tolerating autoantigens. Signaling begins with the binding of a ligand to a specific receptor. The receptors that trigger signaling are mostly (not all) integral membrane proteins on the plasma membrane that upon engagement of their external portion with the ligand, intracellular factors accumulate around their intracellular region. The integral receptors based on their intracellular portion, are divided into two types of tyrosine kinase receptor and non-tyrosine kinase receptors. These two types include cytokine receptors introduced in the previous section, intrinsic immune receptors such as Toll-like receptors (TLR) and Node-like receptors (NLR), epidermal growth factor receptors, and the platelet-derived growth factor receptor. In addition, other signaling receptors include G protein-coupled receptors (GPCRs), *nuclear receptors* such as vitamin D receptor and the glucocorticoid receptor, and *other classes of receptors* such as Notch family receptors, are involved in early events of signaling to perform a variety of reactions. After ligand binding to one of the above-mentioned receptors, a common occurrence in signal transduction is the phosphate addition to the tyrosine, serine, or threonine residues in the cytosolic portion of the receptors, and also to adaptor proteins. The requirement of this event is kinase enzymes that sometimes by several phases of phosphorylation, helps to the signal transmission. In addition to phosphorylation, promotion of signals also needs acetylation, methylation, and addition of ubiquitin molecules to the target proteins. Protein Adapters are physical interfaces for protein–protein interactions to promote the assembly of signaling molecules complexes in creating signal transduction. Some of the protein adaptors such as LAT, BLNK, SLP76 and GADS are involved in immune cell signaling. Totally, specific operating of receptors with adapter proteins and kinase enzymes generates activation of multiple transcription factors. These transcription factors such as NFκB (nuclear factor kappa-B), AP-1 (activator protein-1), and NFAT (Nuclear factor of activated T cells), in immune cells are involved in various immune functions (Fig. 5.1). In the following, the related genes of signaling proteins that are important in the occurrence and pathogenesis of the AS disease are discussed [39].

5.2.1 VDR Gene

The most prominent manifestations of the AS disease are inflammation from immune responses and abnormal bone mineral density (BMD). Vitamin D due to its effect on these manifestations is important in the development of bone inflammatory diseases such as ankylosing spondylitis. Regulating of immune responses through shifting balance of Th1 and Th17 to Th2 and Treg, inhibiting inflammatory cytokines and reducing antigen presentation and also regulating bone activity by creating homeostasis in calcium synthesis and bone metabolism occur by vitamin D. In AS disease, the amounts of active form of vitamin D, 1, 25-OH vit D, in serum is inversely correlated with the level of inflammatory factors ESR and CRP, and the disease severity [40]. Due to the membrane transmission ability of vitamin D, the vitamin D receptor (VDR) is located in the nucleus. This receptor, upon ligation, as a transcription factor, induced the expression of several genes. The ability of this gene to prevent autoimmune diseases can be due to the expression of this gene in

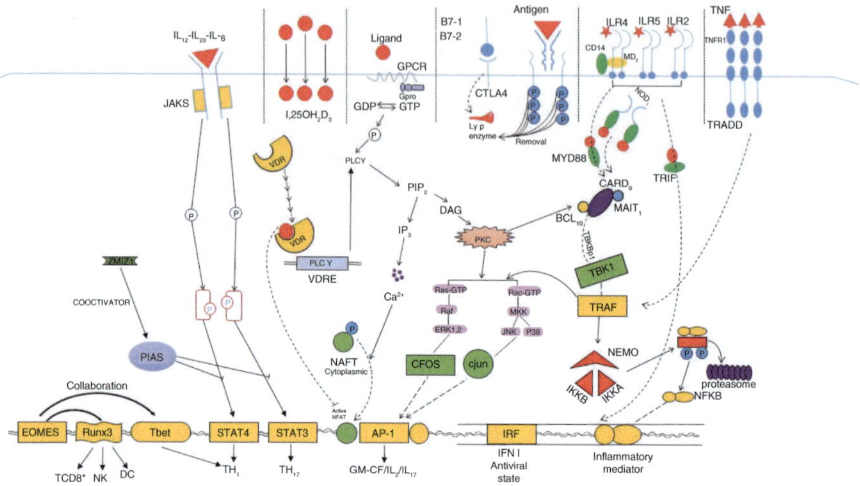

Fig. 5.1 Signal transduction: *An overview of some signaling pathways in which their mediators are involved in AS risks.* TNF receptor after binding to its cytokine ligand recruits the adaptor protein TRADD (TNF receptor-associated death domain), in turn, TRADD can recruit proteins called TRAFs (TNF receptor-associated factors), which possess a unique type of E3 ligase activity that polyubiquitinate NEMO/IKK complex. This event leads to the phosphorylation of NF-κB inhibitor (IκBα) and targets it for proteasomal degradation. IκBα degradation leads to the entry of active NF-κB transcription factors into the nucleus. On the other hand, TRAF molecules can trigger the MAP kinase cascade. In the MAP kinase pathway, Ras-GTP and Rac-GTP leading to parallel kinases enzyme cascade to synthesis Fos and Jun proteins which compose the best characterized AP-1 transcription factor. TLR2, TLR4, and TLR5 are expressed on the cell surface and after binding to their ligands, trigger two different signaling pathways. TLRs by recruiting adaptor protein MyD88 lead to NF-κB and AP-1 transcription factor activation and some of them by using adaptor protein TRIF, activate IRFs transcription factor. NOD2 is a member of the NOD-like receptor cytosolic family, which, by forming a signaling complex, activates the NF-κB transcription factor. CTLA-4 is a member of the CD28 family receptor which inhibits sending a signal from TCR by activating phosphatases enzyme to remove phosphate from the intracellular site of this receptor. A conformational change on GPCR after binding to its ligand permit the activation of heterotrimeric G protein by changing GDP to GTP. The major enzyme which activates by GPCR is PLC. Phosphorylated PLCγ1 catalyzes the hydrolysis of the plasma membrane phospholipid phosphatidylinositol 4,5-bisphosphate (PIP2), giving rise to two breakdown products, namely IP3 and DAG. DAG can activate the PKC enzyme which is involved in both MAP kinase and NF-κB signaling pathways. PKC induces the activation of the CARD9/BCL10/MALT1 complex. This complex by creating a connection with TBKBP1 and in turn TBK1 induces NF-κB transcription factor. IP3 produces a rapid increase in cytosolic-free calcium which activates NFAT and sends it to the nucleus. NFAT, by binding to the AP1 enhancer motif, stimulates the expression of some gene-like IL-2, IL-17, and GM-CSF. VDR, a ligand-dependent transcription regulator molecule belonging to the superfamily of nuclear receptors, after binding to 1,25 (OH)2D3, translocates to the nucleus where it binds to vitamin D response elements (VDRE) and induces some gene expression. Besides regulation through VDRE, VDR can inhibit genes by competition with NFAT transcription factors and inhibiting IL-2 expression. Cytokine receptors, after binding to cytokines by recruiting non-receptor tyrosine kinases called JAK, induce the phosphorylation and activation of the STATs transcription factor. The activated STATs are inhibited by PIAS which prevents STAT interaction with DNA. ZMIZ1 is a coactivator of PIAS. EOMES is a transcription factor that collaborates with T-bet in Th1 induction and RUNX3 in TCD8+, NK, and DC development

many immune cells. The effect of the VDR gene on the incidence of osteoarthritis and its association in the reduction of bone mineralization and increasing inflammation is an evidence of the importance of this gene in AS disease [40]. The *VDR* gene is located on chromosome 12q13. The most known SNPs of this gene include TaqI, BsmI, ApaI at the end of a gene, in the 3′UTR region, and FokI that is in the promoter of VDR. Among them, FokI and TaqI polymorphisms are in exon and directly affect the structure of the VDR protein for binding to vitamin D, while ApaI and BsmI are in the non-translational region and only are effective in transcriptional gene activity [41]. The presence of SNPs in the *VDR* gene not only influences the *VDR* gene's expression but also due to its role as a transcription factor, is responsible for the expression of other immune and inflammatory genes. Also, some of these polymorphisms trigger the activity of VDR protein without the presence of its ligand. Studies about the importance of *VDR* gene polymorphisms in the incidence of AS disease are limited and only in the Chinese population with AS, the relationship between the TaqI SNP alone, and also its presence with BsmI SNP in the form of a haplotype with a risk of AS has been found [42].

5.2.2 TLR4 Gene

Toll-like receptor (TLR) is a subset of innate immune pattern recognition receptor that detects different types of microbes. TLRs are different in terms of function and location in cells, and in humans, they are divided into nine groups named TLR1 to TLR9. These receptors are type I integral membrane glycoproteins which with leucine-rich repeats flanked region detecting a ligand and transmitting signal by intracellular region which is similar to that of IL-1R and IL-18R cytokines. Similar to other innate immune receptors, TLRs distinguish autoantigen from foreigners by detecting repeatable patterns in bacteria and viruses. The TLR attachment is specific to each of these ligands and is sometimes facilitated by other proteins. The TLR4 collaborates with CD14 and MD2 for binding to LPS of the Gram-negative bacteria cell wall. This receptor after binding to the ligand, by using TRIF and MYD88 adapter proteins, activates IRF and NF-κB transcription factors, respectively. Subsequently, IFN-I cytokines expression is induced by the IRF transcription factor for the antiviral defense, and NF-κB transcription factor causes the secretion of inflammatory cytokines and adaptive immune response stimulation. TLR4 is involved in the autoimmune diseases' development with its extensive ability to produce immune responses. In the case of AS, the TLR4 effect is not limited to stimulating the immune response and the incidence of inflammation, but also, this receptor by expressing on mature osteoclast cells and increasing the expression of RANKL on osteoblasts enhances osteoclastogenesis and osteoporosis. This process is followed by bone repairing, which in AS patients leads to deviated bone formation and bony ankylosis. The location of *TLR4* gene is on the long arm of chromosome 9, and the expression of this gene increases in AS patients [43]. In addition to the mRNA of the *TLR4* gene, among these receptors, enhancement of *TLR5* expression and by a lesser extent, *TLR2* expression occurs in AS patients, which are severely reduced during treatment by anti-TNF agents [44].

CD14 by interaction with LBP (lipopolysaccharide-binding protein) on LPS, collaborates with a TLR-4 in the provocation of immune responses. The presence of −159 C > T SNP in the CD14 gene in chromosome 5q31 increases the susceptibility to AS disease [45]. Given the importance of TLR4 in AS disease, several genetic studies have been conducted on this gene located on the large arm of chromosome 9. The two common SNPs in the *TLR4* gene are Asp299Gly and Thr399Ile, which have been shown effective in increasing the risk of inflammatory diseases such as IBD. About the population with AS, basically, there has been no difference in the incidence of these two SNPs in comparison to healthy subjects [46, 47].

The target gene of Let7i microRNA is *TLR4*. Increasing this microRNA expression in AS individuals is associated with a reduction in *TLR4* expression which can be protective for AS [44].

5.2.3 G Protein-Coupled Receptor Gene

G protein-coupled receptors (GPCRs) are plasma membrane receptors that act by activating associated GTP binding proteins. The activated G protein initiates downstream signaling events which mediate several signaling pathways. An association with AS has been identified in three loci encoded G protein-coupled receptors including GPR35, GPR37, and GPR65 located on 2q37, 7q31, and 14q31 chromosomes, respectively. T cell death-associated gene 8 (*TRAG8*) is a GPR65 mouse homolog, leading the inhibition of pro-inflammatory cytokines and also inducing thymocyte apoptosis. GPR37 Over-expression results in misfolded protein, then, the accumulation of these proteins, leading to autophagy process. Transmission of the indoleamine 2, 3- dioxygenase) IDO (signal, which is the major mediator in the immune system and causes tolerance in dendritic cells, is done by GPR35. These receptors play a key role in the development of inflammatory and autoimmune diseases due to their functions in the transmission of different signals, the development of T cells in the thymus, and the induction of tolerance in DC cells, but the study of their exact role in AS, as well as the level of their effectiveness, needs to be investigated in more detail [6, 48].

5.2.4 CTLA-4 Gene

Activation of T cells in responding to antigens, in addition to TCR binding to the peptide, requires a secondary signal that is resulted from the attachment of co-receptors on T cells to ligands on APCs. The importance of these connections is so great that the cells will refrain from responding to the antigens if they are not present or replaced by inhibitory receptors. CTLA-4 is one of the important inhibitors of T cells in generating tolerance to autoantigen, as well as a balance in the response and activity of T cells in the immune system. The CTLA-4 knocked out mice encounters early death because of uncontrolled lymphocytes activity. This receptor is a member of the CD28 family receptor which its ligand, similar to CD28, is B7. This receptor administers its inhibitory activity by interfering in the binding of ligand B7 to CD28 as well as activating phosphatase and removing phosphor from the TCR and CD28 signal transduction molecules. The strong function of CTLA-4 in maintaining tolerance and the balance in T cells activity against pathogens leads to the importance of this receptor in the pathogenesis and therapeutic approaches in autoimmune diseases. Also, the association of *CTLA4* gene polymorphisms with several autoimmune diseases, such as Graves' and type 1 diabetes disease has been proven. Two functional polymorphisms of this gene, +49 A/G and − 318 C/T, have been studied several times in patients with AS. The CTLA-4 + 49 polymorphism that occurs in the first exon of a *CTLA4* gene with the replacement of the nucleic G instead of C, leads to a reduction of CTLA-4 receptor on the cell surface and also its soluble form. The result of this polymorphism is a deficiency in CTLA-4 function and an increase in the amount of CRP in individuals with AS. However, this SNP is not effective in increasing AS risk in Asian populations. The CTLA-4 -138 polymorphism in which, T is located instead of C, induced enhancement of CTLA-4 gene expression. Therefore, the presence of this SNP can be protective against AS diseases. In addition to the above *CTLA4* polymorphism, there are several polymorphisms that have not yet been investigated in association with the risk of AS or also protection against it. It is possible to find the function of CTLA-4 in AS disease more clearly by examination of other polymorphisms and also the investigation of above mentioned two polymorphisms in non-Asian races.

5.2.5 PD-1 Gene

PD-1, similar to CTLA-4 is a member of CD28 family receptors. This receptor inhibits signal transduction in T cells upon binding to PD-L1 (expressed on APC and many other tissue cells) and PD-L2 (expressed on APC) [49]. Despite the name of this receptor, PD-1 does not play a role in the apoptosis of T cells, and it is involved in inhibiting the activity of these cells, and therefore, the elimination of this gene in mice is equal to the incidence of autoimmune diseases. Any change in the PD-1 gene that blocks the interaction of this receptor with its ligand is important in the development of autoimmune diseases, such as type 1 diabetes. The *PD-1* gene is similar to CTLA-4 on the long arm of chromosome 2. The incidence of rs2227982 SNP in the fifth exon of this gene leads to a change in the valine amino acid to alanine and, by changing the interaction of this receptor with its ligand, increases the risk of AS. The risk of AS in accompaniment of rs2227982 with rs2227981 variant and the presence of CT haplotype in the *PD-1* gene is further increased, although the rs2227981 variant alone has no effect on the AS susceptibility [37, 50–54].

5.2.6 PTPN22 Gene

The dominant mechanism of maintaining the immune cell's tolerance against auto-antigens or maintaining the balance in response to pathogens is inhibiting signaling units phosphorylation via the intracellular phosphatase enzymes. Lymphocyte tyrosine phosphatase (LYP) is a non-receptor classical type I phosphatase, which is present in hematopoietic cells. LYP is encoded by the *PTPN22* gene placed on the 1p13 chromosome, and hence, this phosphatase is also called PTPN22. This phosphatase plays a key role in the negative regulation of T cells and the occurrence of some SNPs in the PTPN22 gene resulting in decreased gene expression or LYP function impairment, and is effective in increasing the risk of autoimmune diseases. The incidence of PTPN22 1858 C/T SNP, which is highly related to the risk of T1D, is in equal frequency between AS patients and healthy. In the Taiwanese population with AS, the presence of PTPN22 1123G/C SNP in the promotor of this gene, leads to a decrease in the PTPN22 expression and reduction in inhibition of T cells, thereby increasing the risk of AS. As previously mentioned, the presence of CTLA-4 + 49 A/G does not increase the risk of AS, but the accompaniment of this SNP with PTPN22 1123 G/C further raises the risk of AS. The simultaneous presence of these two SNPs and, thereby, the simultaneous reduction in CTLA-4 and PTPN22's activity, increase the risk of IBD, as well in patients with AS.

5.2.7 CARD9 Gene

Caspase recruitment domain-containing protein 9 (CARD9) functions as an adaptor protein to transduce receptor events to transcription factors. It has a critical role in the innate immune system and has a central role in responses to both intracellular and extracellular bacterial/fungal components through their respective pattern recognition receptors. It is downstream of dectin-1 to response to fungal and cytoplasmic PRR same as NOD2 to response to intracellular pathogens. Signal transporting of these receptors after activation of Syk (splenic tyrosine kinase), occurs by interaction of CARD9 with BCL-10 and MALT1 to induce the canonical NF-κB pathway and also p38 mitogen-activated protein kinase (MAPK) and c-Jun N-terminal kinase (JNK) pathways for pro-inflammatory responses. In addition to innate immunity, CARD9 signaling is also involved in the activation and modulation of adaptive immunity. This protein after stimulation of CARD9 signaling leads to the maturation of dendritic cells into full effector antigen-presenting cells which can prime naive T cells for differentiation to interferon γ-producing Th1 cells and also the generation of IL-17-producing Th17 cells.

The role of CARD9 in inflammatory responses and Th17 differentiation is strong evidence for the functional effect of this protein in the AS disease. The *CARD9* gene is located on chromosome 9q34. There are effective mutations with inflammatory diseases, in the region of this gene and its adjacent genes. Similar to *IL23R* which has some common variants in susceptibility to IBD and AS, *CARD9* as the second common variant is also involved in susceptibility to both IBD and AS. Accordingly, the rs10870077 SNP in *CARD9* is effective in susceptibility to both IBD and AS diseases.

One of the strongest SNPs in the *CARD9* gene is rs4077515 which raises the risk of susceptibility to AS in European ancestry. It could be interesting that this variant cannot be found in the Chinese population, and also in Iranian, just found in HLA-B27 negative Iranian patients as a protective variant. Another SNP in the *CARD9* gene that is independently effective in AS risks in European ancestry is rs10781500 that same as above SNP occurs by presenting C nucleotide instead of G and T nucleotides. There are some SNP in the *CARD9* gene such as rs10781496, rs10781499, rs3812558 that they have a strong linkage disequilibrium (LD) for presenting together, and also each of them individually is associated in susceptibility to AS diseases. In addition to the *CARD9* gene, the adjacent genes are also important in AS development, and this is why this locus is important in AS studies [3, 55–57].

5.2.8 TBKBP1 Gene

TBKBP1, also known as Sintbed and located on the 17q21 chromosome, is an adaptor protein that binds to TBK1. TANK-binding kinase is an enzyme involved in the NF-κB and IRFs signal transduction pathways. The exact function of TBKBP1 in the process of TBK1 activation has not yet been fully defined, but evidences suggest that TBKPB1 plays a role in creating a connection between TBK1-IKK and upstream signaling pathways, possibly by binding to TBK1 and interaction with TRAF. Therefore, TBKBP1 with its role in TNF signaling pathway has attracted great attention in AS pathogenesis studies. An rs8070463 SNP on chromosome 17q21 near *TBKBP1* has been reported to be associated with AS susceptibility in patients of Western European descents but this SNP is not associated with AS susceptibility or even AS severity in Han Chinese AS patients [58, 59].

5.2.9 TRADD Gene

The primary molecule transducing signals in TNFR1 is TNF receptor-associated death domain (TRADD) which is immediately recruited to TNFR1 after activation by TNF. The death domain in both molecules mediates the communication between TNFR1 and TRADD. The binding of TRADD to TNFR1 leads to the recruitment of innumerous associated signaling molecules. TNF by recruitment of FAS-associated death domain (FADD) and in turn caspases enzymes leads to apoptosis. In addition to FADD, TRADD also has a TRAF-binding motif that leads to the use of TRAF1 and 2, and hence can induce the activation of NF-κB and MAP kinases to regulate pro-inflammatory cytokine production. TRADD because of its role in TNF signaling and inflammatory cytokine production is a functional candidate gene in AS disease pathogenesis. *TRADD* gene is located on chromosome 16q22. In this site, there are two strong associated SNP with AS, namely rs9033 and rs868213, in which TRADD is located between them. Near to the *TRADD* gene, there are rs6979 and rs9939768 SNPs, and the association of them with AS has been proved several times [60].

5.2.10 STAT3 Gene

Signaling transducer and activator of transcription-3 (STAT3) is a member of transcription factors, which, in collaboration with Janus kinases, triggers JAK-STAT signaling pathways downstream of cytokine receptors. STAT3 is known as an effective transcription factor for differentiation and maintenance of Th17 cells in response to the IL-6 and IL-23 cytokines. Loss of function of STAT3 mutations results in Job's syndrome, in which an absence of Th17 lymphocytes leads to recurrent severe infections, especially with extracellular bacteria. This gene and its mutations have been shown to be associated with IBD which is clinically associated with AS. According to the association of IL-23R with AS, elevated amounts of circulating Th17 cells in the blood of AS patients and the similarities found in the pathogenesis of IBD and AS disease, *STAT3* is an effective gene in AS susceptibility. *STAT3* gene is located on 17q21 and rs744166 and rs6503695 SNPs of *STAT3* are strongly associated with AS in European Caucasians. In addition to the European ancestry, the association of the rs2293152 variant of *STAT3* with AS has also been found in Chinese. Despite the low association of *IL23R* with AS in the Chinese population, the association of AS with the *STAT3* gene indicates that there are different mechanisms of the disease pathogenesis that have the same impact on Th17 cells. In addition to the mutations listed above, there are some SNPs in the *STAT3* gene such as rs1053008, rs236580, and rs4103200 which have shown a modest association with AS disease.

STAT3 is activated with phosphorylation by JAK2 as an especial kinase for this transcription factor. Despite the importance of JAK2 in IL-23R and its association with Crohn's disease, any relation of JAK2 with AS has not yet been found. In addition to JAK2, another kinase enzyme to STAT3 phosphorylation is TYK2. The rs280518 SNP in the *TYK2* gene happens very rarely but has the strongest relation with susceptibility to AS (OR = 7.7; CI = 95%).

As noted above, the phosphorylated form of STAT3 is an activated form that is inhibited by mir-29b-1-5p. This microRNA as a regulator of the IL-23 pathway has been shown to be increased in the AS patients and induced enhancement of IFNγ and angiogenin but not IL-17A and TNF [34, 61–63].

5.2.11 STAT4 Gene

STAT4 is another cytoplasmic transcription factor that is involved in JAK-STAT pathways in responding to cytokine receptors. STAT4 transmits signals induced by IL-12 and IL-23, which all are important cytokines in the autoimmune diseases' development. Also, it was found that STAT4 plays crucial roles in the differentiation and proliferation of both Th1 and Th17 cells, which are crucial effectors in chronic inflammatory disorders like AS and rheumatoid arthritis (RA). *STAT4* gene that is located on chromosome 2q33 is expressed in activated peripheral blood monocytes, macrophages, and dendritic cells at the inflammation sites. This gene and its SNP have been reported to be correlated with autoimmune diseases like RA, but few studies are performed about the association of STAT4 and AS susceptibility. In the Chinese Han population, this variant is significantly associated with AS susceptibility and severity augmented, but this relation has not been seen in Southwest Chinese people with AS [64, 65].

5.2.12 RUNX3 Gene

Runx3 is a transcription factor that is effective in expressing many genes, including cytokines, proteins related to apoptosis and growth. This transcription factor is important in the development of many immune cells. *RUNX3* is a key gene in CD8 lymphocyte differentiation and therefore, in the event of inhibition or reduction of the expression of this gene, a sharp decline in the number of CD8+ T cells has happened. The differentiation of CD8+ T cells is driven by the binding of IL-7 to IL-7R and inducing of RUNX3 expression. In addition to CD8+ T cells, this transcription factor is also effective in the development of DC and NK cells, and in the event of a damage, Langerhans maturation to DCs is also defected. The *RUNX3* gene, located on the 1p36 chromosome, plays a role in the onset and progression of many diseases, including gastric cancer, as well as autoimmune and inflammatory diseases. The effect of the *RUNX3* gene on inflammatory diseases is so great that knocking out of this gene causes the presence of IBD in mice. Also, due to the presence of the RUNX3 transcription factor in the TGFβ signaling pathway, the role of this gene in the development of autoimmune diseases is justifiable. The occurrence of the rs4648889 variant in the regulatory area above the promotor of the *RUNX3* gene increases the risk of AS by reducing the expression of this gene. Existing of rs11249215, rs7551188, and rs13995621 variants in the *RUNX3* gene, by reducing the gene expression, in addition to increasing the risk of the AS disease, are effective in reducing the patient's activity and increasing the severity of the disease. These RUNX3 SNPs associated with AS are also associated with decreased CD8+ T lymphocytes count that are key cells in AS pathogenesis, likely in response to antigenic peptides presented by HLA-B27. *RUNX3* gene involvement in the severity of AS disease, in addition to the risk of this disease, can be due to the effect of this gene on the inflammation process [58, 66, 67].

5.2.13 TBX21 Gene

TBX21 is located on the 17q21 chromosome and encodes for T-bet. T-bet is a transcription factor that was firstly introduced in CD4+ T cells as the key Th1 lineage-defining transcription factor which controls the IFNγ and CXCR3 expression. However, it is now obvious that T-bet is widely expressed in immune cell subsets and controls the function and differentiation of many cell types including CD8+ T cells, NK cells, and B cells. T-bet directly regulates the transcription of IL-23R which is a pivotal receptor for the survival of Th17 cells. The development and terminal maturation of immature NK cells, especially innate lymphoid cells (ILCs) which are liver residents, are dependent on T-bet. The presence of T-bet in CD8+ T cells is effective in their function. In fact, the existence of T-bet in CD8+ T cells increases the production of inflammatory cytokines such as IFNγ and IL-17 and this type of CD8+ T cells is increased in people with AS. The presence of rs11657479 SNP in the 3′ UTR of *TBX21* gene leads to an increment in the expression of this gene in AS patients, but not in healthy people. This SNP is correlated with AS risks and also weakly with the disease activity. In addition to this variant, rs9901869 that is SNP in the region between *NPEPPS-TBKBP1-TBX21* genes is also important in the increase of AS risk. Anti-TNF treatment in patients with AS cannot be effective in reducing T-bet expression in CD8+ T cells and the inflammation caused by these cells, while the inhibition of T-bet in controlling inflammation of AS disease have attracted much attention [68–70].

5.2.14 Ancillary Mediators Involved in Lymphocyte Differentiation

In addition to the above-mentioned transcription factors or coactivators which are effective in T cells development, and as a result, in ankylosing spondylitis pathogenesis, there are some signaling mediator genes such as EOMES, ZMIZ1, BACH2, and SH2B3 which are involved in CD8+, CD4+ T cells differentiation and probably in AS susceptibility. *EOMES* gene on the short arm of chromosome 3 encodes eomesodermin which is a transcription factor involved in CD8+ T cell differentiation and is stimulated by RUNX3. In addition to RUNX3, eomesodermin also corporates with T-bet to induce IFNγ production by CD8+ T cells and in the event of a defect, CD8+ T cells have been shown to express IL-17. Some variants of this gene can influence the CD8+ T cells count and AS predisposition. *ZMIZ1* (zinc finger MIZ-type containing 1) gene is located on chromosome 10q22 and encodes a transcriptional coactivator of the Protein Inhibitor of Activated STAT (PIAS)-like family, and in addition to its effect on STAT-mediated cytokine signaling, it is probably effective in T cell differentiation. The presence of rs1250550 in this gene is associated with both CD8+ T cells count and AS risk. *BACH2* (B cell-specific transcription factor) and *SH2B3* (SH2B adaptor protein) genes, located on chromosome 6p15 and 12q24, respectively, are associated with both ankylosing spondylitis risk and CD4+ T lymphocyte count. Although the relationship between these factors and AS disease has been noted, further studies of the variants of these genes among healthy people with AS patients, and their effects on the AS predisposition are required.

5.3 Other Associated Genes with AS Disease

In addition to genes of cytokines and involved mediators in signal transduction, some others in association with AS disease have been reported. These genes are linked to the AS disease due to their function on the immune system and inflammation, as well as their effect on bone formation. We discussed these genes in the following paragraphs of this chapter.

5.3.1 ANTXR2

The ANTXR2 (anthrax toxin receptor 2) gene encodes a transmembrane protein that recognizes and binds to the anthrax toxin to allow its attachment to the cells and triggers the disease process. It expresses primarily in macrophages and human tissue including liver, lung, placenta, small intestine, kidney, colon, and skeletal muscles. ANTXR2 is involved in capillary formation and hence, it is also known as capillary morphogenesis protein 2 (CMP2). ANTXR2, in addition to anthrax toxin, binds to type IV collagen and laminin, which shows the ANTXR2 role in extracellular matrix adhesion. *ANTXR2* gene is located on chromosome 4q21 and some recessive mutations in the *ANTXR2* gene are related to two autosomal diseases, including juvenile hyaline fibromatosis and infantile systemic hyalinosis. Although there is no functional justification for linking the *ANTXR2* gene to AS disease, some variants of this gene are associated with increased susceptibility to AS disease. The expression of this gene that can be inhibited by miR-124 has been found to be similar between AS patients and healthy controls, but the presence of rs4333130 and rs4389526 variants in the *ANTXR2* gene is associated with AS in European ancestry from different countries. This association has not been seen in the Han Chinese population and also in the Korean population, rs4333130 SNP is definitely rare. These differences show a substantial distinct genetic background of East Asian populations from Western populations that also have been observed in other variants. The rs4333130 SNP is also related to AS disease in Iranian so that the presence of C allele and CC genotype are found to be significantly protective against AS, and in contrast, patients with CT genotype exhibit significantly higher pain and disease activity scores [3, 33, 71, 72].

5.3.2 SNAPC4

The snRNA-activating protein complex subunit 4 (SNAPC4) is the largest subunit of the SNAP complex, a multi-subunit complex of proteins that consists of at least four stably associated subunits. SNAPC4 is essential for snRNA gene transcription by both RNA polymerases II and III because the promotors of these two polymerases have similar enhancers. The impact of SNAPC4 in autoimmune disorders is difficult to imagine, but in AS disease has been reported that SNAPC4 SNPs are likely in strong LD with *CARD9*-associated SNPs. The *SNAPC4* gene similar to *CARD9* is located on the 9q34 chromosome. The expression of SNAPC4 reduced in peripheral leukocytes of AS patients in comparison with healthy people. The presence of rs11145835 SNP in the intronic region of the SNAPC4 gene is related to a reduction of *CARD9* and *SNAPC4* expression which is associated with increased risk of AS in the Han Chinese population. The rs3812571 SNP in *SNAPC4* is also related to AS risk in Han Chinese and European populations but not in Iranian. This SNP is in strong LD with rs4077515 SNP in the *CARD9* gene. In the European population in addition to the above SNP, the presence of rs11794847 and rs10781507 SNPs are effective in enhancement of AS risk. These strong associations observed with SNPs in *SNAPC4* and AS disease are more likely the result of strong LD between this gene and *CARD9* [73].

5.3.3 KIF21B

Kinesin family member 21B (KIF21B) gene belongs to kinesin motor proteins family, that are involved in the transportation of required components along with the cells. KIFs have a role in mitosis and meiosis by organizing the spindle and moving the chromosome. In neurons, KIF21B is located in dendrites and induces the transportation of components through axonal and dendritic microtubules. In addition to neurons, KIF21B is also expressed in multiple immune cells including CD4+ and CD8+ T cells, CD56 bright natural killer cells, and B cells. This gene due to its function in the structural rearrangement of the cytoskeleton necessary for the formation of the immunological synapse can be effective in exerting a very consequential role in the activation of immune cells and the formation of immune-mediated inflammation. KIF21B has been shown to be associated with IBD, MS, and ulcerative colitis diseases. In white European ancestry from the UK, USA, Canada, and Australia it has been demonstrated that the rs11584383 SNP in downstream of the KIF21B gene is strongly associated with AS. Another SNP in this gene that is related to susceptibility to AS disease in European ancestry is rs2297909 polymorphism. Different variants of the *KIF21B* gene in the Chinese population have been reported to influence the susceptibility to AS disease. The rs2297909 polymorphism is unrelated to AS in a Chinese population, and instead of that the presence of rs502658 and rs10494829 polymorphisms independently are the susceptibility markers for AS. In addition to the above-mentioned variants, two other SNP namely, rs756254 and rs296560, with T allele and TT genotype increase the AS risk significantly [74–76].

5.3.4 PTGER4

Prostaglandins are oxygenated metabolites of arachidonic acid that are produced by cyclooxygenase enzyme and act through 7-transmembrane domain-type receptors. Prostaglandin E2 receptor 4 (PTGER4) gene, which is located on the 5p13 chromosome, encodes EP4 subunit receptor for prostaglandin E2. Prostaglandin E2 exerts its effects on immune regulation and bone metabolism through interaction with this EP4 receptor on the surface of different cells. PTGER4 stimulates dendritic cells to produce IL-23 and in turn, this cytokine increases the expansion of Th17 and IL-17A production. IL-17A and IL-23 levels, and Th17 lymphocyte counts are all known to be effective in ankylosing spondylitis pathogenesis. In addition to immune response,

PTGER4 is involved in bone remodeling including resorption of existing bone and de novo bone formation. Therefore, PTGER4 due to its role in linking inflammation and bone formation is important in AS pathogenesis. The expression of PTGER4 increases in a synovial sample of people with spondyloarthritis. In European ancestry populations from different countries with AS the presence of rs12186979 and rs10440635 SNPs which are near to the *PTGER4* are related to AS susceptibility disease. In East Asian ancestry, the peak of association with AS is different from European, and on them, the rs13354346 SNP in the intronic region of the *PTGER4* gene is related to AS disease [6, 57, 77].

5.3.5 PPARGC1B

The Peroxisome Proliferator-Activated Receptor-Gamma, Coactivator 1, Beta (PPARGC1B) gene, which encodes PGC-1B, is on chromosome 5q32. This genetic region is associated with type 2 diabetes and breast cancer. The exact cause of the association with these diseases is unknown, but with regard to the well-known properties of PGC-1B protein, it is understandable. PPARGC1B plays a critical role in energy metabolism, including gluconeogenesis, thermogenesis, fatty acid β-oxidation, and mitochondrial biogenesis. A central transcription factor in the control of mitochondrial biogenesis is Nuclear Respiratory Factor 1 (NRF1), which is regulated by PPARGC1B. The functions of osteoclasts are inhibited due to reduced oxidative phosphorylation and also oxidative phosphorylation dysfunction plays a pivotal pathogenic role in several human diseases. PGC-1B over-expression can lead to a marked improvement in oxidative phosphorylation defects. Knocking down of *PGC-1B* leads to inhibition in osteoclast differentiation. Whereas, *PPARGC1B* induces the activation of osteoclast by a coordinate in mitochondrial biogenesis. With an imbalance between osteoblasts and osteoclasts and enhancement in osteoclast activation, the action of ossification predominates and leads to osteophyte formation and even ankyloses. These events are the marks characterization of AS disease. The association of this gene with AS disease in the presence of rs11959820 SNP has been shown in patients of Western European descent. In addition to European, PPARGC1B is also associated with susceptibility to AS disease in Chinese and effects on patients' function in the presence of rs7379457 and rs32579 SNPs [58].

5.3.6 ANO6 Gene

In human cells, between the two inner and outer membranes, there are asymmetric phospholipids which under some physiological conditions, these phospholipids are rotated and lead to phosphatidylserine exposure by calcium assist. The anoctamin 6 (ANO6) gene encodes a multipass transmembrane protein belonging to the anoctamin family, which mediates phosphatidylserine exposure. For this reason, this gene which also known as TMEM16F is involved in apoptosis, platelet function, and also mineralization of bone that occur by osteoblast. Knocking out of the *ANO6* gene in mice has resulted in osteoporosis which shows the involvement of this gene in osteoblast phosphatidyl scrambling. This gene due to its role in bone development is probably related to AS disease. In AS patients from the Asian population, the presence of rs17095830 SNP on the 12q12 chromosome within the *ANO6* gene leads to enhancement of AS risk [74–78].

5.3.7 Β-Defensin Gene Clusters

The β-defensin gene clusters on chromosome 8p23 including DEFB4A, DEFB104, DEFB103, and DEFB1, encoded β-defensin peptides which preserve the epithelial cells against microbe-induced injury and is also effective in inflammation and enhancing immune function. This gene region is one of the most copy numbers variable regions of the human genome. The copy number variations of the *DEFB4* gene are related to psoriasis and Crohn's disease which both are inflammatory diseases. About AS disease, a higher copy number (CN) of *DEFB4–2* is related to a decreased AS risk in comparison with a lower copy number. In addition, CN enhancement of *DEFB4–2* is also related to diminished severity of AS. This is while the CN of *DEFB4–1* and *DEFB103* are not associated with AS disease. It can be concluded that the CN of the β-defensin gene may play a different role in multiple autoimmune diseases [79].

5.3.8 Pentraxin3

Pentraxin3 (PTX3) same as CRP and SAP, is a member of the pentraxin superfamily, which participates in the procedures of acute inflammation and immune response against pathogens. This plasma protein is encoded by the *PTX3* gene, located on chromosome 3q25. PTX3 is produced by macrophages, endothelial cells, and dendritic cells in response to TNF and IL-1 inflammatory cytokines. In inflammatory and autoimmune diseases, such as lupus erythematosus, rheumatoid arthritis, and AS, an increase in plasma levels of PTX3 has been observed. PTX3 plasma levels are a biomarker for the diagnosis and prognosis of some diseases, but it is not related to other inflammatory markers including CRP and ESR. Anti TNF therapy in AS patients, is not effective on increased PTX3 levels despite its effect on CRP and ESR levels. PTX3 SNPs are associated with the plasma level of this protein and by that are associated with some diseases' pathogenesis. In AS patients the presence of rs3816527 SNP with C allele and CC genotype, and also rs3845978 SNP carrying T allele and CT genotype are strongly associated with AS risk. These two SNPs with rs2305619 SNP, which is related to increasing PTX3 plasma level, but not AS risk, are in strong LD, and the presence of these three SNPs together, increases AS risk definitely [80, 81].

5.3.9 MIF Gene

MIF gene is located on the 22q11 chromosome and codes a macrophage migration inhibitory factor protein that regulates both the innate and adaptive immune responses and is effective in inflammation and inducing TNF production from monocytes. This protein is associated with several autoimmune conditions including IBD, MS, SLE. About ankylosing spondylitis, this protein gains attention due to its role in inflammation and also inducing mineralization in osteoblast. The level of MIF is increased in serum and synovial fluid of AS patients; and also the presence of MIF -173 G/C genotype in the Indian population with AS, elevates the AS predisposition with OR = 5.00, CI = 95%. This result was not repeated in the population of AS in turkey but the presence of MIF -173 G/G genotype in AS patients, is in relation to age and disease duration in Turkish people [82]. This gene and its variants need to be studied in other races and its relevance to the pathogenesis and risk of the AS disease must be investigated [45].

5.3.10 BCL11B

B-cell chronic lymphocytic leukemia/lymphoma 11B (BCL11B) gene is located on human chromosome 14q32. BCL11B is involved in T cell differentiation, development, and proliferation probably through the regulation of IL-2 expression. Therefore, this gene by elevating IL-2 expression can play a role in increasing the immune responses. The overexpression of this gene has been associated with malignancies in T cell, and the lower expression of that has been seen in AS patients which the hypermethylation of BCL11B promotors can be a reason for this event in an individual with AS. In addition to these regulator epigenetic events, the *BCL11B* gene is targeted by mir-124, mir-363, mir-21, and mir-16 which all are expressed differently between AS patients and healthy people. The *BCL11B* gene expression reduction is not related to AS clinical manifestation so the exact effect of this gene in AS diseases is not clear yet [83–85].

5.3.11 Autophagy-Related Genes

Autophagy is the natural, regulated mechanism of the cell which controlled the digestion of impaired organelles to maintain cellular homeostasis. It plays a pivotal role in programmed cell death, inflammation, and immune systems. The role of the autophagy process in the immune system is its involvement in immune defense against bacterial invasion, the thymic T cell selection process, antigen processing, cross-presentation, and even cytokine responses of immune cells. In addition, autophagy is an essential condition in bone homeostasis and also interacted with osteoporosis. Due to the above effects of this process and its involvement in some autoimmune and inflammatory diseases such as SLE and IBD, it may be effective in AS pathogenesis as well. Some limited studies on autophagy-related genes have shown, their association with AS diseases. The presence of rs9652059 SNP in Unc-51-like kinase 1 (ULK1) gene which is an autophagy-related gene, and also the haplotype of this SNP with rs11616018 and rs4964879, partially increase the AS susceptibility. *ULK1* gene is located on chromosome 12q24 and is the most upstream step of autophagosome formation, and is required for the initiation of autophagy. On the other hand, the immunity-related GTPase family M (IRGM) gene, which locates on chromosome 5q33.1 and encodes a GTP-binding protein, is also related to autophagy. The rs4958846 independently and rs10065172 dependently to rs4958846 are associated with female AS predisposition but not with the clinical phenotype of this disease. For introducing autophagy as an effective process in AS risk, more studies in different races other than Chinese are required [3, 86, 87].

References

1. Rich RR, et al. *Clinical immunology e-book: principles and practice*. Amsterdam: Elsevier Health Sciences; 2012.
2. Jin G, et al. Association between IL-1RN gene polymorphisms and susceptibility to ankylosing spondylitis: a large human genome epidemiology review and meta-analysis. Genet Mol Res. 2013;12(2):1720–30.
3. Momenzadeh P, et al. Determination of IL1R2, ANTXR2, CARD9, and SNAPC4 single nucleotide polymorphisms in Iranian patients with ankylosing spondylitis. Rheumatol Int. 2016;36(3):429–35.
4. Xia Y, et al. Association between cytokine gene polymorphisms and ankylosing spondylitis susceptibility: a systematic review and meta-analysis. Postgrad Med J. 2018;94(1115):508–16.
5. Haibel H, et al. Open label trial of anakinra in active ankylosing spondylitis over 24 weeks. Ann Rheum Dis. 2005;64(2):296–8.
6. Cortes A, et al. Identification of multiple risk variants for ankylosing spondylitis through high-density genotyping of immune-related loci. Nat Genet. 2013;45(7):730.
7. Sieper J, et al. Sarilumab for the treatment of ankylosing spondylitis: results of a phase II, randomised, double-blind, placebo-controlled study (ALIGN). Ann Rheum Dis. 2015;74(6):1051–7.
8. Tsui FW, et al. The genetic basis of ankylosing spondylitis: new insights into disease pathogenesis. Appl Clin Genet. 2014;7:105.
9. Ruan W-F, et al. The diagnostic and prognostic role of interleukin 12B and interleukin 6R gene polymorphism in patients with ankylosing spondylitis. JCR: J Clin Rheumatol. 2018;24(1):18–24.
10. Sieper J, et al. OP0166 tocilizumab (TCZ) is not effective for the treatment of ankylosing spondylitis (AS): results of a phase 2, international, multicentre, randomised, double-blind, placebo-controlled trial. Ann Rheum Dis. 2013;71(Suppl 3):110–1.
11. Sieper J, et al. Assessment of short-term symptomatic efficacy of tocilizumab in ankylosing spondylitis: results of randomised, placebo-controlled trials. Ann Rheum Dis. 2014;73(1):95–100.
12. Oppmann B, et al. Novel p19 protein engages IL-12p40 to form a cytokine, IL-23, with biological activities similar as well as distinct from IL-12. Immunity. 2000;13(5):715–25.
13. Becher B, Durell BG, Noelle RJ. Experimental autoimmune encephalitis and inflammation in the absence of interleukin-12. J Clin Invest. 2002;110(4):493–7.

14. Ivanova M, et al. Genetic variations in the IL-12B gene in association with IL-23 and IL-12p40 serum levels in ankylosing spondylitis. Rheumatol Int. 2019;39(1):111–9.
15. Wong R-H, et al. Association of IL-12B genetic polymorphism with the susceptibility and disease severity of ankylosing spondylitis. J Rheumatol. 2012;39(1):135–40.
16. Zhang L, et al. Association study of IL-12B polymorphisms susceptibility with ankylosing spondylitis in mainland Han population. PLoS One. 2015;10(6):e0130982.
17. Liang SC, et al. An IL-17F/a heterodimer protein is produced by mouse Th17 cells and induces airway neutrophil recruitment. J Immunol. 2007;179(11):7791–9.
18. Fossiez F, et al. T cell interleukin-17 induces stromal cells to produce proinflammatory and hematopoietic cytokines. J Exp Med. 1996;183(6):2593–603.
19. Miossec P. Interleukin-17 in rheumatoid arthritis: if T cells were to contribute to inflammation and destruction through synergy. Arthritis Rheum. 2003;48(3):594–601.
20. Nakae S, et al. Suppression of immune induction of collagen-induced arthritis in IL-17-deficient mice. J Immunol. 2003;171(11):6173–7.
21. Bowness P, et al. Th17 cells expressing KIR3DL2+ and responsive to HLA-B27 homodimers are increased in ankylosing spondylitis. J Immunol. 2011;186(4):2672–80.
22. Chen L, et al. miR-10b-5p is a novel Th17 regulator present in Th17 cells from ankylosing spondylitis. Ann Rheum Dis. 2017;76(3):620–5.
23. Chyuan I-T, Chen J-Y. Role of interleukin-(IL-) 17 in the pathogenesis and targeted therapies in spondyloarthropathies. Mediat Inflamm. 2018;2018:2403935.
24. Wang X, et al. Expression of IL-23 and IL-17 and effect of IL-23 on IL-17 production in ankylosing spondylitis. Rheumatol Int. 2009;29(11):1343–7.
25. Brown M. Breakthroughs in genetic studies of ankylosing spondylitis. Rheumatology. 2008;47(2):132–7.
26. Rueda B, et al. The IL23R Arg381Gln non-synonymous polymorphism confers susceptibility to ankylosing spondylitis. Ann Rheum Dis. 2008;67(10):1451–4.
27. Rahman P, et al. Association of interleukin-23 receptor variants with ankylosing spondylitis. Arthritis Rheum. 2008;58(4):1020–5.
28. Sung I-H, et al. IL-23R polymorphisms in patients with ankylosing spondylitis in Korea. J Rheumatol. 2009;36(5):1003–5.
29. Daryabor G, et al. Determination of IL-23 receptor gene polymorphism in Iranian patients with ankylosing spondylitis. Eur Cytokine Netw. 2014;25(1):24–9.
30. Han R, et al. Interleukin-23 receptor polymorphism (rs10889677 a/C) in ankylosing spondylitis: Meta-analysis in Caucasian and Asian populations. Clin Chim Acta. 2018;477:53–9.
31. Dong H, et al. IL23R gene confers susceptibility to ankylosing spondylitis concomitant with uveitis in a Han Chinese population. PLoS One. 2013;8(6):e67505.
32. Sode J, et al. Genetically determined high activities of the TNF-alpha, IL23/IL17, and NFkB pathways were associated with increased risk of ankylosing spondylitis. BMC Med Genet. 2018;19(1):165.
33. Reveille JD, et al. Genome-wide association study of ankylosing spondylitis identifies non-MHC susceptibility loci. Nat Genet. 2010;42(2):123.
34. Davidson SI, et al. Association of STAT3 and TNFRSF1A with ankylosing spondylitis in Han Chinese. Ann Rheum Dis. 2011;70(2):289–92.
35. Jiang Y, Wang L. Role of histone deacetylase 3 in ankylosing spondylitis via negative feedback loop with microRNA-130a and enhancement of tumor necrosis factor-1α expression in peripheral blood mononuclear cells. Mol Med Rep. 2016;13(1):35–40.
36. Lv C, et al. Association of Interleukin-10 gene polymorphisms with ankylosing spondylitis. Clin Invest Med. 2011;34:E370–6.
37. Lee WY, et al. Polymorphisms of cytotoxic T lymphocyte-associated antigen-4 and cytokine genes in Taiwanese patients with ankylosing spondylitis. Tissue Antigens. 2010;75(2):119–26.
38. Yue Y, et al. Association of long noncoding RNAs polymorphisms with ankylosing spondylitis, Vogt-Koyanagi-Harada disease, and Behcet's disease. Invest Ophthalmol Vis Sci. 2018;59(2):1158–66.

39. Abbas AK, Lichtman AH, Pillai S. Cellular and molecular immunology E-book. Amsterdam: Elsevier Health Sciences; 2014.
40. Kocyigit BF, Akyol A. Vitamin D levels in patients with ankylosing spondylitis: is it related to disease activity? Pakistan J Med Sci. 2018;34(5):1209.
41. Zhang P, et al. Association between vitamin D receptor gene polymorphism and ankylosing spondylitis in Han Chinese. Int J Rheum Dis. 2017;20(10):1510–6.
42. Cai G, et al. Vitamin D in ankylosing spondylitis: review and meta-analysis. Clin Chim Acta. 2015;438:316–22.
43. Assassi S, et al. Whole-blood gene expression profiling in ankylosing spondylitis shows upregulation of toll-like receptor 4 and 5. J Rheumatol. 2011;38(1):87–98.
44. Mohammadi H, et al. MicroRNA implications in the etiopathogenesis of ankylosing spondylitis. J Cell Physiol. 2018;233(8):5564–73.
45. Vishwakarma S, et al. Association of CD14 and macrophage migration inhibitory factor gene polymorphisms with inflammatory microRNAs expression levels in ankylosing spondylitis and polyarthralgia. Int J Immunogenet. 2018;45(4):190–200.
46. Machado NP, et al. Clinical characteristics and frequency of TLR4 polymorphisms in Brazilian patients with ankylosing spondylitis. Rev Bras Reumatol. 2016;56(5):432–40.
47. Adam R, Sturrock R, Gracie J. TLR4 mutations (Asp299Gly and Thr399Ile) are not associated with ankylosing spondylitis. Ann Rheum Dis. 2006;65(8):1099–101.
48. Mahmoudi M, et al. New insights toward the pathogenesis of ankylosing spondylitis; genetic variations and epigenetic modifications. Mod Rheumatol. 2017;27(2):198–209.
49. Soleimanifar N, et al. Study of programmed cell death 1 (PDCD1) gene polymorphims in Iranian patients with ankylosing spondylitis. Inflammation. 2011;34(6):707–12.
50. Huang C-H, et al. Associations of the PTPN22 and CTLA-4 genetic polymorphisms with Taiwanese ankylosing spondylitis. Rheumatol Int. 2014;34(5):683–91.
51. Azizi E, et al. Association of CTLA4 gene polymorphism in Iranian patients with ankylosing spondylitis. J Clin Immunol. 2010;30(2):268–71.
52. Liu X, et al. Programmed cell death 1 gene polymorphisms is associated with ankylosing spondylitis in Chinese Han population. Rheumatol Int. 2011;31(2):209–13.
53. Orozco G, et al. Lack of association between ankylosing spondylitis and a functional polymorphism of PTPN22 proposed as a general susceptibility marker for autoimmunity. Ann Rheum Dis. 2006;65(5):687–8.
54. Chen S, et al. The associations between PD-1, CTLA-4 gene polymorphisms and susceptibility to ankylosing spondylitis: a meta-analysis and systemic review. Rheumatol Int. 2016;36(1):33–44.
55. Ma X, et al. Evidence for genetic association of CARD9 and SNAPC4 with ankylosing spondylitis in a Chinese Han population. J Rheumatol. 2014;41(2):318–24.
56. Pointon JJ, et al. Elucidating the chromosome 9 association with AS; CARD9 is a candidate gene. Genes Immun. 2010;11(6):490–6.
57. Evans DM, et al. Interaction between ERAP1 and HLA-B27 in ankylosing spondylitis implicates peptide handling in the mechanism for HLA-B27 in disease susceptibility. Nat Genet. 2011;43(8):761–7.
58. Liu J, et al. Analysis of clinical indexes and RUNX3, TBKBP1, PPARGC1B polymorphisms in Chinese Han patients with ankylosing spondylitis. Genet Test Mol Biomarkers. 2015;19(1):37–43.
59. Lian Z, et al. Analysis of PPARGC1B, RUNX3 and TBKBP1 polymorphisms in Chinese Han patients with ankylosing spondylitis: a case-control study. PLoS One. 2013;8(4):e61527.
60. Pointon JJ, et al. The chromosome 16q region associated with ankylosing spondylitis includes the candidate gene tumour necrosis factor receptor type 1-associated death domain (TRADD). Ann Rheum Dis. 2010;69(6):1243–6.
61. Lai N-S, et al. Aberrant expression of interleukin-23-regulated miRNAs in T cells from patients with ankylosing spondylitis. Arthritis Res Ther. 2018;20(1):1–10.
62. Chen C, Zhang X, Wang Y. Analysis of JAK2 and STAT3 polymorphisms in patients with ankylosing spondylitis in Chinese Han population. Clin Immunol. 2010;136(3):442–6.

63. Danoy P, et al. Association of variants at 1q32 and STAT3 with ankylosing spondylitis suggests genetic overlap with Crohn's disease. PLoS Genet. 2010;6(12):e1001195.
64. Liu Z, Zhang P, Dong J. Genetic variants of STAT4 are associated with ankylosing spondylitis susceptibility and severity in a Chinese Han population. Int J Clin Exp Med. 2014;7(12):5877.
65. Liu X, et al. Association of HLA-DP/DQ and STAT4 polymorphisms with ankylosing spondylitis in Southwest China. Int Immunopharmacol. 2016;39:10–5.
66. Cho S-M, Jung S-H, Chung Y-J. A variant in RUNX3 is associated with the risk of ankylosing spondylitis in Koreans. Genomics Inform. 2017;15(2):65.
67. Vecellio M, et al. The genetic association of RUNX3 with ankylosing spondylitis can be explained by allele-specific effects on IRF4 recruitment that alter gene expression. Ann Rheum Dis. 2016;75(8):1534–40.
68. Vecellio M, et al. RUNX3 and T-bet in Immunopathogenesis of ankylosing spondylitis—novel targets for therapy? Front Immunol. 2019;9:3132.
69. Gocke AR, et al. T-bet regulates the fate of Th1 and Th17 lymphocytes in autoimmunity. J Immunol. 2007;178(3):1341 8.
70. Lau MC, et al. Genetic association of ankylosing spondylitis with TBX21 influences T-bet and pro-inflammatory cytokine expression in humans and SKG mice as a model of spondyloarthritis. Ann Rheum Dis. 2017;76(1):261–9.
71. Chen C, Zhang X, Wang Y. ANTXR2 and IL-1R2 polymorphisms are not associated with ankylosing spondylitis in Chinese Han population. Rheumatol Int. 2012;32(1):15–9.
72. Bang S-Y, et al. Genetic studies of ankylosing spondylitis in Koreans confirm associations with ERAP1 and 2p15 reported in white patients. J Rheumatol. 2011;38(2):322–4.
73. Wong MW, et al. The large subunit of basal transcription factor SNAPc is a Myb domain protein that interacts with Oct-1. Mol Cell Biol. 1998;18(1):368–77.
74. Lin Z, et al. A genome-wide association study in Han Chinese identifies new susceptibility loci for ankylosing spondylitis. Nat Genet. 2012;44(1):73–7.
75. Liu Y, et al. Association of common variants in KIF21B and ankylosing spondylitis in a Chinese Han population: a replication study. Immunogenetics. 2013;65(12):835–9.
76. Yang X, et al. Association of KIF21B genetic polymorphisms with ankylosing spondylitis in a Chinese Han population of Shandong Province. Clin Rheumatol. 2015;34(10):1729–36.
77. Reveille JD. Genetics of spondyloarthritis—beyond the MHC. Nat Rev Rheumatol. 2012;8(5):296.
78. Gao S, et al. Association of rs4552569 and rs17095830 single-nucleotide polymorphisms with susceptibility to ankylosing spondylitis in east Asian population: a meta-analysis. J Genet. 2018;97(4):825–33.
79. Ding N, et al. Association of β-defensin gene copy number variations with ankylosing spondylitis in Chinese population: a case–control study. Mod Rheumatol. 2016;26(1):146–50.
80. Deyab G, et al. Anti-rheumatic treatment is not associated with reduction of pentraxin 3 in rheumatoid arthritis, psoriatic arthritis and ankylosing spondylitis. PLoS One. 2017;12(2):e0169830.
81. Zhang X, Ding W. Association of genetic variants in pentraxin 3 gene with ankylosing spondylitis. Med Sci Monit: International Medical Journal of Experimental and Clinical Research. 2016;22:2911.
82. Gürel Ç, et al. Evaluation of MIF-173 G/C polymorphism in Turkish patients with ankylosing spondylitis. Balkan Med J. 2016;33(6):614.
83. Karami J, et al. Promoter hypermethylation of BCL11B gene correlates with downregulation of gene transcription in ankylosing spondylitis patients. Genes Immun. 2017;18(3):170–5.
84. Shi Z, et al. Gene expression profiling analysis of patients with ankylosing spondylitis: retracted. J Spin Disord Tech. 2015;28(4):E244–50.
85. Pimentel-Santos FM, et al. Whole blood transcriptional profiling in ankylosing spondylitis identifies novel candidate genes that might contribute to the inflammatory and tissue-destructive disease aspects. Arthritis Res Ther. 2011;13(2):1–8.

86. Zhang X, et al. Association between the autophagy-related gene ULK1 and ankylosing spondylitis susceptibility in the Chinese Han population: a case–control study. Postgrad Med J. 2017;93(1106):752–7.
87. Xia Q, et al. Autophagy-related IRGM genes confer susceptibility to ankylosing spondylitis in a Chinese female population: a case–control study. Genes Immun. 2017;18(1):42–7.

Part IV

Environmental Factors

6 Spondyloarthropathies and Gut Microbiota

Narjes Soleimanifar and Sara Assadiasl

6.1 Introduction

Human being has used to live with a countless number of microbes inside and outside of his body including skin, gastrointestinal tract, lung, saliva, oral mucosa, conjunctiva, biliary tract, mammary glands, placenta, seminal fluid, and uterus. The most vivid example of these is the gut microbiota. Our gut has been colonized by an enormous number of microbes from diverse species, which protect us from pathogenic strains and provide rare elements like vitamin K, receiving habitat and nutrients in return. It is estimated that 10% of all the metabolites in the human body are produced by the commensal microbiome [1]. Since years, the role of microbiota in health and disease has been investigated, but recently there have been further efforts to define its implication in triggering and/or progression of certain diseases and to manipulate it for treating the infectious, hepatic, metabolic, respiratory, psychological, and autoimmune diseases as well as gastrointestinal cancers [2].

Spondyloarthropathies (SpA) a family of autoimmune inflammatory disorders including ankylosing spondylitis (AS), psoriatic arthritis (PsA), reactive arthritis (ReA), juvenile spondyloarthritis (JSpA), and undifferentiated SpAs (uSpAs) have also been shown to be affected by gut microbiome as some differences have been demonstrated between the microbiota of SpA patients and healthy population [3]. This finding was supported by the theory of disrupted gut environment in SpA, due to the eventual dysregulated immune responses and vice versa. Herein, we describe the impact of gut microbiota on developing gut immunity, dysbiosis in Spondyloarthropathies, SpAs association with inflammatory bowel diseases and finally, the possible interventions that could be applied to restore the healthy microbiota in SpA patients.

N. Soleimanifar · S. Assadiasl (✉)
Molecular Immunology Research Center, Tehran University of Medical Sciences, Tehran, Iran
e-mail: assadiasl@sina.tums.ac.ir

M. H. Nicknam (ed.), *Ankylosing Spondylitis - Axial Spondyloarthritis*, https://doi.org/10.1007/978-981-16-4733-8_6

6.2 Gut Microbiome

During recent years, the growing evidence about the association of gut microbiome with several disorders, particularly autoimmune and metabolic diseases, in addition to the technical advancements (e.g., DNA sequencing, metabonomics, proteomics, and computation-based bioinformatics), have encouraged the meticulous study of human commensal microbes. In fact, human being provides the habitat of trillions of microbes which their impact on his health and disease is inevitable. However, there are differences between microbe colonization in different sites of the body as well as interpersonal variations. For instance, anaerobic Firmicutes and Bacteroidetes species flourish the intestine, while Actinobacteria and Proteobacteria species are aggregated on the skin [4]. Notably, the gut microbiota has been shown to be profoundly involved in the development and regulation of the immune system in particular T helper 17 and T regulatory lymphocytes [5]. Although the microbiome varies between individuals, there are similarities among healthy people. Gut microbiome analysis in healthy populations revealed approximately 1150 species of bacteria, the majority of which (50–75%) were Firmicutes, followed by Bacteroidetes (10–50%) and Actinobacteria (1–10%), and less than 1% Proteobacteria [6].

The microbiota is rapidly developed after birth according to the surrounding environment, breastfeeding, nutritional habits, hygiene level and antibiotics consumption, thus a three-year-old child could possess a complete set of microbiota similar to that of an adult. Moreover, human microbiota is usually volatile because of nutritional diversity, illness, hormonal fluctuations, hygiene, exposing to various environments and climates, and particularly antibiotics administration; nonetheless, there is a general colonization which is dominant in each individual, tending to be preserved once the intrinsic or extrinsic interfering factor is resolved [7]. Accordingly, it is hypothesized that a failure to return to the normal microbiome after a transient disturbance might predispose the individuals to certain diseases such as autoimmune disorders. In effect, maintaining the healthy balance between host and microbiota, so-called symbiosis, is an essential requirement for preventing illness, whereas microbiome dysregulation, known as dysbiosis, could be considered as a risk factor for various disorders [8]. For instance, it has been demonstrated that the microbiota in patients with chronic inflammatory diseases show lower bacterial diversity compared to the healthy controls as microbiota of patients suffering from inflammatory bowel diseases (IBD) consists of 25% less genes than healthy people [9].

To define the differences between microbiota composition of healthy population and patients, the normal gut microbiome should be described properly; however, the result of studies indicate considerable variations in the microbiota composition of the normal population, for example, a study of the European MetaHIT consortium identified three different enterotypes in fecal samples from four European countries including enterotype 1, 2, and 3 dominated by the genus Bacteroides, Prevotella, and Ruminococcus, respectively. These types were neither nation- nor gender-specific but associated with life conditions (e.g., nutrition, hygiene, environment, climate) [10].

6.3 Spondyloarthropathies and Microbes

Regarding the distinct role of microbiota in induction, chronicity, and progression of inflammatory disorders, there are many studies highlighting the microbiome differences between AS patients and the healthy population. One of the first studies comparing ileal samples of AS patients and healthy individuals showed no significant difference between the number of microbes but more microbial diversity in AS gut with anincreased number of several families of Clostridiales, including Lachnospiraceae from Coprococcus and Roseburia genera and Ruminococcaceae, or Bacteroidales, including Rikenellaceae, Porphyromonadaceae from Parabacteroides genus and Bacteroidaceae while the decreased frequency of Veillonellaceae, Prevotellaceae, Actinomycetaceae, and Streptococcaceae families [11]. Similarly, a group found the decreased amount of Streptococcus and Actinomyces in AS patients' gut in comparison to healthy controls [12], while others observed an increased abundance of sulfate reducing Bacteroides in AS [13]. One study comparing the microbiota composition of stool samples between patients with juvenile SpA classified as enthesitis-related arthritis (ERA) and healthy adolescents demonstrated an elevated number of Bacteroides, including *B. fragilis*, *B. plebeius* and *B. eggerthii* species and Enterococcus genera, while the decreased frequency of the Prevotella genus, including Prevotella copri and Prevotella stercorea species in ERA patients [14]; whereas, in two preceding studies, ERA patients exhibited decreased amounts of Clostridium leptum [15] and *Faecalibacterium prausnitzii* compared to the healthy adolescents. Despite these differences, serum IgA and IgG antibody *against Faecalibacterium prausnitzii* were similar between controls and patients. There was also some evidence of aberrant cellular immune responses to the membrane proteins of Salmonella typhimurium in juvenile SpA patients [16].

One recent study analyzing fecal samples of treated and untreated AS patients, as well as healthy individuals using metagenomic shotgun sequencing, demonstrated increased number of *B. coprophilus*, Eubacterium siraeum, Parabacteroides distasonis, *A. fermentans* and *Prevotella copri* species in AS patients' gut microbiota; moreover, pathway analysis revealed increased oxidative phosphorylation, glycosaminoglycan degradation and lipopolysaccharide biosynthesis in AS. Notably, in vitro experiments revealed elevated amounts of IFN-γ-producing cells triggered by a bacterial peptide of AS-enriched species, mimicking type II collagen. Overall findings indicated gut microbiota perturbation in untreated AS patients and showed some AS-related species which exhibited molecular mimicry to autoantigens [17].

In psoriatic arthritis reduced number of many bacterial species such as Coprococcus, together with a lower microbial diversity, has been reported [18]. Other example of microbiome association with SpAs is reactive arthritis which is assumed to be emerged following gastrointestinal infections by Yersinia, Salmonella, Shigella, and Campylobacter, or urinary tract infections by Chlamydia tracomatis. Approximately 20% of the patients with ReA develop AS within 10–20 years [19, 20]; moreover, bacterial products from the previous infection have been detected in the joints of ReA patients [21].

In addition to the altered number of certain microbes in the gut, it seems to be functional deviations in response to the bacteria in AS patients, as it was shown that their peripheral blood monocytes (PBMCs) produce less IL-10 when stimulated with autologous Bacteroides [22]. Interestingly, Klebsiella pneumonia which has been recognized as a triggering or perpetuating factor for AS showed no difference in the gut microbiome of AS and healthy cases [12, 23]. Previous studies had indicated the involvement of klebsiella generally regarding elevated levels of anti-klebsiella IgA in AS patients' plasma [24, 25]. Taken together, some alterations in number, composition, and function of gut microbiota have been reported in SpA patients comparing to healthy individuals; nonetheless, there is barely any consensus between these findings, and they could not be supposed as conclusive.

6.4 Spondyloarthropathies and Inflammatory Bowel Diseases

In addition to the abovementioned diseases, SpAs include the inflammatory bowel disease (IBD)-related arthritis. In this category, gut inflammation is considered as an extra-articular symptom of Spondyloarthropathies. IBDs comprise ulcerative colitis (UC) and Crohn's disease (CD) both of them accompanied with dysbiosis of the gut microbiome, while there is a significant overlap between microbes associated with IBD and SpA. In addition, 5–10% of SpA patients develop concomitant IBD, corresponding to an increased risk of 10- to 20-fold [26]. This can be explained at least in part by shared genetic factors predisposing a person to both of these inflammatory disorders; gene polymorphisms in cytokines, their receptors and downstream pathways have been shown to be implicated in SpAs and IBD [27].

An old study showed that approximately 50% of SpA patients without any intestinal symptoms had microscopic signs of bowel inflammation in colonoscopy. Two inflammatory types were observed on morphological alterations: an acute type similar to the infectious enterocolitis and a chronic type resembling early Crohn's disease [28]. Consequently, the same group demonstrated that remission of joint inflammation was correlated with resolving gut inflammation and vice versa, indicating a strong link between joint and gut inflammation [29]. One ileocolonoscopy survey on a group of patients with axial and peripheral arthritis revealed that 46.2% of the patients had microscopic gut inflammation, including 16.9% acute and 29.2% chronic inflammations. Male sex, younger age, high Bath Ankylosing Spondylitis Disease Activity Index (BASDAI) score and restricted spinal mobility measured by the Bath Ankylosing Spondylitis Metrology Index (BASMI) were independently associated with gut involvement. The prevalence of gut inflammation in axial SpA was higher than peripheral type, but it was similar in non-radiographic-axSpA and AS [30]. One study performing 30-years of follow-up demonstrated that nearly 19% of Crohn's' disease patients develop a type of spondyloarthritis [31]. Likewise, evaluation of 626 IBD cases (57% with ulcerative colitis (UC)) showed a 17% prevalence of joint pain; among them, 12% had AS, 43% peripheral arthritis, 32% chronic back pain, and 13% showed other types of joint pain. Moreover, the diagnosis of AS occurred after the initial diagnosis of IBD in 80% of affected patients within a mean (SD) period of 5.6 (±6) years [32]. Furthermore, investigating 68 patients with axial SpA using ileocolonoscopy and MRI of sacroiliac joints showed a significant higher SPondylo Arthritis Research Consortium of Canada (SPARCC) score in patients with chronic gut inflammation compared to those with normal gut histology. Besides, chronic gut inflammation and male sex were independently associated with the Degree of bone marrow edema [33]. In addition to the clinical evidence, shared polymorphisms in some genes, for instance, IL-12B, IL-27A, IL-1R2, IL-23R, TYK2, STAT3, and CARD9, have been detected in AS, Crohn's disease and PsA, all of them involved in inflammatory IL-23/IL-17 axis [34, 35]. According to these findings, it could be supposed that a significant association exists between gut and joint inflammations suggesting the gut microbiome and its dysregulation as a predisposing factor for intra- and extra-intestinal inflammatory disorders.

6.5 Animal Models of SpA and Gut Immunity

One of the most striking findings from an animal study of SpA models was the absence of arthritis and colitis in germ-free HLA-B27-transgenic rats, which were supposed to exhibit SpA and IBD symptoms [36]; however, subsequent transfer of microbiome to the gut of these rats restored inflammatory features [37]. Later, subtle differences were demonstrated between normal and HLA-B27-transgenic rats, as it was found that an increased proportion of certain microbial species such as Prevotellaceae and Rikenellaceae was associated with inflammatory responses [38].

IL-23 and its receptor polymorphisms have been demonstrated to be significantly implicated in the immunopathogenesis of both IBD and SpA. IL-23 promotes differentiation and activation of Th17 cells and subsequent IL-17 secretion [39]. *C. trachomatis*, the bacteria associated with ReA has been shown to promote IL-23 production in vitro and in animal models, inducing IL-23/IL-17 inflammatory axis [40]. The SpA animal model SKG mice have augmented Th17 responses because of ZAP-70 mutation in the signaling pathway. One study found that the activity of SKG Th17 cells is further enhanced when treated with microbial derivate such as curdlan, leading to severe ileitis. On the other hand, germ-free environment could reduce gut and joint inflammation of these animals [41].

A group of important bacterial derivates studied in animal models of SpA are short chain fatty acids (SCFAs) such as butyrate, which is a fermentation product of microbes [42]. It has been found that in the mice fed with SCFA-rich diet (butyrate), naïve TCD4+ cells would preferentially differentiate from Treg cells [43, 44]. In addition, the gnotobiotic mice colonized with *Clostridium leptum* and Clostridium coccoides which produce SCFA exhibited more Treg cells and higher levels of TGF-B in the colon [45]. The potential anti-inflammatory effects of SCFAs are still under investigation.

It has already been shown that germ-free animals fail to develop secondary lymphoid organs [46]; subsequently, it was found that certain species in gut microbiome influence adaptive immunity responses, for instance, segmented filamentous bacteria (SFB) such as Citrobacter rodentium which is attached to the microvilli of intestinal epithelial lymphocytes (IELs) could induce Th17 differentiation in secondary lymphoid organs via antigen presentation by intestinal CD11c + dendritic cells [47]. Moreover, SFB attachment to IELs induces morphological changes and upregulation of the inflammation-associated genes such as serum amyloid A (SAA) in IELs. It was shown that the presence of recombinant SAA in co-cultures of naïve CD4+ T cells with dendritic cells of lamina propria (LP) induces differentiation of Th17 lymphocytes in vitro; hence, it could be presumed that SFB attachment to the IELs provides antigenic and chemical signals for developing Th17 cells in LP and extra-intestinal lymph nodes [48]. In addition to SAA, SFB could enhance the expression of MHC-II, defensins, and fucosyl transferase in IELs, and they also trigger isotype switching towards IgA and recruit IgA-producing plasma cells to the intestinal epithelium [49]. Moreover, colonization of germ-free K/BxN mice intestine with segmented filamentous bacteria resulted in autoimmune arthritis following the excessive expansion of Th17 cells [50]. Therefore, SFBs play a considerable role in the development and regulation of mice's gut immunity. Although SFBs have not yet been identified in the human intestine, their immunomodulatory role may be played by similar species. Recent efforts to genome sequencing of the gut microbiota might help recognize SFBs counterparts in humans [51].

6.6 Dysbiosis and Inflammation in SpA

The epithelium of the intestine is protected by many secretory elements separating the microbiome from the layer beneath, including mucus, secretory IgA, and antimicrobial peptides (AMPs), which might be disrupted in SpA patients' gut. Since the gut mucus acts as a nutritional source for intestinal commensal microbiota, any dysregulation in mucus production might result in dysbiosis. Animal studies have shown that mucus-deficient mice develop colitis and arthritis resembling the transgenic HLA-B27 phenotype [52, 53]. Moreover, it has been reported that the major mucus protein, muc2, could elicit tolerogenic responses in intestinal epithelial cells and dendritic cells, which indicates the implication of the mucus layer in maintaining intestinal tolerance and integrity [54].

Antimicrobial peptides such as defensins, C-type lectins and cathelicidins are produced mainly by Paneth cells. The expression of AMPs is regulated by recognition of microbial products via innate immunity receptors, given that the NOD2 polymorphisms are associated with decreased production of defensins and increased risk of Crohn's disease [55]. Contrarily, AMP expression appears to be increased in ileal biopsies of AS patients and myeloid cells from SpA-susceptible B27 rats [56]. The precise role of IgA in gut dysbiosis is not clear. There are many reports about elevated IgA levels in blood circulation of AS patients particularly against Klebsiella; on the other hand, severe forms of AS are seen in selective IgA-deficient cases [57].

Apart from secretory agents, gut epithelium as a principal physical barrier has been found to be disrupted in AS patients. In fact, the gut microbiome stimulates epithelial cells proliferation and differentiation, expression of tight junction proteins and adhesion molecules through stimulation of signaling pathways such as nuclear factor kappa B(NF-κB) and mitogen-activated protein (MAP) kinase; therefore, the blunted and fused villi in the ileum of AS patients might be suggestive of impaired proliferative responses in intestinal epithelial cells due to the altered microbiome [58]. On the other hand, enhanced E-cadherin expression has been observed in IECs of SpA cases with subclinical bowel inflammation [59]. Moreover, T cells from AS patients' colon biopsies showed augmented expression of αEb7, an E-cadherin ligand; whereas, an old study had reported disturbed N-cadherin function in IBD mice suggesting a reduced expression of adhesion molecules in the gut epithelium [60].

The other alteration reported in SpA patients and HLA-B27 mice gut is increased intestinal permeability or so-called "leaky gut," in which intestinal epithelium permits the microorganisms to invade the beneath tissue, break the tolerance and induce inflammation [61]. This phenomenon explains the failure of some studies in describing microbiota differences between SpA patients and healthy controls. In fact, leaky gut supposes increased tissue accessibility, not different microbial load or diversity, as the initial cause of inflammation. As a result of the epithelial permeablization, the microbe-associated molecular patterns (MAMPs) of invading microbes would be recognized by pathogen recognition receptors (PRRs) such as Toll-like receptors (TLRs), NOD-like receptors (NLRs), RIG-Iike receptors (RLRs), and C-type lectin receptors (CLRs) which trigger the signaling pathways leading to the inflammatory activation of innate immune cells and IELs [3]. Consequent to the MAMPs activation of immune cells in gut epithelium and tissue injury, damage-associated molecular patterns (DAMPs) might cause further activation of the innate immunity, inflammation expansion and eventual transfer of activated cells to the extra-intestinal tissues such as joint.

The autophagy and endoplasmic reticulum (ER) response have also been shown to be dysregulated in IBD and SpA patients. Many autophagy proteins such as LC3II, ATG5, and ATG12 are overexpressed in intestinal inflammatory lesions of AS cases, augmenting IL-23 expression [62]. Moreover, since the autophagy of epithelial cells limits the dissemination of pathogenic bacteria and commensal microbes to extra-intestinal tissues, its dysregulation could result in inefficient antibacterial defense [63]. Polymorphisms of the genes involved in ER stress pathways such as XBP-1 and IRE1 appear to be associated with AS and Crohn's disease. Furthermore, HLA-B27, as a large protein susceptible to misfolding and ER accumulation, could trigger ER stress responses [64]. Bacterial lipopolysaccharides (LPS) might enhance ER responses in HLA-B27+ macrophages and induce Th17 responses accompanied by IL-23 production. ER-stress-induced IL-1α production could stimulate osteoclast formation, which leads to the subsequent pathologic events in joints [65].

There is also evidence of migration of primed intestinal innate and adoptive immune cells to SpA-affected sites, for instance, CD163+ macrophages, which increase in the gut of IBD and SpA patients are selectively increased in the SpA synovium [66]. Moreover, T lymphocytes isolated from SpA synovial tissue express high amounts of integrin α4β7, the ligand of intestinal addressing molecule MadCAM-1 on gut vascular endothelium, and integrin αEβ7 which binds to E-cadherin expressed on IECs, suggesting an intestinal origin for these T cells [67]. Furthermore, T cell clones specific for enteric pathogens *Yersinia enterocolitica* and *Salmonella typhimurium* have been detected in the synovial tissue of ReA patients [68, 69]. These findings suggest a considerable correlation between dysbiosis, gut inflammation and extra-intestinal inflammatory responses in SpA patients.

6.7 HLA-B27

HLA-27 has already been shown to associate with Spondyloarthropathies strongly, and its footprints could be followed in the involvement of the microbiome in SpAs pathogenesis. There are some theories explaining the implication of HLA-B27 in microbes' effect. One theory is the structural similarity between HLA-B27 and many Gram negative bacteria. Long ago, it was found that antibodies specific for some Klebsiella species were cytotoxic for HLA-B27+ lymphocytes [70]; later, it was shown that monoclonal antibodies to HLA-B27 could detect cross-reactive antigens in *Klebsiella pneumonia, Yersinia enterocolitica,* and Shigella flexneri [71]. Subsequently, a six-amino-acid sequence was identified in HLA-B27 structure, which was very similar to a sequence in the nitrogenase enzyme of klebsiella [72]. Then, other amino acid sequences were found in HLA-B27 identical to those from Gram negative bacteria, a unique characteristic for this HLA subtype [73].

The other theory is the inefficiency of HLA-B27+ monocytes in eradicating Gram negative bacteria such as Salmonella [74]. Dendritic cells of mice with a high copy number of HLA-B27 exhibited diminished reactivity in mixed lymphocyte reaction with T cells; moreover, they showed reduced proliferative capacity against LPS [75]; on the other hand, secretion of tumor necrosis factor-alpha (TNF-α) and IL-10 has been induced significantly in the HLA-B27+ cells infected with Salmonella [76]. It has also been shown that recolonization of germ-free HLA-B27 rats with Bacteroides would result in gut inflammation, but when recolonized with Lactobacillus and Fusiform bacteria, there was no inflammatory response [77]. These and other findings suggest that HLA-B27 phenotype due to the molecular mimicry and failure to eradicating inflammatory species might be involved in developing a distinct microbiome and subsequent inflammatory responses in SpA and IBD patients.

6.8 Cytokines Induction by Microbiome

Cytokines like IL-17, IL-22, and IL-17 have been recognized to be implicated in SpAs pathogenesis, expressing in blood, gut, and synovium of these patients. Th17 cells are induced in intestinal lamina propria through segmented filamentous bacteria and microbiota-derivates such as LPS and flagellin, which initiate the expression of IL-6, IL-1, and IL-23 by monocytes [78]. Infectious bacteria like *Salmonella enteritidis* has also been demonstrated to induce Th17 development in animal model's gut [79]. Th17 cells reside abundantly in the intestinal lamina propria of mice; however, in germ-free or antibiotic-treated mice, the number of LP Th17 cells is significantly decreased [80]. Besides, intestinal Th17 cells appear to be able to migrate to the other parts of the body, especially to the spleen [81]. One experiment has shown that autoimmune arthritis was alleviated in the K/BxN mouse model under germ-free conditions, due to the reduced amounts of autoantibodies, decreased number of splenic autoantibody-secreting cells, impaired germinal center formation, and diminished splenic Th17 cell population subsequent to the disappearance of Th17 cells from the intestinal lamina propria. The introduction of segmented filamentous bacteria into the germ-free animals restored Th17 cell compartment in lamina propria and enhanced autoantibody production; therefore, arthritis symptoms were back [50]. Nonetheless, the expansion of IL-17-producing T cells has not yet been approved in gut samples of AS patients, and it seems that IL-23 producing cells are dominating the site [82].

Notably, differentiation of Th17 cells in vitro could be improved by the addition of TLR5 ligand, flagellin [83]. Moreover, Tlr9-deficient mice exhibit reduced percentages of Th17 cells in lamina propria [84]. It was also demonstrated that bacteria-infected apoptotic IECs trigger dendritic cells to produce Th17-differentiating cytokines IL-6 and TGF-B by expression of phosphatidylserine and other TLR ligands [85]. Therefore, it could be suggested that besides intrinsic factors such as extracellular ATP binding to purinergic receptors expressed on CD70highCD11c + dendritic cells, the development of Th17 cells is markedly dependent on microbiota-derived stimulations [86].

The other source of producing inflammatory cytokines in SpA patients are NKp44+ innate lymphoid cells (ILCs) which release IL-22 [87]. NKp44 ligands could recognize the microbial products from Mycobacterium, Nocardia farcinica, and Pseudomonas aeruginosa; hence, these cells could be directly activated by the gut microbiome [88]. The engagement of NKp44 ligand on RORγt+ILCs has been shown to elicit the secretion of TNF-α and other inflammatory cytokines [89].

T regulatory cells have also been shown to contribute to shaping the cytokine environment of the gastrointestinal tract by producing IL-10 and TGF-B cytokines. Certain bacterial species such as Lactobacilli and Bifidobacteria are involved in Treg cells development in the colon. Mice treated with Lactobacillus reuteri or the probiotic mixture VSL#3 (a mixture of Bifidobacteria, Lactobacilli, and *Streptococcus salivarius*) exhibited the elevated number of intestinal Treg cells [90]. B. fragilis, is the other strain implicated in functional maturation of Treg cells and IL-10 production in mice [91]. This process is mediated by polysaccharideA (PSA), a surface polysaccharide of *B. fragilis* which binds to TLR2 on CD4+ T cells and triggers IL-10 production. Interestingly, PSA suppresses Th17 cell responses, which further indicates its anti-inflammatory properties [92].

The other species implicated in Treg induction in mice intestine are spore-forming bacteria, such as Clostridium (e.g., *Clostridium leptum*) and Coccoides groups. These species could induce colonic Treg cells accumulation in germ-free mice. They colonize preferentially and form a thick layer on the epithelial surface, where they induce the production of indoleamine 2, 3-dioxygenase (IDO) and matrix metalloproteinases (MMPs) from IEC. IDO possesses immunomodulatory potentials, and MMP converts TGF-β from inactive form to the active one, which promotes Treg cell differentiation and survival. The population of colon Treg cells in mice colonized with Clostridium consists of a considerable number of Helios-negative cells, suggesting Treg-inducing stimulations mediated by Clostridium species. Moreover, Treg cells induced by Clostridium express higher levels of IL-10 cytokine [93]. Therefore, some species affecting the quantity and quality of Treg cells in the colon could modulate the anti-inflammatory cytokines level, a property that could be used for tolerance induction in inflammatory circumstances such as autoimmune and allergic disorders.

6.9 Probiotics and Prebiotics

Probiotics are live microbes that, when consumed in sufficient quantities, confer health benefits to the host [94]. The word Probiotic comes from the Greek word "pro" meaning "promoting" and "biotic" meaning "life." "Probiotics" term was coined in the early twentieth century, when Elie Metchnikoff, the "Father of Probiotics," observed that rural people in Bulgaria lived to very old ages despite poverty and hard life. He theorized that beneficial bacteria found in nutritional sources such as sour milk could reside in the intestinal tract and promote the health condition. Although almost all Probiotics are categorized as bacteria, especially Lactobacillus and Bifidobacterium, some fungi could act as Probiotics, such as *Saccharomyces boulardii* variety Cerevisiae [95].

Probiotics exist in many food resources, particularly in old traditional types, including yogurt, kefir, kombucha, sauerkraut, tempeh, kimchi, pickles, miso, sourdough bread and some cheeses. Probiotics help food digestion, vitamin synthesis, maintaining gut pH and preventing pathogen colonization. They are also involved in the development and establishing healthy gut immunity [96]. Nowadays, the probiotics are gaining more interest because of their ability to dampen inflammation and regulating immune responses. Their presence in alimentary products could affect the gut microbiome significantly as it has been demonstrated that even a single bacterial species can deviate the homeostatic balance of the immune system to a healthy direction. For instance, in animal models, *B. fragilis* exerts anti-inflammatory responses by inducing the production of IL-10 from Tregs cells and inhibiting Th17 responses [91]. Similarly, Clostridia species were shown to promote Treg development, thus provided partial protection against colitis and systemic IgE responses [45]. These and other findings suggest the idea of inducing Treg cells in the gut environment of IBD and SpA patients with these probiotics. Accordingly, administration of heat-killed or live *Lactobacillus rhamnosus* GG to the rats caused amelioration of experimental arthritis probably through inhibition of the p38 MAPK pathway, which regulates COX2 expression and prevents cytokine-induced apoptosis [97, 98]. Similarly, VSL#3, a commercially available probiotic-containing eight strains of bacteria including Lactobacillus and Bifidobacterium species, when given to IL-10-deficient mice, reduces TNF-α and IFN-α production in the gut mucosa, both of which are involved in the pathogenesis of SpA and IBD [99]. Moreover, Probiotic Lactobacillus casei has been found to decrease arthritis scores and levels of pro-inflammatory cytokines in rat models of Rheumatoid Arthritis. Its effectiveness was revealed to be more than indomethacin [100]. However, despite all the encouraging results from animal studies, human studies were not so successful. One randomized controlled trial of giving a probiotic-containing *Lactobacillus acidophilus*, *B. lactis*, and *Streptococcus salivarius* to SpA patients did not show any significant benefit [101]; likewise, another randomized controlled trial failed to show any considerable improvement in SpA cases receiving a probiotic-containing Lactobacillus salivarius, *Lactobacillus paracasei*, *B. infantis*, and *B. bifidum* species [102]. Obviously, further investigations are required to elucidate the efficacy or inefficiency of probiotics in SpAs patients.

Prebiotics are food components that induce the growth and activity of beneficial microorganisms such as bacteria and fungi in the gastrointestinal tract. The influence of dietary habits on the gut microbiome is undeniable because digested food is the main source of alimentation for the resident microorganisms. One study demonstrated the effect of a prebiotic regimen containing oligofructose and inulin in changing gut microbiota, reducing inflammatory cytokines and consequently alleviating colitis in HLA-B27-transgenic rats [103]. In the same way, the mice fed with apples high in polyphenols had decreased inflammatory mediators and exhibited significant amelioration of colitis [104]. It has also been demonstrated that there is a significant association between consumption of dietary fat and outgrowth of microbes implicated in developing IBD [7]. However, the role of prebiotics in treating spondyloarthropathies remains to be understood.

6.10 Antibiotics and Fecal Transplant

Antibiotics might be helpful in managing ReA by eliminating the source of pathogenic species, including certain Gram negative microbes. On the other hand, they are profoundly implicated in microbiota disturbance [105]. Moreover, the adverse effect of antibiotics in predisposing the gut to flourish *Clostridium difficile* has already been shown; meanwhile there have been efforts to cure this situation with fecal transplantation from healthy individuals [106]. Therefore, the fecal transplant might be suggested as an accessory option in the treatment of diseases associated with reduced biodiversity of the gut, such as SpA [107].

6.11 Conclusion

Several studies have been conducted to discover the association of gut microbiota with spondyloarthropathies. There have also been progressions in describing the role of the microbiome in developing gut immunity and determining the cytokines combination and level in the gastrointestinal tract. Moreover, despite inconsistent findings of microbial alterations in SpA, there have been attempts to manipulate gut microbiota for suppressing dysregulated immune responses. Obviously, this issue stands at the beginning because a large proportion of evidence has been obtained from animal studies and controversial results, probably due to the population and technical variations that make it difficult to come to a conclusion. Therefore, large-scale studies in different healthy populations using comparable techniques should be conducted to describe the normal microbiota or at least normal entrotypes. Thereafter, the microbiota of patients has to be analyzed in comparison to the healthy individuals, and once the most significant disparities were detected, therapeutic interventions could be performed to "normalize" the composition and amount of microorganisms in SpA patients. Finally, the impact of this "normalization" has to be evaluated on the clinical and paraclinical manifestation of disease as well as patients' quality of life.

References

1. Huttenhower C, Gevers D, Knight R, Abubucker S, Badger JH, Chinwalla AT, et al. Structure, function and diversity of the healthy human microbiome. Nature. 2012;486(7402):207.
2. Wang B, Yao M, Lv L, Ling Z, Li L. The human microbiota in health and disease. Engineering. 2017;3(1):71–82.
3. Asquith M, Elewaut D, Lin P, Rosenbaum JT. The role of the gut and microbes in the pathogenesis of spondyloarthritis. Best Pract Res Clin Rheumatol. 2014;28(5):687–702.
4. Wikoff WR, Anfora AT, Liu J, Schultz PG, Lesley SA, Peters EC, et al. Metabolomics analysis reveals large effects of gut microflora on mammalian blood metabolites. Proc Natl Acad Sci U S A. 2009;106(10):3698–703.
5. Soichi T. The effect of probiotics and gut microbiota on Th17 cells. Int Rev Immunol. 2013;32(5–6):511–25.
6. Manichanh C, Borruel N, Casellas F, Guarner F. The gut microbiota in IBD. Nat Rev Gastroenterol Hepatol. 2012;9(10):599–608.
7. David LA, Maurice CF, Carmody RN, Gootenberg DB, Button JE, Wolfe BE, et al. Diet rapidly and reproducibly alters the human gut microbiome. Nature. 2014;505(7484):559–63.
8. Atarashi K, Honda K. Microbiota in autoimmunity and tolerance. Curr Opin Immunol. 2011;23(6):761–8.
9. Qin J, Li R, Raes J, Arumugam M, Burgdorf KS, Manichanh C, et al. A human gut microbial gene catalogue established by metagenomic sequencing. Nature. 2010;464(7285):59–65.
10. Arumugam M, Raes J, Pelletier E, Le Paslier D, Yamada T, Mende DR, et al. Erratum: enterotypes of the human gut microbiome (Nature (2011) 473 (174–180)). 2011;474(7353).
11. Costello ME, Ciccia F, Willner D, Warrington N, Robinson PC, Gardiner B, et al. Brief report: intestinal dysbiosis in ankylosing spondylitis. Arthritis Rheumatol. 2015;67(3):686–91.
12. Ebringer R, Cooke D, Cawdell D, Cowling P, Ebringer A. Ankylosing spondylitis: klebsiella and HL-A B27. Oxford: Oxford University Press; 1977.
13. Stebbings S, Munro K, Simon M, Tannock G, Highton J, Harmsen H, et al. Comparison of the faecal microflora of patients with ankylosing spondylitis and controls using molecular methods of analysis. Rheumatology. 2002;41(12):1395–401.
14. Aggarwal A, Sarangi A, Gaur P, Shukla A, Aggarwal R. Gut microbiome in children with enthesitis-related arthritis in a developing country and the effect of probiotic administration. Clin Exp Immunol. 2017;187(3):480–9.
15. Stoll ML, Kumar R, Morrow CD, Lefkowitz EJ, Cui X, Genin A, et al. Altered microbiota associated with abnormal humoral immune responses to commensal organisms in enthesitis-related arthritis. Arthritis Res Ther. 2014;16(6):486.

16. Singh YP, Singh AK, Aggarwal A, Misra R. Evidence of cellular immune response to outer membrane protein of Salmonella typhimurium in patients with enthesitis-related arthritis subtype of juvenile idiopathic arthritis. J Rheumatol. 2011;38(1):161–6.
17. Zhou C, Zhao H, Xiao X-Y, Guo R-J, Wang Q, Chen H, et al. Metagenomic profiling of the pro-inflammatory gut microbiota in ankylosing spondylitis. J Autoimmun. 2020;107:102360.
18. Scher JU, Ubeda C, Artacho A, Attur M, Isaac S, Reddy SM, et al. Decreased bacterial diversity characterizes the altered gut microbiota in patients with psoriatic arthritis, resembling dysbiosis in inflammatory bowel disease. Arthritis Rheumatol. 2015;67(1):128–39.
19. Keat A, Maini R, Nkwazi G, Pegrum G, Ridgway G, Scott JT. Role of *Chlamydia trachomatis* and HLA-B27 in sexually acquired reactive arthritis. Br Med J. 1978;1(6113):605–7.
20. Granfors K, Jalkanen S, Mäki-Ikola O, Lahesmaa-Rantala R, Saario R, Toivanen A, et al. Salmonella lipopolysaccharide in synovial cells from patients with reactive arthritis. Lancet. 1990;335(8691):685–8.
21. Merilahti-Palo R, Söderström K, Lahesmaa-Rantala R, Granfors K, Toivanen A. Bacterial antigens in synovial biopsy specimens in yersinia triggered reactive arthritis. Ann Rheum Dis. 1991;50(2):87–90.
22. Stebbings SM, Taylor C, Tannock GW, Baird MA, Highton J. The immune response to autologous bacteroides in ankylosing spondylitis is characterized by reduced interleukin 10 production. J Rheumatol. 2009;36(4):797–800.
23. Stone M, Payne U, Schentag C, Rahman P, Pacheco-Tena C, Inman RD. Comparative immune responses to candidate arthritogenic bacteria do not confirm a dominant role for Klebsiella pneumonia in the pathogenesis of familial ankylosing spondylitis. Rheumatology (Oxford). 2004;43(2):148–55.
24. Tani Y, Tiwana H, Hukuda S, Nishioka J, Fielder M, Wilson C, et al. Antibodies to Klebsiella, Proteus, and HLA-B27 peptides in Japanese patients with ankylosing spondylitis and rheumatoid arthritis. J Rheumatol. 1997;24(1):109–14.
25. Rashid T, Ebringer A. Ankylosing spondylitis is linked to Klebsiella—the evidence. Clin Rheumatol. 2007;26(6):858–64.
26. Stolwijk C, Boonen A, van Tubergen A, Reveille JD. Epidemiology of spondyloarthritis. Rheum Dis Clin. 2012;38(3):441–76.
27. Ellinghaus D, Jostins L, Spain SL, Cortes A, Bethune J, Han B, et al. Analysis of five chronic inflammatory diseases identifies 27 new associations and highlights disease-specific patterns at shared loci. Nat Genet. 2016;48(5):510–8.
28. Mielants H, Veys E, Cuvelier C, De Vos MJR. Ileocolonoscopic findings in seronegative spondylarthropathies. Br J Rheumatol. 1988;27(Suppl_2):95–105.
29. Mielants H, Veys E, Cuvelier C, De MV, Goemaere S, De LC, et al. The evolution of spondyloarthropathies in relation to gut histology. III. Relation between gut and joint. J Rheumatol. 1995;22(12):2279–84.
30. Van Praet L, Van den Bosch FE, Jacques P, Carron P, Jans L, Colman R, et al. Microscopic gut inflammation in axial spondyloarthritis: a multiparametric predictive model. Ann Rheum Dis. 2013;72(3):414–7.
31. Shivashankar R, Loftus EV, Tremaine WJ, Bongartz T, Harmsen WS, Zinsmeister AR, et al. Incidence of spondyloarthropathy in patients with Crohn's disease: a population-based study. J Rheumatol. 2012;39(11):2148–52.
32. Malaty HM, Lo GH-W, Hou JK. Characterization and prevalence of spondyloarthritis and peripheral arthritis among patients with inflammatory bowel disease. Clin Exp Gastroenterol. 2017;10:259–63.
33. Van Praet L, Jans L, Carron P, Jacques P, Glorieus E, Colman R, et al. Degree of bone marrow oedema in sacroiliac joints of patients with axial spondyloarthritis is linked to gut inflammation and male sex: results from the GIANT cohort. Ann Rheum Dis. 2014;73(6):1186–9.
34. Nanda S. Novel genetic variants link ankylosing spondylitis and Crohn disease: evidence of a shared pathogenesis? Nat Rev Rheumatol. 2011;7(2):70.
35. Danoy P, Pryce K, Hadler J, Bradbury LA, Farrar C, Pointon J, et al. Association of variants at 1q32 and STAT3 with ankylosing spondylitis suggests genetic overlap with Crohn's disease. PLoS Genet. 2010;6(12):e1001195.

36. Taurog JD, Richardson JA, Croft J, Simmons WA, Zhou M, Fernández-Sueiro JL, et al. The germfree state prevents development of gut and joint inflammatory disease in HLA-B27 transgenic rats. J Exp Med. 1994;180(6):2359–64.
37. Rath HC, Herfarth HH, Ikeda JS, Grenther WB, Hamm TE, Balish E, et al. Normal luminal bacteria, especially Bacteroides species, mediate chronic colitis, gastritis, and arthritis in HLA-B27/human beta2 microglobulin transgenic rats. J Clin Invest. 1996;98(4):945–53.
38. Lin P, Bach M, Asquith M, Lee AY, Akileswaran L, Stauffer P, et al. HLA-B27 and human β2-microglobulin affect the gut microbiota of transgenic rats. PLoS One. 2014;9(8):e105684.
39. McGeachy MJ, Cua DJ. The link between IL-23 and Th17 cell-mediated immune pathologies. Seminars in immunology. Seminars Immunol. 2007;19:372–6. Elsevier
40. Ausiello CM, Fedele G, Palazzo R, Spensieri F, Ciervo A, Cassone AJM, et al. 60-kDa heat shock protein of *Chlamydia pneumoniae* promotes a T helper type 1 immune response through IL-12/IL-23 production in monocyte-derived dendritic cells. Microbes Infect. 2006;8(3):714–20.
41. Rehaume LM, Mondot S, Aguirre de Cárcer D, Velasco J, Benham H, Hasnain SZ, et al. ZAP-70 genotype disrupts the relationship between microbiota and host, leading to spondyloarthritis and ileitis in SKG mice. Arthritis Rheumatol. 2014;66(10):2780–92.
42. Bäckhed F, Ding H, Wang T, Hooper LV, Koh GY, Nagy A, et al. The gut microbiota as an environmental factor that regulates fat storage. Proc Natl Acad Sci U S A. 2004;101(44):15718–23.
43. Smith PM, Howitt MR, Panikov N, Michaud M, Gallini CA, Bohlooly YM, et al. The microbial metabolites, short-chain fatty acids, regulate colonic Treg cell homeostasis. Science. 2013;341(6145):569–73.
44. Furusawa Y, Obata Y, Fukuda S, Endo TA, Nakato G, Takahashi D, et al. Commensal microbe-derived butyrate induces the differentiation of colonic regulatory T cells. Nature. 2013;504(7480):446–50.
45. Atarashi K, Tanoue T, Shima T, Imaoka A, Kuwahara T, Momose Y, et al. Induction of colonic regulatory T cells by indigenous Clostridium species. Science. 2011;331(6015):337–41.
46. Hill DA, Artis D. Intestinal bacteria and the regulation of immune cell homeostasis. Annu Rev Immunol. 2009;28:623–67.
47. Lécuyer E, Rakotobe S, Lengliné-Garnier H, Lebreton C, Picard M, Juste C, et al. Segmented filamentous bacterium uses secondary and tertiary lymphoid tissues to induce gut IgA and specific T helper 17 cell responses. Immunity. 2014;40(4):608–20.
48. Ivanov II, Atarashi K, Manel N, Brodie EL, Shima T, Karaoz U, et al. Induction of intestinal Th17 cells by segmented filamentous bacteria. Cell. 2009;139(3):485–98.
49. Umesaki Y, Okada Y, Matsumoto S, Imaoka A, Setoyama H. Segmented filamentous bacteria are indigenous intestinal bacteria that activate intraepithelial lymphocytes and induce MHC class II molecules and fucosyl asialo GM1 glycolipids on the small intestinal epithelial cells in the ex-germ-free mouse. Microbiol Immunol. 1995;39(8):555–62.
50. Wu H-J, Ivanov II, Darce J, Hattori K, Shima T, Umesaki Y, et al. Gut-residing segmented filamentous bacteria drive autoimmune arthritis via T helper 17 cells. Immunity. 2010;32(6):815–27.
51. Kuwahara T, Ogura Y, Oshima K, Kurokawa K, Ooka T, Hirakawa H, et al. The lifestyle of the segmented filamentous bacterium: a non-culturable gut-associated immunostimulating microbe inferred by whole-genome sequencing. DNA Res. 2011;18(4):291–303.
52. Faure M, Moennoz D, Mettraux C, Montigon F, Schiffrin E, Obled C, et al. The chronic colitis developed by HLA-B27 transgenic rats is associated with altered in vivo mucin synthesis. Dig Dis Sci. 2004;49(2):339–46.
53. Van der Sluis M, De Koning BA, De Bruijn AC, Velcich A, Meijerink JP, Van Goudoever JB, et al. Muc2-deficient mice spontaneously develop colitis, indicating that MUC2 is critical for colonic protection. Gastroenterology. 2006;131(1):117–29.
54. Shan M, Gentile M, Yeiser JR, Walland AC, Bornstein VU, Chen K, et al. Mucus enhances gut homeostasis and oral tolerance by delivering immunoregulatory signals. Science. 2013;342(6157):447–53.

55. Laukens D, Peeters H, Marichal D, Vander Cruyssen B, Mielants H, Elewaut D, et al. CARD15 gene polymorphisms in patients with spondyloarthropathies identify a specific phenotype previously related to Crohn's disease. Ann Rheum Dis. 2005;64(6):930–5.
56. Fert I, Cagnard N, Glatigny S, Letourneur F, Jacques S, Smith JA, et al. Reverse interferon signature is characteristic of antigen-presenting cells in human and rat spondyloarthritis. Arthritis Rheumatol. 2014;66(4):841–51.
57. Gomes MM, Herr AB. IgA and IgA-specific receptors in human disease: structural and functional insights into pathogenesis and therapeutic potential. Springer Semin Immunopathol. 2006;28(4):383–95. Springer
58. Cuvelier C, Barbatis C, Mielants H, De Vos M, Roels H, Veys E. Histopathology of intestinal inflammation related to reactive arthritis. Gut. 1987;28(4):394–401.
59. Demetter P, Baeten D, De Keyser F, De Vos M, Van Damme N, Verbruggen G, et al. Subclinical gut inflammation in spondyloarthropathy patients is associated with upregulation of the E-cadherin/catenin complex. Ann Rheum Dis. 2000;59(3):211–6.
60. Hermiston ML, Gordon JI. Inflammatory bowel disease and adenomas in mice expressing a dominant negative N-cadherin. Science. 1995;270(5239):1203–7.
61. Mielants H, De Vos M, Goemaere S, Schelstraete K, Cuvelier C, Goethals K, et al. Intestinal mucosal permeability in inflammatory rheumatic diseases. II Role of disease. J Rheumatol. 1991;18(3):394–400.
62. Ciccia F, Accardo-Palumbo A, Rizzo A, Guggino G, Raimondo S, Giardina A, et al. Evidence that autophagy, but not the unfolded protein response, regulates the expression of IL-23 in the gut of patients with ankylosing spondylitis and subclinical gut inflammation. Ann Rheum Dis. 2014;73(8):1566–74.
63. Benjamin JL, Sumpter R Jr, Levine B, Hooper LV. Intestinal epithelial autophagy is essential for host defense against invasive bacteria. Cell Host Microbe. 2013;13(6):723–34.
64. Kaser A, Adolph TE, Blumberg RS. The unfolded protein response and gastrointestinal disease. Seminars in immunopathology. Cham: Springer; 2013.
65. Colbert RA, Tran TM, Layh-Schmitt G. HLA-B27 misfolding and ankylosing spondylitis. Mol Immunol. 2014;57(1):44–51.
66. Baeten D, Demetter P, Cuvelier CA, Kruithof E, Van Damme N, De Vos M, et al. Macrophages expressing the scavenger receptor CD163: a link between immune alterations of the gut and synovial inflammation in spondyloarthropathy. J Pathol. 2002;196(3):343–50.
67. Jacques P, Elewaut D. Joint expedition: linking gut inflammation to arthritis. Mucosal Immunol. 2008;1(5):364–71.
68. Hermann E, Mayet W-J, Poralla T, Zum Büschenfelde K-HM, Fleischer B. Salmonella-reactive synovial fluid T-cell clones in a patient with post-infectious Salmonella arthritis. Scand J Rheumatol. 1990;19(5):350–5.
69. Probst P, Hermann E, Fleischer B. Multiclonal synovial T cell response to *Yersinia enterocolitica* in reactive arthritis: the Yersinia 61-kDa heat-shock protein is not the major target antigen. J Infect Dis. 1993;167(2):385–91.
70. Geczy A, Alexander K, Bashir HV, Edmonds JJN. A factor (s) in Klebsiella culture filtrates specifically modifjies an HLA-B27-associated cell-surface component. Nature. 1980;283(5749):782–4.
71. Van Bohemen CG, Grumet F, Zanen HJI. Identification of HLA-B27M1 and-M2 cross-reactive antigens in Klebsiella. Shigella and Yersinia. 1984;52(4):607.
72. Schwimmbeck PL, Oldstone MB. Molecular mimicry between human leukocyte antigen B27 and klebsiella: consequences for spondyloarthropathies. Am J Med. 1988;85(6):51–3.
73. Scofield R, Warren W, Koelsch G, Harley JB. A hypothesis for the HLA-B27 immune dysregulation in spondyloarthropathy: contributions from enteric organisms, B27 structure, peptides bound by B27, and convergent evolution. Proc Natl Acad Sci USA. 1993;90(20):9330–4.
74. Penttinen MA, Heiskanen KM, Mohapatra R, DeLay ML, Colbert RA, Sistonen L, et al. Enhanced intracellular replication of *Salmonella enteritidis* in HLA–B27–expressing human monocytic cells: dependency on glutamic acid at position 45 in the B pocket of HLA–B27. Arthritis Rheum. 2004;50(7):2255–63.

75. Stagg A, Breban M, Hammer RE, Knight S, Taurog JD. Defective dendritic cell (DC) function in a HLA-B27 transgenic rat model of spondyloarthropathy (SpA). In: Dendritic cells in fundamental and clinical immunology. Cham: Springer; 1995. p. 557–9.
76. Ge S, He Q, Granfors KJPO. HLA-B27 modulates intracellular growth of Salmonella pathogenicity island 2 mutants and production of cytokines in infected monocytic U937 cells. PLoS One. 2012;7(3):e34093.
77. Huttenhower C, Kostic AD, Xavier RJ. Inflammatory bowel disease as a model for translating the microbiome. Immunity. 2014;40(6):843–54.
78. Goto Y, Panea C, Nakato G, Cebula A, Lee C, Diez MG, et al. Segmented filamentous bacteria antigens presented by intestinal dendritic cells drive mucosal Th17 cell differentiation. Immunity. 2014;40(4):594–607.
79. Schulz SM, Köhler G, Holscher C, Iwakura Y, Alber G. IL-17A is produced by Th17, γδ T cells and other CD4– lymphocytes during infection with *Salmonella enterica* serovar Enteritidis and has a mild effect in bacterial clearance. Int Immunol. 2008;20(9):1129–38.
80. Ivanov II, de Llanos FR, Manel N, Yoshinaga K, Rifkin DB, Sartor RB, et al. Specific microbiota direct the differentiation of IL-17-producing T-helper cells in the mucosa of the small intestine. Cell Host Microbe. 2008;4(4):337–49.
81. Morton AM, Sefik E, Upadhyay R, Weissleder R, Benoist C, Mathis D. Endoscopic photoconversion reveals unexpectedly broad leukocyte trafficking to and from the gut. Proc Natl Acad Sci U S A. 2014;111(18):6696–701.
82. Ciccia F, Bombardieri M, Principato A, Giardina A, Tripodo C, Porcasi R, et al. Overexpression of interleukin-23, but not interleukin-17, as an immunologic signature of subclinical intestinal inflammation in ankylosing spondylitis. Arthritis Rheum. 2009;60(4):955–65.
83. Uematsu S, Fujimoto K, Jang MH, Yang B-G, Jung Y-J, Nishiyama M, et al. Regulation of humoral and cellular gut immunity by lamina propria dendritic cells expressing toll-like receptor 5. Nat Immunol. 2008;9(7):769–76.
84. Hall JA, Bouladoux N, Sun CM, Wohlfert EA, Blank RB, Zhu Q, et al. Commensal DNA limits regulatory T cell conversion and is a natural adjuvant of intestinal immune responses. Immunity. 2008;29(4):637–49.
85. Torchinsky MB, Garaude J, Martin AP, Blander JM. Innate immune recognition of infected apoptotic cells directs Th 17 cell differentiation. Nature. 2009;458(7234):78–82.
86. Atarashi K, Nishimura J, Shima T, Umesaki Y, Yamamoto M, Onoue M, et al. ATP drives lamina propria TH 17 cell differentiation. Nature. 2008;455(7214):808–12.
87. Ciccia F, Accardo-Palumbo A, Alessandro R, Rizzo A, Principe S, Peralta S, et al. Interleukin-22 and interleukin-22–producing NKp44+ natural killer cells in subclinical gut inflammation in ankylosing spondylitis. Arthritis Rheum. 2012, 64(6):1869–78.
88. Esin S, Batoni G, Counoupas C, Stringaro A, Brancatisano FL, Colone M, et al. Direct binding of human NK cell natural cytotoxicity receptor NKp44 to the surfaces of mycobacteria and other bacteria. Infect Immun. 2008;76(4):1719–27.
89. Glatzer T, Killig M, Meisig J, Ommert I, Luetke-Eversloh M, Babic M, et al. RORγt+ innate lymphoid cells acquire a proinflammatory program upon engagement of the activating receptor NKp44. Immunity. 2013;38(6):1223–35.
90. Karimi K, Inman MD, Bienenstock J, Forsythe P. *Lactobacillus reuteri*–induced regulatory T cells protect against an allergic airway response in mice. Am J Respir Crit Care Med. 2009;179(3):186–93.
91. Round JL, Mazmanian SK. Inducible Foxp3+ regulatory T-cell development by a commensal bacterium of the intestinal microbiota. Proc Natl Acad Sci U S A. 2010;107(27):12204–9.
92. Round JL, Lee SM, Li J, Tran G, Jabri B, Chatila TA, et al. The Toll-like receptor pathway establishes commensal gut colonization. Science (New York, NY). 2011;332(6032):974.
93. Atarashi K, Tanoue T, Shima T, Imaoka A, Kuwahara T, Momose Y, et al. Induction of colonic regulatory T cells by indigenous Clostridium species. Science. 2011;331(6015):337–41.
94. Hill C, Guarner F, Reid G, Gibson GR, Merenstein DJ, Pot B, et al. Expert consensus document: the international scientific Association for Probiotics and Prebiotics consensus state-

ment on the scope and appropriate use of the term probiotic. Nat Rev Gastroenterol Hepatol. 2014;11(8):506.

95. Banik A, Halder SK, Ghosh C, Mondal KC. Fungal probiotics: opportunity, challenge, and prospects. Recent advancement in white biotechnology through fungi. Cham: Springer; 2019. p. 101–17.
96. Singh N, Yadav H, Marotta F, Singh V. Probiotics-a probable therapeutic agent for spondyloarthropathy. Int J Probiotics Prebiotics. 2017;12(2):57.
97. Baharav E, Mor F, Halpern M, Weinberger A. Lactobacillus GG bacteria ameliorate arthritis in Lewis rats. J Nutr. 2004;134(8):1964–9.
98. Yan F, Polk DB. Probiotic bacterium prevents cytokine-induced apoptosis in intestinal epithelial cells. J Biol Chem. 2002;277(52):50959–65.
99. Madsen K, Cornish A, Soper P, McKaigney C, Jijon H, Yachimec C, et al. Probiotic bacteria enhance murine and human intestinal epithelial barrier function. Gastroenterology. 2001;121(3):580–91.
100. Bedaiwi MK, Inman RD. Microbiome and probiotics: link to arthritis. Curr Opin Rheumatol. 2014;26(4):410–5.
101. Jenks K, Stebbings S, Burton J, Schultz M, Herbison P, Highton J. Probiotic therapy for the treatment of spondyloarthritis: a randomized controlled trial. J Rheumatol. 2010;37(10):2118–25.
102. Brophy S, Burrows CL, Brooks C, Gravenor MB, Siebert S, Allen SJ. Internet-based randomised controlled trials for the evaluation of complementary and alternative medicines: probiotics in spondyloarthropathy. BMC Musculoskeletal Dis. 2008;9(1):4.
103. Hoentjen F, Welling GW, Harmsen HJ, Zhang X, Snart J, Tannock GW, et al. Reduction of colitis by prebiotics in HLA-B27 transgenic rats is associated with microflora changes and immunomodulation. Inflamm Bowel Dis. 2005;11(11):977–85.
104. Castagnini C, Luceri C, Toti S, Bigagli E, Caderni G, Femia AP, et al. Reduction of colonic inflammation in HLA-B27 transgenic rats by feeding Marie Ménard apples, rich in polyphenols. Br J Nutr. 2009;102(11):1620–8.
105. Barber CE, Kim J, Inman RD, Esdaile JM, James MT. Antibiotics for treatment of reactive arthritis: a systematic review and metaanalysis. J Rheumatol. 2013;40(6):916–28.
106. Wortelboer K, Nieuwdorp M, Herrema H. Fecal microbiota transplantation beyond Clostridioides difficile infections. EBioMedicine. 2019;44:716–29.
107. Choi RY, Asquith M, Rosenbaum JT. Fecal transplants in spondyloarthritis and uveitis: ready for a clinical trial? Curr Opin Rheumatol. 2018;30(4):303–9.

7 Spondyloarthropathies and Food Intake

Bahareh Mohebbi and Narjes Soleimanifar

7.1 Introduction

7.1.1 Spondyloarthropathies

Spondyloarthropathies (SpA) is an "umbrella term" that refers to an extended group of heterogeneous diseases that includes ankylosing spondylitis (AS) as one of the important disorders in this category, psoriatic arthritis (PsA), reactive arthritis (ReA), inflammatory bowel disease (IBD) associated spondyloarthritis (IBD-SpA), and undifferentiated spondyloarthritis (uSpA) which share some clinical manifestations, genetic predisposition, and some pathogenic pathways [1, 2]. These interrelated disorders have several distinguishing features in common such as enthesitis, dactylitis, peripheral arthritis, inflammatory back pain, and some extraarticular features such as IBD, uveitis, psoriasis, and HLA-B27 positivity which considered as the prototypical manifestations of SpA [2].

From the genetics vision, there is a strong association between the presence of a special allele of the major histocompatibility complex (MHC) class 1 antigen gene, called human leukocyte antigen-B27 (HLA-B27) gene, and spondyloarthropathy disorders [3–5]. HLA-B27 is a kind of surface marker specifically encoded by HLA class 1 in humans or MHC class 1 in general. A large number of existing studies have shown the prevalence of HLA-B27 in general population and SpA patients so that it is approximately about 6–10% in general healthy ones and 74–89% in SpA patients, and the highest association has been demonstrated in patients suffering from AS disease [6]. MHC class I molecules play an important role in presenting antigens and endogenous peptides to CD 8+ cytotoxic T lymphocytes through T cell surface receptors. The antigen presentation through improper HLA-B27 leads to

B. Mohebbi · N. Soleimanifar (✉)
Molecular Immunology Research Center, Tehran University of medical sciences, Tehran, Iran
e-mail: n-soleimanifar@farabi.tums.ac.ir

M. H. Nicknam (ed.), *Ankylosing Spondylitis - Axial Spondyloarthritis*,
https://doi.org/10.1007/978-981-16-4733-8_7

immune dysregulation at intestinal and entheseal barriers as the primary site of immune cascade activation through altering T cell responses and increasing the rate of apoptotic cell death and inflammation [7]. As, entheseal CD 4+ and CD 8+ T cells with the accompany of interleukin 23 activate the pro-inflammatory immune cascade and also produce interleukin 17 in animal models [8].

7.1.2 Ankylosing Spondylitis

Among all these critical rheumatologic disorders which were mentioned above, ankylosing spondylitis attracts a lot of attention. There is a close correlation between the axial skeleton inflammation and the presence of HLA-B27, which results in making differences in some chronic autoimmune arthritis, for example, differentiating AS from RA disease [9, 10]. AS disease is described by a significant sign in the patient's bones which is called new bone formation and osteoporosis simultaneously; also, it contains the syndesmophytes formation and making ankylosis in the sacroiliac joints and the spine [2, 9]. The AS prevalence differs between the various regions of the world because of many unknown and known reasons, such as genetics, environmental, microbial, and dietary factors. Recent developments have revealed that bowel involvement and inflammation is one of the most critical extraarticular manifestations in SPA, especially in AS patients. Studies reported that both silent and clinically evident IBD occurred more in AS patients contrary to the other arthritis disorders which is associated with AS disease activity [11]. The prevalence of the different types of IBD, including Crohn's disease (CD) and ulcerative colitis (UC), is frequently much more in AS (approximately 6%–14%) than other types of SpA, and most of the patients with AS do not exhibit the symptomatic signs of IBD, consequently, AS disease considered as asymptomatic ones [12, 13]. Malnutrition and improper food intake may be cause or effect of these gastrointestinal manifestation. Decreased level of certain nutrients, including vitamins or mineral elements are detected in SpAs. However some studies have reported the assotiatiaon between AS disease activity and some foods intake, further studies are still needed [14].

7.2 Vitamins

7.2.1 Vitamin D

There is little evidence on the pathophysiology of osteoporosis in AS patients but several studies have been increasingly identified various factors that may be associated with the osteoporosis pathophysiological process, such as drug intake, involvement of some inflammatory procedures, and mobility reduction [2, 15, 16]. Moreover, one of the most important factors that have been discussed in several studies for its benefits in osteoporosis, which is present in AS patients, is the role of vitamin D [15, 16].

Vitamin D or cholecalciferol is a kind of hormone that belongs to steroid groups, is obtained from the special diet in the inactive precursors 25-hydroxy vitamin D (25 (OH) D3). In the external tissues and kidneys, 25-hydroxy vitamin D turned to the active 1, 25 hydroxyvitamin D [1].

In recent years, vitamin D has attracted a lot of attention due to the important modulating role in the innate and adaptive immune system. Also, the pivotal role in the regulation of the balance between phosphorus and calcium in the blood circulation, bones, skeletal and dental health is cosidered a lot lately [17, 18]. A number of epidemiological findings have been demonstrated an association between vitamin D deficiency and susceptibility to some severe autoimmune diseases and inflammatory disorders, such as systemic lupus erythematosus (SLE), multiple sclerosis (MS), oral aphthous ulcer, and type 1 diabetes mellitus [1]. Moreover, it may also lead to developing some of the rheumatic diseases, like rheumatoid arthritis (RA) and Behcet's disease (BD) [19, 20].

Vitamin D receptors are expressed on the innate and adaptive immune cells, such as macrophages, dendritic cells (Dc), and lymphocytes. The active form of vitamin D precursors, 1, 25 hydroxyvitamin D, plays a critical role in the adaptive immune system so that it reduces the proliferation and differentiation of B cells; it also declines the activity of pro-inflammatory T helper 1 (Th1) and T helper 17 (Th17) cells. On the other hand, 1, 25 hydroxyvitamin D enhances the activity of T helper 2 (Th2) and regulatory T (Treg) cells in anti-inflammatory pathways in order to support immune tolerance [21, 22]. In addition, it can affect some cytokine pathways involved in the pathogenesis of SpA, especially AS patients through altering the production of interleukin 17 (IL-17), interleukin 12 (IL-12)/interleukin 23 (IL-23) in T cells [22, 23]. Moreover, current studies have been demonstrated that vitamin D has a vital role in some critical subsets of cells involving in the innate immune system, like monocytes and macrophages lineage as well [24]. One described role of vitamin D on monocytes and macrophages as important player cells involving in the pathogenesis of SpA disorders is inhibiting the mRNA synthesis of some macrophage derived pro-inflammatory and inflammatory cytokines, such as interleukin 1 (IL-1), interleukin 6 (IL-6), IL-12, and tumor necrosis factor alpha (TNF-α), also, decreasing the special activity of macrophages which is called antigen presenting activity to lymphocytes [23, 25].

In order to investigate the vitamin D status and its role in patients with spondyloarthritis, such as AS some different studies have been designed. Consequently, they have demonstrated some alteration in levels of vitamin D in these patients' serums, comparatively to their controls [26, 27].

Several studies have suggested that the serum levels of vitamin D in SpA disorders, especially AS patients are lower than control groups. In 2017, Erten et al. demonstrated that vitamin D deficiency is more frequent in 161 patients with SpA disorders [29], also, in 2011, Arends S et al. demonstrated significant relationships between pathophysiology of osteoporosis in AS patients and low levels of vitamin D copmared with controls. Consequently, vitamin D deficiency in AS patients have been suggested by increasing inflammatory process that leads to osteoporosis indirectly [15, 28, 29]. In another study in 2017, Fernandes et al. showed lower levels of vitamin D in 51.2% of 1030 SpA patients. They found that this deficiency was independently related to seasonal variation and the presence of sacroiliitis. Also, no association between serum levels of vitamin D and comorbidities has been found [27]. Conversely, Klingberg et al. do not exert any data showing the association between serum levels of 25 (OH) vitamin D and seasonal dosing, physical movements, and stiffness. Moreover, Sukran Erten et al. have evaluated the vitamin D levels and their relation with the disease activity rate in both AS and uSpA patients plasma contrary to healthy controls [28, 29]. The vitamin D levels in both AS and uSpA patients were significantly lower than controls. Notably, it has been demonstrated that the lower levels of vitamin D were much more prominent in the plasma of AS males. On the other hand, females in the uSpA group have been shown more decrease in the plasma levels of vitamin D in contrast to control group subjects. Furthermore, Sukran Erten et al. demonstrated a negative correlation between serum levels of vitamin D, pain, and disease activity of AS patients [29]. Although there are some associations between high disease activity and some alterations in the metabolism of vitamin D, there are no correlations between Bath Ankylosing Spondylitis Disease Activity Index (BASDAI) and vitamin D in AS patients. Besides, it has been found that the vitamin D levels are inversely associated with both C reactive protein (CRP) rate and erythrocyte sedimentation rate (ESR) in AS patients but this correlation was not associated with uSpA patients [30].

7.2.2 Other Vitamins

In addition to vitamin D and its critical function, some scientists have been attracted to find the role of antioxidant vitamins, such as vitamin E and A in order to find some components decreasing the level of various symptoms of different rheumatologic disorders [31, 32].

7.2.2.1 Vitamin E

Vitamin E is a common term used for a group of four tocotrienols (α, β, γ, and σ tocotrienols) and of four tocopherols (α, β, γ, and σ tocopherols). Although all these compounds can be used as the antioxidant, only alpha tocopherol can be absored by human cells and make its antioxidant function [32]. Vitamin E is one of the critical fat soluble antioxidant components in the lipid phase of the cells that can be transformed to its active form through the function of the free radical's scavenger, vitamin C. Vitamin E can be used against some oxidative metabolites and some free radicals, such as peroxyl radicals, reactive oxygen species, and reactive nitrogen species. Moreover, vitamin E has an impact on protecting the polyunsaturated fatty acids and modulating signal transduction [33].

It is well known that the best dietary sources of vitamin E are consist of vegetable oils and nuts, such as soybean, corn, walnut, and wheat germ oils which contain higher levels of vitamin E [34]. In fact, peroxyl radicals mostly react with lipid hydroperoxide, but in the presence of vitamin E, peroxyl radicals tend to react with alpha tocopherol, consequently, the production of peroxyl radicals and polyunsaturated fatty acids oxidation is inhibited. Vitamin E is increasingly identified for its critical role in the modulation of the innate, humoral, and cellular responses by focusing on the role of various cells, like macrophages, dendritic cells, natural killer cells, and T cells. However vitamin E deficiency is rare in humans, limited studies reported impaired delayed type hypersesitivity (DTH) in intestinal malabsorption patients and impaired bactericidal and phagocytic capacity in preterm vitamin E deficient infants [32, 35]. On the other hand, vitamin E supplements improve Natural Killer (NK) cells and neutrophiles activity in elderly subjects compare to adult controls [35].

7.2.2.2 Vitamin A

Vitamin A known as a micronutrient belongs to the monohydric alcohol groups. Retinol, retinoic acid, and retinal are the various forms of vitamin A, among which the active metabolite of vitamin A, retinoic acid, is a critical component for accompanying several biological functions, such as cell growth, differentiation, apoptosis, hormone function, tissue homeostasis, embryonic development, and organogenesis [36, 37].

Vitamin A, E, and vitamin D have been considered as antioxidants with anti-inflammatory factors [38, 39]. An increasing number of studies have found that retinoic acid has many essential roles in maturation, differentiation, and function of the innate immune cells, comprising monocytes and macrophages [40]. Hiemstra, I.H. et al. demonstrated that vitamin A acts as an important factor in order to differentiate and develop the colonic CD169 positive macrophages [41, 42]. Moreover, Pereira, W.F. et al. and Vellozo, N.S. et al. proved that it can also inhibit monocyte differentiation toward inflammatory macrophages which is called “M1 macrophages” through suppressing the activation of inflammatory pathways and cytokines, also, transform them into anti-inflammatory or M2 macrophages [43, 44].

In adaptive immune cells, Mucidal et al. displayed a controversial role of retinoic acids in T cell differentiation and their responses. All-transretinoic acid (ATRA) can induce the naïve T cell differentiation into Th2 cells and suppress the differentiation through inducing the expression of interleukin 4 (IL-4) gene as an anti-inflammatory cytokine, also modulating an inflammatory cytokine, IL-12 production by antigen presenting cells (APCs). In AS patients ATRA could decreased the number of Th17 cells which is one of the arised pathologic cells in this disease and this vitamin could decreased the level of IL-17 in the As patients who were not using Non-steroidal anti-inflammatory drugs (NSAIDs). On the other hand, retinoic acid is capable to differentiate naïve T cells toward Th1 cells by inducing signal transduction and activator of transcription 6 (STAT 6) and GATA binding protein 3 (GATA 3) gene expression [45, 46].

Moreover, Vitamin A is considered as the important retinoid prohormone with the critical roles in signal transduction at cytoplasmic and membrane sites. In addition, some studies exhibited that vitamin A is a crucial antioxidant factor involving in suppressing the reactive oxygen species induced hypoxia [47, 48]. Various studies demonstrated improving production and levels of reactive oxygen species in most inflammatory conditions, such as AS disease. Consequently, reactive oxygen species and oxidative stress lead to an increase of inflammatory cells and cytokines production. Also inflammatory cytokines are capable to enhance the rate of oxidative stress markers such as malondial dehydrate (MDA) and myeloperoxidase in return [49]. In the last decade, there has been a great attention on the role of inflammation on producing more reactive oxygen species and the decrease the levels of antioxidant vitamins. However, the definite role of oxidant stress and reactive oxygen species in the progression of the inflammatory AS disease is poorly understood [50].

There have not been a large number of studies investigating the relationship between levels of lipid peroxidation and antioxidant vitamins in plasma and erythrocyte properties in AS patients and healthy controls. Mustafa Nazıroğlu et al. focused on the relationship between plasma and erythrocytes of AS patients and demonstrated that there is a positive relationship between them, so that the plasma and erythrocytes levels of lipid peroxidation were enhanced, though the levels of vitamin C, vitamin A, and vitamin E were reduced. Also, glutathione (GSH) and glutathione peroxidase (GSH-Px) activities were decreased contrary to healthy controls [50–52]. Ozgocmen et al.'s studies showed the same results as those reported by Mustafa Nazıroğlu et al., the plasma and erythrocytes levels of lipid peroxidation were increased in patients suffering from active AS [53, 54]. Contrarily, Mézes et al. and Stanek et al. demonstrated no significant differences in lipid peroxidation concentrations and antioxidants vitamins in AS patients comparing to the control group [50].

7.3 Low Starch Diet and Klebsiella

Another dietary habit that leads to lower disease activity in AS patients is a low starch consumption diet that has been suggested by some researchers. Klebsiella pneumonia is a special bacterium that can be influenced through starch diet and has an important role in the initiation and development of AS disease and related gastrointestinal problems [55].

Microbes from bowel flora are dependent on dietary starch for their growth and therefore a reduction in starch intake might be beneficial in AS disease. As, some patients have reported severe gastrointestinal problems when using special foodstuffs such as low consumption of milk and high consumption of vegetable which contains rich starch. Also, patients who suffer from gastrointestinal problems were reported to have low functional and high disease activity through displaying lower Bath Ankylosing Spondylitis Functional Index (BASFI) and higher BASDAI scores which were related to some inflammatory processes induced in the bowel mucosa instead of the direct effect of dietary products and vitamins [56–58].

As mentioned before, one of the most important microorganisms and microbes involved in the development of AS is Klebsiella pneumonia. These microorganisms were isolated from the intestinal tract of active AS patients and Klebsiella microbes were associated with enhancement of the clinical manifestations of the AS disease [56, 59].

Moreover, there is another type of bacteria among 42 isotypes of Klebsiella microbes called Klebsiella oxytoca which were observed and isolated significantly more in the stool samples of patients suffering from AS contrary to patients suffering from rheumatoid arthritis and osteoarthritis. The level of Klebsiella microbes depend on the various collections, culture methods, and disease activity stages of the disease from which stool samples were obtained. A series of recent studies in 15 different countries have reported the enhancement of Klebsiella antibodies in the serum of 1330 AS patients, contrary to 1191 healthy subjects, moreover, the levels of anti-Klebsiella antibodies in the jejunal fluids of AS patients have elevated. Also, there are some similarities between some microbes and genetic markers or different types of collagen that could delay the diagnosis of patients, such as the similarities between HLA-B27 and Klebsiella nitrogenase reductase or collagen types I, III, and IV and Klebsiella pullulanase [56, 60].

7.4 Fatty Acids

Lipid components can directly or indirectly regulate immune system, some toward immunosuppressive conditions and others in proinflammatory effects. Several clinical trials and epidemiological studies have demonstrated the positive role of polyunsaturated fatty acids such as Omega 3 in the diet of AS patients suffering from abnormalities in nervous and cardiovascular systems. In addition to pharmacological treatments, Omega 3 supplementation in AS patient's dietary habits should be considered due to the anti-inflammatory characteristics in the immune system. Reduction of the catabolic activity of enzymes, production of alternative eicosanoids, decreasing the inflammatory cytokines, and descending the activated T cells are the important anti-inflammatory processes of polyunsaturated fatty acids in AS patients. Studies demonstrated that Omega 3 fatty acids intake in proper doses has an influence on AS patients in order to decrease their disease activity and improvement of some cardiac abnormalities [61–63]. On the other hand, saturated fatty acids (SFA) play pivotal role in inflammation through induction of the inflammatory cytokines like TNF-α, IL-6 and IL-8 in macrophages [81]. Also the lipemia as the effect of saturated fatty acids can evoke the secretion of IL-1b one of the most triggers of inflammation. In AS patients the FFQ analysis has shown a positive correlation between consumption of SFA and BASMI and BASDFI indeces [80].

7.5 Obesity

Recently, obesity has been known as a major worldwide problem that attracted a lot of attention in autoinflammatory disease like spondyloarthropathies. In the case of rheumatoid and inflammatory disorders, the obese status and weight loss play critical roles in the progression and activity of the disease, and the responses to some therapeutics methods and drugs. Although obesity and weight loss are poorly studied, some studies indicated the relation between obese status and the risk of cardiovascular issues, like low and high density lipoproteins, hypertension, insulin resistance, and metabolic syndrome in the RA, AS, and PsA patients [64, 65].

There have not been numerous studies to investigate the obesity, and weight loss status in the AS disease. Sari et al. demonstrated that the percentage of body fat indexes such as BMI was decreased in patients suffering from AS contrary to control groups. Although decreasing body fat indexes in AS patients are not fully understood, several studies mentioned that up-regulation of various enzymes involved in fatty acid oxidation could be considered as the main reason for decreasing body fat of patients suffering from AS [66, 67].

Moreover, some studies indicated the low level of triglyceride (TG) in the fibroblast-like synoviocytes (FLSs) of the AS patients. A recent study by Wei dong et al. concluded that both oxidations of high fatty acids and insulin signaling pathways might be the main reasons for decreasing the body fat level. Metabolic switching from glucose to fatty acid was detected in the ligaments of patients with AS [67]. A series of studies have indicated that increasing in the expression of some regulating genes are critical in fatty acid oxidation mechanisms. For instance, a significant increase in phosphatidylinositide 3-kinases (PI3K) and the especial mediator of many receptor tyrosine kinases called, Insulin Receptor (INSR), and the up-regulation of the beta (β) oxidation enzymes which are involved in the fatty acid oxidation in INSR/PI3K/Protein Kinase C (PKC) pathway [67–69].

7.6 Food Allergy

In recent decade, food allergies and various allergens have attracted a lot of attention due to their pivotal role in developing allergic diseases spreadly. Previous studies have shown that approximately 20% of the general population suffer from various types of food allergens, such as eggs, crabs, cow's milk, etc. with different severity of symptoms [70, 71]. Food allergens exhibited a various range of symptoms, from non-symptomatic changes to mild and severe ones, such as skin rash, vomiting, inflammation in the intestinal mucosa, even death. Several studies demonstrated the diverse relationship between allergic disorders, and infectious disease. In addition, correlation between food allergies and intestinal microorganisms are known widely to date however the relation between allergens and AS disease are not fully illustrated yet [72].

In this regard, Ling et al. indicated significant differences in the microbiome composition in the intestine of infants suffering from allergies contrary to healthy ones. The serum levels of some antibodies such as Immunoglobulin E (IgE) levels are in line with the specific microorganism called Clostridium sensu stricto in this study [73, 74]. Another study by Hua et al. demonstrated that each allergen leads to an increase or decrease in the levels of the specific microbes in the gut microbiota. As a prime example, American adults participating in this research suffering from allergies to nuts and seasonal pollen show low diversity in their gut microbiota toward decreasing the amount of Clostridiales, and increasing the amount of Bacteroidales species [75].

In order to investigate the food allergy status and its role in patients with AS some different auto antibodies against food stuff have been find in the serum of AS patients. Wigglesworth et al. demonstrated a close relation between binding of galactose-alpha-1,3-galactose (alpha-Gal) as an antigen and anti-agalactosyl antibodies (anti-Gal) in AS patients that this interaction can lead to the complement system activation and prime the immune system toward allergic reaction [76]. It has been reported that producing pro-inflammatory cytokines and chemokines, macrophage recruitment, and activation has occurred as the result of the alpha-Gal / anti-Gal binding. The disturbed immune system in AS patient can affect the wound healing, tissue regeneration, and finally cause the pathogenesis and progression of AS [77, 78]. Moreover, another study concluded that pork-related food allergy (alpha-Gal) has a critical role in the pathogenesis and progression of patients with AS due to the significant relation between the pork-specific Immunoglobulin G (IgG) and CRP levels in the serum of AS patients. Qian et al. indicated that the levels of specific IgG antibodies against food intakes such as beef, crab, and pork are significantly more in the serum of AS patients compare to the control. Interestingly, a positive correlation between natural antigens like alpha-Gal and AS disease activity, made the alpha-Gal as a key point in the development of AS disease [76]. These findings suggested that the patients suffering from AS avoid using allergic substances and nutrients like some allergens mentioned above to reduce the severity and progress of AS disease [79].

7.7 Conclusion

In conclusion, dietary habits and food intake, can affect the pathogenesis and symptoms of AS patients. Some useful compounds like vitamins can be used to reduce inflammatory problems, however, others like saturated fatty acids have negative correlation to the disease activity in AS patients food intake. Overall, well designed studies of dietary patterns and nutrients are required to determine the precise role of food intake in susceptibilty and pathogenesis of AS.

References

1. Kolahi S, Khabbazi A, Kazemi N, Mahdavi AM. Does vitamin D deficiency contribute to higher disease activity in patients with spondyloarthritis? Immunol Lett. 2019;212:1–5.
2. Mitulescu T-C, Trandafir M, Dimăncescu M-G, Ciuluvică R-C, Popescu V, Predeţeanu D, et al. Advances in the treatment of uveitis in patients with spondyloarthritis-is it the time for biologic therapy? Romanian J Ophthalmol. 2018;62(2):114.
3. Gill T, Rosenbaum JT. Putative pathobionts in HLA-B27-associated spondyloarthropathy. Front Immunol. 2020;11.
4. Rysnik O, McHugh K, van Duivenvoorde L, van Tok M, Guggino G, Taurog J, Kollnberger S, Ciccia F, Baeten D, Bowness P. Non-conventional forms of HLA-B27 are expressed in spondyloarthritis joints and gut tissue. J Autoimmun. 2016;70:12–21.
5. Soleimanifar N, Amirzargar AA, Mahmoudi M, Pourfathollah AA, Azizi E, Jamshidi AR, Rezaei N, Tahoori MT, Bidad K, Nikbin B, Nicknam MH. Study of programmed cell death 1

(PDCD1) gene polymorphims in Iranian patients with ankylosing spondylitis. Inflammation. 2011;34(6):707–12.
6. Taurog JD, Chhabra A, Colbert RA. Ankylosing spondylitis and axial spondyloarthritis. N Engl J Med. 2016;374(26):2563–74.
7. Pathak H, Gaffney K. Spectrum of spondyloarthritis. Indian J Rheumatol. 2020;15(5):34.
8. Furst DE, Louie JS. Targeting inflammatory pathways in axial spondyloarthritis. Arthritis Res Ther. 2019;21(1):135.
9. Ritchlin C, Adamopoulos IE. Axial spondyloarthritis: new advances in diagnosis and management. BMJ. 2021;372:m4447.
10. Jah N, Jobart-Malfait A, Ermoza K, Noteuil A, Chiocchia G, Breban M, et al. HLA–B27 subtypes predisposing to ankylosing spondylitis accumulate in an endoplasmic reticulum–derived compartment apart from the peptide-loading complex. Arthritis Rheumatol. 2020;72(9):1534–46.
11. Fragoulis GE, Liava C, Daoussis D, Akriviadis E, Garyfallos A, Dimitroulas T. Inflammatory bowel diseases and spondyloarthropathies: from pathogenesis to treatment. World J Gastroenterol. 2019;25(18):2162.
12. Karreman MC, Luime JJ, Hazes JM, Weel AE. The prevalence and incidence of axial and peripheral spondyloarthritis in inflammatory bowel disease: a systematic review and meta-analysis. J Crohn's Colitis. 2017;11(5):631–42.
13. Kelly OB, Li N, Smith M, Chan J, Inman RD, Silverberg MS. The prevalence and clinical associations of subclinical sacroiliitis in inflammatory bowel disease. Inflamm Bowel Dis. 2019;25(6):1066–71.
14. Jethwa H, Prince M, Bukhari M, Abraham S. The evidence for dietary manipulation in inflammatory arthritis. Int J Clin Rheumatol. 2019;14(5):190.
15. Arends S, Spoorenberg A, Bruyn GA, Houtman PM, Leijsma MK, Kallenberg CG, et al. The relation between bone mineral density, bone turnover markers, and vitamin D status in ankylosing spondylitis patients with active disease: a cross-sectional analysis. Osteoporos Int. 2011;22(5):1431–9.
16. Kocyigit BF, Akyol A. Vitamin D levels in patients with ankylosing spondylitis: Is it related to disease activity? Pakistan journal of medical sciences. 2018;34(5):1209.
17. Chang S-W, Lee H-C. Vitamin D and health-the missing vitamin in humans. Pediatrics Neonatol. 2019;60(3):237–44.
18. Medrano M, Carrillo-Cruz E, Montero I, Perez-Simon JA. Vitamin D: effect on haematopoiesis and immune system and clinical applications. Int J Mol Sci. 2018;19(9):2663.
19. Khabbazi A, Rashtchizadeh N, Ghorbanihaghjo A, Hajialiloo M, Ghojazadeh M, Taei R, et al. The status of serum vitamin D in patients with active Behcet's disease compared with controls. Int J Rheum Dis. 2014;17(4):430–4.
20. Vanherwegen A-S, Gysemans C, Mathieu C. Regulation of immune function by vitamin D and its use in diseases of immunity. Endocrinology and Metabolism Clinics. 2017;46(4):1061-94.
21. Alhassan Mohammed H, Mirshafiey A, Vahedi H, Hemmasi G, Moussavi Nasl Khameneh A, Parastouei K, et al. Immunoregulation of inflammatory and inhibitory cytokines by vitamin D 3 in patients with inflammatory bowel diseases. Scandinavian journal of immunology. 2017;85(6):386-94.
22. Colotta F, Jansson B, Bonelli F. Modulation of inflammatory and immune responses by vitamin D. Journal of autoimmunity. 2017;85:78–97.
23. Sassi F, Tamone C, D'Amelio P. Vitamin D: nutrient, hormone, and immunomodulator. Nutrients. 2018;10(11):1656.
24. Guła Z, Stec M, Rutkowska-Zapała M, Lenart M, Korkosz M, Gąsowski J, et al. The absolute number of circulating nonclassical (CD14^{+} CD16^{++}) monocytes negatively correlates with DAS28 and swollen joint count in patients with peripheral spondyloarthritis. Polskie Archiwum Medycyny Wewnętrznej= Polish Arch Int Med. 2017;127(12):846–53.
25. Martens P-J, Gysemans C, Verstuyf A, Mathieu C. Vitamin D's effect on immune function. Nutrients. 2020;12(5):1248.
26. Zhao S, Duffield SJ, Moots RJ, Goodson NJ. Systematic review of association between vitamin D levels and susceptibility and disease activity of ankylosing spondylitis. Rheumatology. 2014;53(9):1595–603.

27. Fernandes S, Etcheto A, van der Heijde D, Landewé R, van den Bosch F, Dougados M, et al. Vitamin D status in spondyloarthritis: results of the ASAS-COMOSPA international study. Clin Exp Rheumatol. 2018;36(2):210–4.
28. Crotti C, Becciolini A, Biggioggero M, Favalli EG. Vitamin D and spondyloarthritis: review of the literature. Open Rheumatol J. 2018;12(1):214–25.
29. Erten S, Kucuksahin O, Sahin A, Altunoglu A, Akyol M, Koca C. Decreased plasma vitamin D levels in patients with undifferentiated spondyloarthritis and ankylosing spondylitis. Internal Medicine. 2013;52(3):339–44.
30. Zhao SZ, Thong D, Duffield S, Goodson N. Vitamin D deficiency in axial spondyloarthritis is associated with higher disease activity. Archives of rheumatology. 2017;32(3):209.
31. Apostu D, Lucaciu O, Mester A, Oltean-Dan D, Baciut M, Baciut G, et al. Systemic drugs with impact on osteoarthritis. Drug Metab Rev. 2019;51(4):498–523.
32. Lee GY, Han SN. The role of vitamin E in immunity. Nutrients. 2018;10(11):1614.
33. Carr A, Maggini S. Vitamin C and immune function. Nutrients. 2017;9(11):1211.
34. Mène-Saffrané L. Vitamin E biosynthesis and its regulation in plants. Antioxidants. 2018;7(1):2.
35. Lewis ED, Meydani SN, Wu D. Regulatory role of vitamin E in the immune system and inflammation. IUBMB Life. 2019;71(4):487–94.
36. Zinder R, Cooley R, Vlad LG, Molnar JA. Vitamin a and wound healing. Nutr Clin Pract. 2019;34(6):839–49.
37. Molano A, Meydani SN. Vitamin E, signalosomes and gene expression in T cells. Mol Asp Med. 2012;33(1):55–62.
38. Drabińska N, Krupa-Kozak U, Abramowicz P, Jarocka-Cyrta E. Beneficial effect of oligofructose-enriched inulin on vitamin D and E status in children with celiac disease on a long-term gluten-free diet: a preliminary randomized, placebo-controlled nutritional intervention study. Nutrients. 2018;10(11):1768.
39. Masri OA, Chalhoub JM, Sharara AI. Role of vitamins in gastrointestinal diseases. World J Gastroenterol: WJG. 2015;21(17):5191.
40. Wirth JP, Petry N, Tanumihardjo SA, Rogers LM, McLean E, Greig A, et al. Vitamin a supplementation programs and country-level evidence of vitamin a deficiency. Nutrients. 2017;9(3):190.
41. Hiemstra IH, Beijer MR, Veninga H, Vrijland K, Borg EG, Olivier BJ, et al. The identification and developmental requirements of colonic CD 169+ macrophages. Immunology. 2014;142(2):269–78.
42. Huang Z, Liu Y, Qi G, Brand D, Zheng SG. Role of vitamin a in the immune system. J Clin Med. 2018;7(9):258.
43. Pereira WF, Ribeiro-Gomes FL, Guillermo LVC, Vellozo NS, Montalvão F, DosReis GA, et al. Myeloid-derived suppressor cells help protective immunity to Leishmania major infection despite suppressed T cell responses. J Leukoc Biol. 2011;90(6):1191–7.
44. Vellozo NS, Pereira-Marques ST, Cabral-Piccin MP, Filardy AA, Ribeiro-Gomes FL, Rigoni TS, et al. All-trans retinoic acid promotes an M1-to M2-phenotype shift and inhibits macrophage-mediated immunity to Leishmania major. Front Immunol. 2017;8:1560.
45. Bidad K, Salehi E, Jamshidi A, Saboor-Yaraghi AA, Oraei M, Meysamie A, Mahmoudi M, Nicknam MH. Effect of alltransretinoic acid on Th17 and T regulatory cell subsets in patients with ankylosing spondylitis. The Journal of rheumatology. 2013;40(4):476–83.
46. Liang Y, Yi P, Wang X, Zhang B, Jie Z, Soong L, et al. Retinoic acid modulates hyperactive T cell responses and protects vitamin A–deficient mice against persistent lymphocytic Choriomeningitis virus infection. J Immunol. 2020;204(11):2984–94.
47. Milani A, Basirnejad M, Shahbazi S, Bolhassani A. Carotenoids: biochemistry, pharmacology and treatment. Br J Pharmacol. 2017;174(11):1290–324.
48. Jakubczyk K, Dec K, Kałduńska J, Kawczuga D, Kochman J, Janda K. Reactive oxygen species-sources, functions, oxidative damage. Polski Merkur Lekarski: organ Polskiego Towarzystwa Lekarskiego. 2020;48(284):124–7.
49. Wójcik P, Gęgotek A, Wroński A, Jastrząb A, Żebrowska A, Skrzydlewska E. Effect of redox imbalance on protein modifications in lymphocytes of psoriatic patients. J Biochem. 2020;167(3):323–31.

50. Nazıroğlu M, Akkuş S, Çelik H. Levels of lipid peroxidation and antioxidant vitamins in plasma and erythrocytes of patients with ankylosing spondylitis. Clinical biochemistry. 2011;44(17-18):1412–5.
51. Pishgahi A, Abolhasan R, Danaii S, Amanifar B, Soltani-Zangbar MS, Zamani M, et al. Immunological and oxidative stress biomarkers in ankylosing spondylitis patients with or without metabolic syndrome. Cytokine. 2020;128:155002.
52. Ugan Y, Nazıroğlu M, Şahin M, Aykur M. Anti-tumor necrosis factor alpha (infliximab) attenuates apoptosis, oxidative stress, and calcium ion entry through modulation of cation channels in neutrophils of patients with ankylosing spondylitis. J Membr Biol. 2016;249(4):437–47.
53. Feng X, Yang Q, Wang C, Tong W, Xu W. Punicalagin exerts protective effects against ankylosing spondylitis by regulating NF-κB-TH17/JAK2/STAT3 signaling and oxidative stress. Biomed Res Int. 2020;2020:4918239.
54. Baykara RA, Tuzcu A, Omma A, Acet GK, Dogan E, Aydin A, et al. Evaluation of serum thiol/disulfide homeostasis in patients with ankylosing spondylitis by a novel method. Northern Clin Istanbul. 2019;6(4):348.
55. Rashid T, Wilson C, Ebringer A. The link between ankylosing spondylitis, Crohn's disease, Klebsiella, and starch consumption. Clin Dev Immunol. 2013;2013:872632.
56. Breban M, Tap J, Leboime A, Said-Nahal R, Langella P, Chiocchia G, et al. Faecal microbiota study reveals specific dysbiosis in spondyloarthritis. Ann Rheum Dis. 2017;76(9):1614–22.
57. Garcia-Ribera S, Amat-Bou M, Climent E, Llobet M, Chenoll E, Corripio R, et al. Specific dietary components and gut microbiota composition are associated with obesity in children and adolescents with prader–willi syndrome. Nutrients. 2020;12(4):1063.
58. Livovsky DM, Pribic T, Azpiroz F. Food, eating, and the gastrointestinal tract. Nutrients. 2020;12(4):986.
59. Simone D, Al Mossawi MH, Bowness P. Progress in our understanding of the pathogenesis of ankylosing spondylitis. Rheumatology. 2018;57(suppl_6):vi4–9.
60. Zhang L, Zhang Y-J, Chen J, Huang X-L, Fang G-S, Yang L-J, et al. The association of HLA-B27 and *Klebsiella pneumoniae* in ankylosing spondylitis: a systematic review. Microb Pathog. 2018;117:49–54.
61. Gutiérrez S, Svahn SL, Johansson ME. Effects of omega-3 fatty acids on immune cells. Int J Mol Sci. 2019;20(20):5028.
62. Innes JK, Calder PC. Omega-6 fatty acids and inflammation. Prostaglandins Leukot Essent Fat Acids. 2018;132:41–8.
63. Sundström B, Stålnacke K, Hagfors L, Johansson G. Supplementation of omega-3 fatty acids in patients with ankylosing spondylitis. Scand J Rheumatol. 2006;35(5):359–62.
64. Chen CH, Chen HA, Liu CH, Liao HT, Chou CT, Chen CH. Association of obesity with inflammation, disease severity and cardiovascular risk factors among patients with ankylosing spondylitis. Int J Rheum Dis. 2020;23(9):1165–74.
65. Ortega FB, Lavie CJ, Blair SN. Obesity and cardiovascular disease. Circ Res. 2016;118(11):1752–70.
66. Toy S, Ozbag D, Altay Z. The effects of pre-obesity on quality of life, disease activity, and functional status in patients with ankylosing spondylitis. Northern Clin Istanbul. 2017;4(1):52.
67. Daïen CI, Sellam J. Obesity and inflammatory arthritis: impact on occurrence, disease characteristics and therapeutic response. RMD Open. 2015;1(1):e000012.
68. Pettersen IKN, Tusubira D, Ashrafi H, Dyrstad SE, Hansen L, Liu X-Z, et al. Upregulated PDK4 expression is a sensitive marker of increased fatty acid oxidation. Mitochondrion. 2019;49:97–110.
69. Xie Z, Zhang J, Ma S, Huang X, Huang Y. Effect of Chinese herbal medicine treatment on plasma lipid profile and hepatic lipid metabolism in Hetian broiler. Poult Sci. 2017;96(6):1918–24.
70. Heine RG. Food allergy prevention and treatment by targeted nutrition. Ann Nutr Metab. 2018;72(3):33–45.
71. Yu W, Freeland DMH, Nadeau KC. Food allergy: immune mechanisms, diagnosis and immunotherapy. Nat Rev Immunol. 2016;16(12):751.

72. Bastan I, Ge XN, Dileepan M, Greenberg YG, Guedes AG, Hwang SH, et al. Inhibition of soluble epoxide hydrolase attenuates eosinophil recruitment and food allergen-induced gastrointestinal inflammation. J Leukoc Biol. 2018;104(1):109–22.
73. Ling Z, Li Z, Liu X, Cheng Y, Luo Y, Tong X, et al. Altered fecal microbiota composition associated with food allergy in infants. Appl Environ Microbiol. 2014;80(8):2546–54.
74. Iweala OI, Choudhary SK, Commins SP. Food allergy. Curr Gastroenterol Rep. 2018;20(5):1–6.
75. Hua X, Goedert JJ, Pu A, Yu G, Shi J. Allergy associations with the adult fecal microbiota: analysis of the American gut project. EBioMedicine. 2016;3:172–9.
76. Niu Q, Wei W, Huang Z, Zhang J, Yang B, Wang L. Association between food allergy and ankylosing spondylitis: an observational study. Medicine. 2019;98(6):e14421.
77. Hodde JP, Hiles MC, Metzger DW. Characterization of the local wound environment following treatment of chronic leg ulcers with SIS wound matrix. J Tissue Viability. 2020;29(1):42–7.
78. Zhang W, Zhang Y, He Y, Wang X, Fang Q. Lipopolysaccharide mediates time-dependent macrophage M1/M2 polarization through the Tim-3/Galectin-9 signalling pathway. Exp Cell Res. 2019;376(2):124–32.
79. Yu J, Zhu R, Yu K, Wang Y, Ding Y, Zhong Y, et al. Galectin-9: a suppressor of atherosclerosis? Front Immunol. 2020;11:604265.
80. Soleimanifar N, Nicknam MH, Bidad K, Jamshidi AR, Mahmoudi M, Mostafaei S, Hosseini-Khah Z, Nikbin B. Effect of food intake and ambient air pollution exposure on ankylosing spondylitis disease activity. Advances in Rheumatology. 2019 Jul 29;59.
81. Rocha DM, Caldas AP, Oliveira LL, Bressan J, Hermsdorff HH. Saturated fatty acids trigger TLR4-mediated inflammatory response. Atherosclerosis. 2016;244:211–15.

8 Spondyloarthropathies and Environmental Stresses

Hanieh Mojtahedi and Narjes Soleimanifar

8.1 Introduction

The Seronegative Spondyloarthropathies (SpA) are a group of overlapping disorders that share certain clinical features and genetic associations. The patients suffer from chronic, intermittent pain and inflammation that affects the connecting or supporting structures of the body like the joints, tendons, ligaments, and bones. The most common features are axial arthritis and oligoarthritis, asymmetrical presentation, sacroiliitis, enthesitis, and spondylitis. There are also extra-articular features, such as the involvement of eyes (anterior uveitis), skin, and genitourinary tract [1].

SpA pathogenesis is not fully understood; however, with respect to the presence of chronic inflammation and immune system dysfunction, recent classification has specified spondyloarthropathies as the transitional between autoimmunity and autoinflammatory disease. The primary member of the SpA family is Ankylosing spondylitis (AS) which is the main focus of this chapter, followed by implying Psoriatic Arthritis (PsA), Reactive Arthritis (ReA), juvenile SpA, and undifferentiated forms of SpA (uSpAs) in appropriate cases.

Studies have shown that genetic predisposition is considered for approximately 30% of autoimmune diseases through a positive familial history and the presence of HLA-B27 in most SpA patients. Genes alone cannot account for diseases, and the rest 70% of nongenetic triggers may be developed by environmental factors [2, 3]. Environmental factors are the diverse kinds of stressors that may occur as an intense, short-lived event of destruction like Physical and mechanical stressors or may exert

H. Mojtahedi
Department of Immunology, School of Medicine, Shahid Beheshti University of Medical Sciences, Tehran, Iran

N. Soleimanifar (✉)
Molecular Immunology Research Center, Tehran University of Medical Sciences, Tehran, Iran
e-mail: n-soleimanifar@farabi.tums.ac.ir

M. H. Nicknam (ed.), *Ankylosing Spondylitis - Axial Spondyloarthritis*,
https://doi.org/10.1007/978-981-16-4733-8_8

their influence over an extended period in a chronic manner like smoking or alcohol addiction. Both are associated with human activities and have the most critical influence on the health and immune system [4].

Generally, the immune system is the first organ that encounters environmental hazards, and autoimmunity happens when a chronic irritation disturbs the immune system tolerance and leads to attack the tissues. The environmental risk factors are the most mediators that can worsen or speed up the onset of the disease [5, 6]. Additionally, risk factors are convoluted with cause-and-effect relationships, making it challenging to find the source and overcome the problem. For instance, smoking and obesity are related to the growth of depression, and depression triggers more smoking with less physical activity in return. Less physical activity and an unhealthy diet lead to oxidative stress and systemic inflammation, consequently provoking many immune dysregulations.

In the present study, we review the effects of environmental factors like smoking, mechanical, psychological, and oxidative stresses, which have been studied more in SpA.

8.2 Biomechanical Stress

The musculoskeletal system is responsible for providing the body stability and forms its structure, whereas making it flexible enough for tiny movement. This system, which is classified as dense connective tissues, is highly responsive to mechanical forces. The condition is evidenced by the fact that many musculoskeletal organs are capable of adjusting their biochemical composition and molecular architecture in response to mechanical demands. Both the intrinsic and extrinsic forces are formed by the contraction of muscles or the elasticity of connective tissues. The extrinsic types of forces can arise from outside the body, whereas the intrinsic ones originated from the inside [7].

Spondyloarthropathy (SpA) is a complex group of rheumatic diseases that exhibit typical clinical and genetic features and are classified as either peripheral or axial (axSpA) depending on which part of the body is primarily affected. In Axial spondyloarthritis (AxSpA) and by extension in other forms of SpA, the most prominent sites of involvement are the spine and the sacroiliac joints [8]. Ankylosing spondylitis (AS), the main feature of SpA, is an autoinflammatory disease that primarily involves the spinal joints, sacroiliac joints (SIJ), and adjacent soft tissues such as ligaments and tendons [9]. The main clinical symptoms contain low back pain and progressive spinal stiffness, together with inflammation of the hip, shoulders, peripheral joints like toes and fingers. In progressive conditions, this inflammation can result in fibrosis and calcification, leading to inflexibility, similar to a "bamboo" in which the spine is fused and immobile. There are also extra-articular symptoms like inflammatory bowel disease (IBD) and uveitis [10]. In contrast to RA, which the extensive joint damage is rarely along with tissue repair, in AS, joint and spine destruction is characterized by the new bone formation and cartilage repair, so chronic inflammation and bony ankylosis are two primary symptoms of AxSpA [11].

Several reasons suggest that mechanical stress plays an essential role in the AxSpA pathogenesis. As described before, the axial skeleton carries the burden of body mass that is subject to significant stress. Besides, in SpA, the principal involved joints belong to the lower limbs compared to the upper ones, pointing to the fact that transitional forces pass from the spine accumulate in the sacroiliac joints make them exposed to higher mechanical loading [12]. Moreover, enthesitis is the primary and common sign of most SpA diseases. Enthesitis refers to the inflammation and pain in the site where bone and tendon, and ligaments join together [13]. It seems that these effectual sites are prone to such recurrent microtrauma resulting in microdamage. Any abnormal process such as stress and injury occurring at insertion sites of muscle, ligaments, and tendons into joint capsules or bones may contribute to the pathogenesis of enthesopathy; therefore, chronic inflammation may be driven by mechanical stress [14]. Besides, microanatomical features in SpA-related enthesitis show that the erosion and new bone formation of superficial fibrocartilage are observed at various topographical locations and are usually at the distal part of the enthesis where the bone is under more tension, strongly suggesting a role for mechanical factors [15].

Additional evidence suggests that chronic biomechanical stress may cause infiltration of capillary-like blood vessels through the enthesis from the bone marrow, providing a site for inflammatory tissue entry, osteoblast initiation, and the development of bone spurs (enthesophytes) [16]. WL Zhou et al. have shown that the extent of sonographic enthesitis in spondyloarthritis and the severity of radiographic peripheral and axial joint damage in AS and psoriatic arthritis (PsA) are related to the innate immunity function [17]. The presence of inflammatory cells in the milieu of the enthesis supports the theory that mechanical micro damages make danger signals or neo-epitopes in the environment conduct recruiting the innate immune cells [12]. Generally, the inflammation in tendinopathy involves stromal tenocytes and immune-sensing and infiltrating cells affecting tendon homeostasis [18]. Macrophage and mast cells-derived immune mediators moderate matrix metaloprotease (MMP) expression in tenocytes and collagen synthesis.

Moreover, the presence of T lymphocytes and NK cells and subsequent downstream cytokine production determines the extra cellular matrix (ECM) crosstalk reparation versus degeneration. The in vitro study on tendinopathy biopsy samples showed the increased expression of IL-1β, which decreases significantly the expression of type I collagen, and increased expression IL-17F, which regulates ECM changes toward a type III collagen phenotype [19, 20]. The availability of secukinumab and ixekizumab (anti-IL-17A monoclonal antibodies), as an incredibly intriguing potential target for axial ankylosing spondylitis (SpA) and psoriatic arthritis enthesopathy, makes the role of inflammatory cytokines more clear [20, 21]. Besides, phosphorylation of kinases such as ERK and p38 MAPK can be started with mechanical stresses, resulting in a higher IL-17, IL-23, TNF-α expression and the joint inflammation of PsA [14, 22].

In terms of physical activity, most AS patients reported physical stress within 3 months before the onset [23]. Among 1026 AS patients, 44% recalling an instance of injury or trauma as a potential trigger for their AS. 1.7% of them reported physical trauma, and 0.7% had performed surgery within the first 3 months of initial diagnosis [24]. Also, an association between exercises exacerbated symptoms, including 55% modified sporting activities and 28% exacerbated symptoms after physical activity was reported after AS symptom onset. Although mechanical stress is regularly considered destructive or damaging, it is worthy to notice the benefits of physical activity apart from other mechanical forces on general human health toward regulating cardiovascular condition, weight, and metabolism synchronization [25]. By conditioning ligaments and tendons, physical exercise has a direct effect on the joint. Physical activity indirectly strengthens muscles, regulating joint extension and flexion and thereby preserving joint stability [26]. This principle of stability is critical because muscles around affected joints are stiffer and less used in SpA [27]. This condition also explains why, despite appearing contradictory at first glance, physical therapy is beneficial in SpA and recommended for AS by several international guidelines [28].

8.3 Psychological Stress

The spondyloarthropathies, especially AS, are chronic rheumatic conditions and progressive diseases restricting spinal mobility and functional disability. Persistence of pain, deformities, and physical inactivity make the patients reluctant to social activities, and a decrease in life quality may result in productivity loss in their working environment; thus, they are prone to experience some psychiatric complications which may influence disease activity and outcome in return [29]. Therefore, assessing psychological status throughout the disease is as essential as the clinical evaluation of the condition [30].

In a study by Zochling et al., stress was shown to be a potential trigger for the onset of AS, so that 7% of AS patients reported emotional stress, which leads to initial symptoms of AS disease. It was also observed that AS patients had work stressors within 3 months before the onset [31]. Stressful symptoms that are most commonly observed in AS patients are anxiety and depression. Depression and anxiety have been reported in 28% to 32% of patients with AS [32, 33]. In the literature, several studies investigated psychiatric symptoms and quality of life in AS patients [34–36]. Barlow et al. have determined that one-third of AS patients point to some features and symptoms of depression. High internal locus of control and low reliance on powerful others were common amongst AS patients [37]. In another study, Gunther et al. have determined that apart from the disease duration, the coping strategies of AS males make the stressful situations playing down [38].

Moreover, prolonged stressful condition contributes to chronic inflammation and adversely driven autoimmune disorders. The principal concept implies that stress affects the immune system directly or indirectly via the nervous system. Psychological stresses typically activate the hypothalamic–pituitary–adrenal (HPA) axis by releasing the catecholamines and corticosteroids from the adrenal gland [39]. At the same time, an excess of sympathetic activation produces noradrenaline which activates NF-kB through TLRs signaling pathways which consequently triggers the release of pro-inflammatory cytokines such as interleukin IL-1, IL-6, and tumor necrosis factor (TNF) [40].

8.4 Oxidative Stress

Oxidative stress arises when the oxidative and antioxidative systems balance disturbed and lead to the reactive oxygen species (ROS) increase [41, 42]. ROS, including oxygen-containing neutral and free radical molecules, radical hydroxyl anion, superoxide anion, and nitric oxide, can be produced in normal cellular metabolism. Despite their destructive potential, ROS in low concentration plays important roles as signaling molecules that are crucial for cell differentiation, proliferation, apoptosis, and signal transduction [42]. When the speed of the ROS production exceeds, and there is an insufficient capacity of antioxidants to remove them, oxidative stress triggering oxidative damage to DNA, proteins, and lipids and makes inflammation the pathologic hallmark of AS and other SpA [43, 44].

Inflammatory cells can stimulate various enzyme production to induce oxidative stress. Mutually several ROS presence at the site of inflammation can enhance pro-inflammatory cytokines by activating the inflammatory signal pathways [43, 45]. This state of persistent cause and effect can help the durability of inflammation in the environment, one of the basic principles of chronic inflammatory diseases, and initiate various research on the SpA patients through this subject [46–48]. In the study of Dilek Solmazis et al., on more than 80 AS patients, total antioxidant status (TAS) versus total oxidant status (TOS) was measured, and it was shown that the patients with active AS patients (BASDAI ≥4) had significantly higher TOS levels than the inactive group. Also, there was a significant correlation between TOS and ESR, CRP, BASMI, BASDAI, and BASFI, and interestingly the BASMI was positively correlated to TAS [49].

In another study by Yousefi et al., the immunological biomarkers in Ankylosing spondylitis were assessed along with oxidative stress. Data revealed that the severity of the inflammation and disease symptoms are increased in AS patients compared to healthy controls following elevated levels of oxidative stress like TOS, GPX, SOD, NO, and CAT. A significant increase in Th17 cells, the critical stimulator of autoimmune-inflammatory disorders, and a decrease in Treg cells, immune system suppressors, may affect the intensification of symptoms in the active phase patients. Besides, an increase in expression of inflammatory cytokines like TNF-α, IL-1β, and IL-6 and chemokines like the CCL2, CCL3, and CXCL8 were reported in AS patients compared to the healthy group [47].

Moreover, signaling pathways activated by pro-inflammatory cytokines and oxidative stress products, both cause, and effect, can evoke the formation and activation of osteoclasts resulting in the progression of bone loss in AS [9]. Le Wang et al. investigate the relationship of oxidants/antioxidants and bone turnover markers (BTMs) in AS. In this study, the serum levels of the oxidative stress markers, the advanced oxidation protein products (AOPPs), and malondialdehyde (MDA) were significantly higher in the AS patients whereas, the levels of the antioxidant markers in erythrocytes, superoxide dismutase (SOD), glutathione peroxidase (GSH-Px), and catalase (CAT) were significantly lower. Analyses of bone mineral density (BMD) showed that the lumbar spine or femoral neck BMD were negatively correlated with the oxidative status, BASMI, inflammatory marker, and disease activity, and interestingly it was positively correlated with the antioxidant status [50]. Moreover, it is illustrated that ROS is related to the Wnt/Beta-catenin and BMP/Smad pathways activation. These pathways are involved in the progression of new bone formation in AS [51, 52].

8.5 Smoking

As a combination of thousands of chemical components, cigarette smoke can have unfavorable effects on the immune system. Smoking weakens immune responses and helps in the onset of autoimmunity through prolonging long-term infections [53]. Studies imply that smoking can evoke both innate and adaptive immunity through NFκB and MAPK signaling. Cigarette smoking triggers local immunity via induction of pattern recognition receptors (TLR4) and the MyD88 signaling pathway resulting in the generation of pro-inflammatory cytokines like IL-1, IL-6, and TNF and chronic inflammation [54]. The chronic inflammation disturbed the T cell population's balance toward Th1 and Th17 subsets, leading to the elevated production of IFN-γ, IL-10, IL-17, and IL-21. Smoking may also induce autoimmunity through activation of antigen-presenting cells (APCs) and autoreactive pro-inflammatory TCD4 + cells [55]. These distinct effector T cell subsets play a leading role in the formation of autoantibodies, RANKL-independent osteoclastogenesis, and synovial neoangiogenesis in SpA [55, 56].

However, many factors related to smoking like BMI, manual occupations, lower physical activity, etc., make the matter more complex to clarify the pivotal role of smoking on Spondyloarthropathies, the higher prevalence of current smokers among SpA patients compared to healthy adults (29% versus 15%) in UK cohort study were considered a lot. Also, among the SpA smokers, the highest prevalence of smoking belongs to young adults (19 versus 8%) who had more severe symptoms, which can imply the smoking effect on both the incidence and severity of SpA [57, 58].

A meta-analyze study by Sizheng Steven Zhao et al. among 18 cross-sectional studies has determined that ever smokers had significantly higher BASDAI, BASFI, and spinal pain, and poorer quality of life than never smokers [59]. These differences remained significant after adjusting for education, deprivation, BMI, comorbidities, and alcohol status; however, in longitudinal studies, results were too heterogeneous to perform analysis [56]. Concerning the physical mobility and stiffness, a British cohort of 53 AS patients demonstrated that smokers had reduced mobility through the measurement of finger ground distance, Schober test, total spinal motion, and distance between the occiput to walls. In addition, Irène Kona Kaut et al. evaluated the spinal stiffness at the cervical level in 214 patients over time, which was significantly decreased in the Menton-sternum in flexion and extension distance, Menton-acromion distance, tragus -acromion distance, occiput-wall and C7-Wall distance [60]. In another study of 48 AS patients in Turkey, a significant decrease in the modified lumbar Schober test and chest expansion were determined in non-smokers [61]. Moreover, many radiographic progression studies reported significant associations between smoking and spinal progression or syndesmophyte progression as well. In Poddubnyy et al. study in 210 mostly non-TNFi treated axSpA patients, current smokers had over twice the odds of radiologic progression compared with non-current smokers [62]. Similarly, Kim et al. reported three times higher odds of progression in axSpA patients; however, Deminger et al., no significant effect was observed over 5 years. Although the odds of progression were increased in male ever smokers, the condition was reversed in females [63]. Despite these findings, it is hard to clarify the role of smoking in radiographic progression in SpA because of the confounding factors mingled with smoking like occupation, physical activity, and mechanical stress in parallel [64–66].

Smoking impacts on Psoriatic Arthritis (PsA) is nearly associated with the impact on psoriasis through the incitement of oxidative stress, signaling pathways like mitogen-activated protein kinase (MAPK), NF-κB pathway, and Janus kinase/signal transducers and activators of transcription (JAK-STAT), and production of different cytokines including IL-2, IL-12, TNF [67]. Some studies suggested that smoking has a protective effect on psoriasis; however, smoking increases the risk of PsA in the general population appears "protective" of demonstrating Psoriatic arthritis symptoms among people with psoriasis [59].

8.6 Vaccination

Vaccination is a type of biological acquired immunity intended for impeding specific diseases, but vaccines also are incorporated in antigen overload and possible triggering of autoimmunity through cytokine production, HLA expression, molecular mimicry, B cells polyclonal activation, antigens induction, and modification mechanisms [68].

Arthritis is a more common feature associated with vaccination. However, the underlying mechanisms are not yet clear; a cross-reaction between synovial antigen and bacterial lipopolysaccharide epitopes, enhanced by HLA-B27 expression, may provide circumstance [69]. HLA-B27 expression, on the other hand, is not a requirement for vaccine-related arthritis, though it may predict a more prolonged and severe incident. Vaccines can also cause autoimmune reactions by binding to critical antigen binding clefts on the major histocompatibility complex class II molecule, causing T cell proliferation. Their ingredients, such as pathogenic antigens and adjuvants (e.g., aluminum compounds), may lead to autoimmunity through similar mechanisms in activation of immune responses following molecular mimicry and induction of autoantibodies [68]. The autoimmunity induced by adjuvant-containing vaccinations is associated with the activation of APCs, production of pro-inflammatory cytokines, enhancement of innate immune-mediated responses, and clonal expansion of autoreactive T cells to self-antigens that surpass tolerance [70]. It is clear that these mechanisms do not indicate the definite existence of autoimmunity after vaccination. For such an event to occur, additional conditions must be met, such as the presence of stimulating cytokines to activate a critical mass of autoreactive clones and the absence of effective regulatory mechanisms [71]. Since the experimental models may provide biological plausibility to the hypothesis of a link between vaccine administration and the onset of autoimmune disease, these studies are generally based on case reports.

Among the spondyloarthropathies member, Reactive Arthritis (ReA) and psoriatic arthritis (PsA) are more likely to have emerged after different vaccinations. The Incidence of ReA manifestation in a healthy 79-year-old man induced by influenza vaccination was reported by Junichi Asakawa. The negative rheumatoid factor shows no evidence for microbial infections such as Streptococci, Chlamydia, or Parvovirus B19. Human leukocyte antigen (HLA) typing analysis revealed positive results for HLA-B54, one of the cross-reactive antigens to HLA-B27. This phenomenon was repeated years ago in a 32 years old man with positive HLA-B27 who presented a typical onset of reactive arthritis 2 weeks after influenza vaccination [72]. However, ReA after vaccination is a rare event; a few cases such as Hepatitis B, Bacillus Calmette-Guerin (BCG), MMR, influenza, tetanus, typhoid, and pertussis have been reported [72–74].

Although the relationship between rubella vaccination and PsA has been reported, most challenges in this area are related to the risk of vaccination on disease activity related to immunosuppressor administration [75–77]. This subject is more related to immunogenicity and safety of vaccination which is far from this chapter concept.

References

1. Kataria RK, Brent LH. Spondyloarthropathies. Am Fam Physician. 2004;69(12):2853–60.
2. Reveille JD, Ball EJ, Khan MA. HLA-B27 and genetic predisposing factors in spondyloarthropathies. Curr Opin Rheumatol. 2001;13(4):265–72.
3. Ehrenfeld M. Geoepidemiology: the environment and spondyloarthropathies. Autoimmun Rev. 2010;9(5):A325–A9.
4. Mangino M, Roederer M, Beddall MH, Nestle FO, Spector TD. Innate and adaptive immune traits are differentially affected by genetic and environmental factors. Nat Commun. 2017;8(1):1–7.
5. Rogler G, Vavricka S. Exposome in IBD: recent insights in environmental factors that influence the onset and course of IBD. Inflamm Bowel Dis. 2015;21(2):400–8.
6. Nolte H, Backer V, Porsbjerg C. Environmental factors as a cause for the increase in allergic disease. Ann Allergy Asthma Immunol. 2001;87(6):7–11.
7. Bliss S. Musculoskeletal structure and physiology. In: Zink C, Van Dyke J, editors. Canine sports medicine and rehabilitation. 2nd ed. New York: John Wiley & Sons; 2018. p. 43–71.
8. Ehrenfeld M. Spondyloarthropathies. Best Pract Res Clin Rheumatol. 2012;26(1):135–45.
9. Van Der Linden S, Brown M, Kenna T, Maksymowych W, Robinson P. Ankylosing spondylitis. Kelley and Firestein's textbook of rheumatology (Tenth Edition). 2017;2:1256–79.
10. Rudwaleit M, Baeten D. Ankylosing spondylitis and bowel disease. Best Pract Res Clin Rheumatol. 2006;20(3):451–71.

11. Vosse D, De Vlam K. Osteoporosis in rheumatoid arthritis and ankylosing spondylitis. Clinical & Experimental Rheumatology. 2009;27(4):S62.
12. Van Mechelen M, Lories RJ. Microtrauma: no longer to be ignored in spondyloarthritis? Curr Opin Rheumatol. 2016;28(2):176–80.
13. Soliman E. Enthesitis in spondyloarthritis: role of musculoskeletal ultrasound. Br J Medical Health Sci (BJMHS). 2021;3(3):875–84.
14. McGonagle D, Lories RJ, Tan AL, Benjamin M. The concept of a "synovio-entheseal complex" and its implications for understanding joint inflammation and damage in psoriatic arthritis and beyond. Arthritis Rheum. 2007;56(8):2482–91.
15. Jacques P, McGonagle D. The role of mechanical stress in the pathogenesis of spondyloarthritis and how to combat it. Best Pract Res Clin Rheumatol. 2014;28(5):703–10.
16. Binks D, Matzelle M, Bergin D, Hodgson R, Gravallese E, McGonagle D, et al. OP0121 the frequency of bone erosion and oedema in inflammatory and degenerative arthropathies proximal to the peri-entheseal cruciate ligament vascular channels. Ann Rheum Dis. 2013;72(Suppl 3):A92-A.
17. Zhou W, Chandran V, Cook R, Gladman DD, Eder L. The association between occupational-related mechanical stress and radiographic damage in psoriatic arthritis. In: Seminars in arthritis and rheumatism. Amsterdam: Elsevier; 2019.
18. Millar NL, Murrell GA, McInnes IB. Inflammatory mechanisms in tendinopathy–towards translation. Nat Rev Rheumatol. 2017;13(2):110.
19. Archambault J, Tsuzaki M, Herzog W, Banes AJ. Stretch and interleukin-1β induce matrix metalloproteinases in rabbit tendon cells in vitro. J Orthop Res. 2002;20(1):36–9.
20. Millar NL, Akbar M, Campbell AL, Reilly JH, Kerr SC, McLean M, et al. IL-17A mediates inflammatory and tissue remodelling events in early human tendinopathy. Sci Rep. 2016;6(1):1–11.
21. McInnes IB, Mease PJ, Kirkham B, Kavanaugh A, Ritchlin CT, Rahman P, et al. Secukinumab, a human anti-interleukin-17A monoclonal antibody, in patients with psoriatic arthritis (FUTURE 2): a randomised, double-blind, placebo-controlled, phase 3 trial. Lancet. 2015;386(9999):1137–46.
22. De Vlam K, Gottlieb AB, Mease PJ. Current concepts in psoriatic arthritis: pathogenesis and management. Acta Derm Venereol. 2014;94(6):627–37.
23. Jun J-B, Kim T-H, Jung S, Yoo D-H, Kim T-Y, Kim S. Seronegative spondyloarthropathy initiated by physical trauma. Clin Rheumatol. 2000;19(5):348–51.
24. Ansell R, Shuto T, Busquets-Perez N, Hensor E, Marzo-Ortega H, McGonagle D. The role of biomechanical factors in ankylosing spondylitis: the patient's perspective. Reumatismo. 2015;67(3):91–6.
25. Murphy RM, Watt MJ, Febbraio MA. Metabolic communication during exercise. Nat Metab. 2020;2(9):805–16.
26. Loos H, Sulzer SH, Atisme K. Exercise tips for chronic pain management. Logan: Utah State University Extension; 2019.
27. Debusschere K, Cambré I, Gracey E, Elewaut D. Born to run: the paradox of biomechanical force in spondyloarthritis from an evolutionary perspective. Best Pract Res Clin Rheumatol. 2017;31(6):887–94.
28. Martey C, Sengupta R. Physical therapy in axial spondyloarthritis: guidelines, evidence and clinical practice. Curr Opin Rheumatol. 2020;32(4):365–70.
29. Mustur D, Vesović-Potić V, Stanisavljević D, Ille T, Ille M. Assessment of functional disability and quality of life in patients with ankylosing spondylitis. Srp Arh Celok Lek. 2009;137(9–10):524–8.
30. Martindale J, Smith J, Sutton CJ, Grennan D, Goodacre L, Goodacre J. Disease and psychological status in ankylosing spondylitis. Rheumatology. 2006;45(10):1288–93.
31. Zochling J, Bohl-Bühler MH, Baraliakos X, Feldtkeller E, Braun J. Infection and work stress are potential triggers of ankylosing spondylitis. Clinical rheumatology. 2006;25(5):660–6.

32. Lim J-M, Cho O-H. The influence of disease activity and uncertainty on anxiety and depression in patients with ankylosing spondylitis. J Korean Acad Soc Home Health Care Nursing. 2017;24(1):61–8.
33. Özkan Y. Anxiety, depression, problem solving and stress management in patients with ankylosing spondylitis. Meandros Medical and Dental Journal. 2018;19(1):57.
34. Bostan EE, Borman P, Bodur H, Barça N. Functional disability and quality of life in patients with ankylosing spondylitis. Rheumatol Int. 2003;23(3):121–6.
35. Ward MM. Health-related quality of life in ankylosing spondylitis: a survey of 175 patients. Arthritis Care Res. 1999;12(4):247–55.
36. Ward MM. Quality of life in patients with ankylosing spondylitis. Rheum Dis Clin N Am. 1998;24(4):815–27.
37. Barlow JH, Macey SJ, Struthers GR. Health locus of control, self-help and treatment adherence in relation to ankylosing spondylitis patients. Patient Educ Couns. 1993;20(2–3):153–66.
38. Günther V, MuR E, Traweger C, Hawel R. Stress coping of patients with ankylosing spondylitis. J Psychosom Res. 1994;38(5):419–27.
39. Jara LJ, Navarro C, Medina G, Vera-Lastra O, Blanco F. Immune-neuroendocrine interactions and autoimmune diseases. Clin Dev Immunol. 2006;13(2–4):109–23.
40. Skopouli FN, Katsiougiannis S. How stress contributes to autoimmunity—lessons from Sjögren's syndrome. FEBS Lett. 2018;592(1):5–14.
41. Joffre J, Hellman J. Oxidative stress and endothelial dysfunction in sepsis and acute inflammation. Antioxid Redox Signal. 2021; https://doi.org/10.1089/ars.2021.0027.
42. Niu L, Han D. Oxidation and antioxidation. Chemical analysis of antioxidant capacity: De Gruyter; 2020. p. 1–19.
43. Stanek A, Cieślar G, Romuk E, Kasperczyk S, Sieroń-Stołtny K, Birkner E, et al. Decrease in antioxidant status of plasma and erythrocytes from patients with ankylosing spondylitis. Clin Biochem. 2010;43(6):566–70.
44. Li J, Liu S, Cui Y. Oxidative and Antioxidative stress linked biomarkers in ankylosing spondylitis: a systematic review and Meta-analysis. Oxidative Med Cell Longev. 2020;2020:4759451.
45. Hoffmann MH, Griffiths HR. The dual role of reactive oxygen species in autoimmune and inflammatory diseases: evidence from preclinical models. Free Radic Biol Med. 2018;125:62–71.
46. Karakoc M, Altindag O, Keles H, Soran N, Selek S. Serum oxidative–antioxidative status in patients with ankylosing spondilitis. Rheumatol Int. 2007;27(12):1131–4.
47. Danaii S, Abolhasani R, Soltani-Zangbar MS, Zamani M, Mehdizadeh A, Amanifar B, et al. Oxidative stress and immunological biomarkers in ankylosing spondylitis patients. Gene Rep. 2020;18:100574.
48. Pishgahi A, Abolhasan R, Danaii S, Amanifar B, Soltani-Zangbar MS, Zamani M, et al. Immunological and oxidative stress biomarkers in ankylosing spondylitis patients with or without metabolic syndrome. Cytokine. 2020;128:155002.
49. Solmaz D, Kozacı D, İsmail Sarı AT, Önen F, Akkoç N, Akar S. Oxidative stress and related factors in patients with ankylosing spondylitis. Eur J Rheumatol. 2016;3(1):20.
50. Wang L, Gao L, Jin D, Wang P, Yang B, Deng W, et al. The relationship of bone mineral density to oxidant/antioxidant status and inflammatory and bone turnover markers in a multicenter cross-sectional study of young men with ankylosing spondylitis. Calcif Tissue Int. 2015;97(1):12–22.
51. D-y Z, Pan Y, Zhang C, B-x Y, Yu S-s, Wu D-l, et al. Wnt/β-catenin signaling induces the aging of mesenchymal stem cells through promoting the ROS production. Mol Cell Biochem. 2013;374(1):13–20.
52. Susperregui AR, Gamell C, Rodríguez-Carballo E, Ortuño MJ, Bartrons R, Rosa JL, et al. Noncanonical BMP signaling regulates cyclooxygenase-2 transcription. Mol Endocrinol. 2011;25(6):1006–17.
53. Qiu F, Liang C-L, Liu H, Zeng Y-Q, Hou S, Huang S, et al. Impacts of cigarette smoking on immune responsiveness: up and down or upside down? Oncotarget. 2017;8(1):268.

54. Semlali A, Witoled C, Alanazi M, Rouabhia M. Whole cigarette smoke increased the expression of TLRs, HBDs, and proinflammory cytokines by human gingival epithelial cells through different signaling pathways. PLoS One. 2012;7(12):e52614.
55. Lee J, Taneja V, Vassallo R. Cigarette smoking and inflammation: cellular and molecular mechanisms. J Dent Res. 2012;91(2):142–9.
56. Zhao S, Jones GT, Macfarlane GJ, Hughes DM, Dean LE, Moots RJ, et al. Associations between smoking and extra-axial manifestations and disease severity in axial spondyloarthritis: results from the BSR biologics register for ankylosing spondylitis (BSRBR-AS). Rheumatology. 2019;58(5):811–9.
57. Moreno-Gómez C, Romaguera-Bosch D, Tauler-Riera P, Bennasar-Veny M, Pericas-Beltran J, Martinez-Andreu S, et al. Clustering of lifestyle factors in Spanish university students: the relationship between smoking, alcohol consumption, physical activity and diet quality. Public Health Nutr. 2012;15(11):2131–9.
58. Kurtze N, Eikemo TA, Kamphuis CB. Educational inequalities in general and mental health: differential contribution of physical activity, smoking, alcohol consumption and diet. Eur J Public Health. 2013;23(2):223–9.
59. Zhao SS, Goodson NJ, Robertson S, Gaffney K. Smoking in spondyloarthritis: unravelling the complexities. Rheumatology. 2020;59(7):1472–81.
60. Kaut IK. Axial spondyloarthritis and cigarette smoking. Open Rheumatol J. 2017;11:53.
61. Kaan U, Ferda Ö. Evaluation of clinical activity and functional impairment in smokers with ankylosing spondylitis. Rheumatol Int. 2005;25(5):357–60.
62. Poddubnyy D, Haibel H, Listing J, Märker-Hermann E, Zeidler H, Braun J, et al. Baseline radiographic damage, elevated acute-phase reactant levels, and cigarette smoking status predict spinal radiographic progression in early axial spondylarthritis. Arthritis Rheum. 2012;64(5):1388–98.
63. Deminger A, Klingberg E, Geijer M, Göthlin J, Hedberg M, Rehnberg E, et al. A five-year prospective study of spinal radiographic progression and its predictors in men and women with ankylosing spondylitis. Arthritis Res Ther. 2018;20(1):1–14.
64. Ramiro S, van Tubergen A, Landewé R, Stolwijk C, Dougados M, van den Bosch F, et al. THU0103 disease activity in male smokers has a> 10-fold amplified effect on radiographic damage in comparison with female non-smokers in ankylosing spondylitis. Ann Rheum Dis. 2014;73(Suppl 2):212–3.
65. Soleimanifar N, Nicknam MH, Bidad K, Jamshidi AR, Mahmoudi M, Mostafaei S, Hosseini-Khah Z, Nikbin B. Effect of food intake and ambient air pollution exposure on ankylosing spondylitis disease activity. Advances in Rheumatology. 2019;59:1–9.
66. Maksymowych W, Zheng Y, Wichuk S, Chiowchanwisawakit P, Lambert R. OP0144 the effect of TNF inhibition on radiographic progression in ankylosing spondylitis: an observational cohort study of 384 patients. London: BMJ Publishing Group Ltd; 2015.
67. Pezzolo E, Naldi L. The relationship between smoking, psoriasis and psoriatic arthritis. Expert Rev Clin Immunol. 2019;15(1):41–8.
68. Schattner, A. and B. Rager-Zisman, Virus-induced autoimmunity. Reviews of infectious diseases. 1990;12(2):204–22.
69. Kennedy J. Reactive arthritis: the result of an anti-idiotypic immune response to a bacterial lipopolysaccharide antigen where the idiotype has the immunological appearance of a synovial antigen. Med Hypotheses. 2000;54(5):723–5.
70. Israeli E, Agmon-Levin N, Blank M, Shoenfeld Y. Adjuvants and autoimmunity. Lupus. 2009;18(13):1217–25.
71. Wraith DC, Goldman M, Lambert P-H. Vaccination and autoimmune disease: what is the evidence? Lancet. 2003;362(9396):1659–66.
72. Biasi D, Carletto A, Caramaschi P, Tonoli M, Bambara L. A case of reactive arthritis after influenza vaccination. Clin Rheumatol. 1994;13(4):645.
73. Gross K, Combe C, Krüger K, Schattenkirchner M. Arthritis after hepatitis B vaccination: report of three cases. Scand J Rheumatol. 1995;24(1):50–2.

74. Asakawa J, Kobayashi S, Kaneda K, Ogasawara H, Sugawara M, Yasuda M, et al. Reactive arthritis after influenza vaccination: report of a case. Mod Rheumatol. 2005;15(4):283–5.
75. Caso F, Ramonda R, Del Puente A, Darda MA, Cantarini L, Peluso R, et al. Influenza vaccine with adjuvant on disease activity in psoriatic arthritis patients under anti-TNF-α therapy. Clin Exp Rheumatol. 2016;34(3):507–12.
76. Mease PJ, Ritchlin CT, Martin RW, Gottlieb AB, Baumgartner SW, Burge DJ, et al. Pneumococcal vaccine response in psoriatic arthritis patients during treatment with etanercept. J Rheumatol. 2004;31(7):1356–61.
77. Furer V, Zisman D, Kaufman I, Arad U, Berman M, Sarbagil-Maman H, et al. Immunogenicity and safety of vaccination against seasonal influenza vaccine in patients with psoriatic arthritis treated with secukinumab. Vaccine. 2020;38(4):847–51.

Index

M. H. Nicknam (ed.), *Ankylosing Spondylitis - Axial Spondyloarthritis*, https://doi.org/10.1007/978-981-16-4733-8

FSC
www.fsc.org
MIX
Papier aus verantwortungsvollen Quellen
Paper from responsible sources
FSC® C105338

If you have any concerns about our products,
you can contact us on
ProductSafety@springernature.com

In case Publisher is established outside the EU,
the EU authorized representative is:
Springer Nature Customer Service Center GmbH
Europaplatz 3, 69115 Heidelberg, Germany

Printed by Libri Plureos GmbH
in Hamburg, Germany